Interventional Treatment of Wounds

Dennis P. Orgill
Editor

Interventional Treatment of Wounds

A Modern Approach for Better Outcomes

Springer

Editor
Dennis P. Orgill, MD, PhD
Division of Plastic Surgery,
Brigham and Women's Hospital Harvard Medical School
Boston, MA, USA

Additional material to this book can be downloaded from
https://link.springer.com/book/10.1007/978-3-319-66990-8

ISBN 978-3-319-66989-2 ISBN 978-3-319-66990-8 (eBook)
https://doi.org/10.1007/978-3-319-66990-8

Library of Congress Control Number: 2017962421

Printed on acid-free paper

This Springer imprint is published by Springer Nature
The registered company is Springer International Publishing AG
The registered company address is: Gewerbestrasse 11, 6330 Cham, Switzerland

Foreword

The Interventional Treatment of Wounds: A Modern Approach for Better Outcomes emphasizes the proper use of surgical techniques. Most wounds are addressed conservatively with medical care rather than surgery and have a 75% chance of healing. The role of surgery in massive traumatic wounds and after cancer ablation is well-defined. Its role for the chronic wound is underappreciated.

Surgery for the chronic wound involves a multidisciplinary approach that includes vascular surgery, general surgery, plastic surgery, orthopedics, and podiatric surgery. There are also many medical specialties involved including infectious disease, rheumatology, dermatology, internal medicine, and hyperbaric medicine.

The most important factor is to define the etiology of the wound. Addressing both arterial and venous blood flow and achieving a clean wound are the first step. The next is to assess the biomechanical causes of the wound. The goal is to achieve maximal function within each patient's physical and medical capacity. The chapters elegantly deal with each of the possible reconstructive options for lower extremity salvage and pressure ulcers. They also deal with amputations that can lead to a very functional foot when done using sound biomechanical principles. Finally they deal with the surgical treatment of pressure sore, a continual and frustrating wound.

By emphasizing biomechanics and soft tissue reconstructive options, the reader quickly understands what needs to be done to avoid wound recidivism as well as restore function. The lower extremity chapters focus on the foot and ankle and include details on how to optimize the outcome. The chapters on soft tissue options discuss multiple flap options as well as the easier skin graft and the proper use of biologics.

Negative pressure wound therapy's role is also discussed for its ability to both prepare a wound for closure and allow a wound to heal by secondary intention.

Dr. Orgill is a renowned expert in wound healing and has put together a wonderful series of chapters written by experts in their fields. This section should give any surgeon all the tools necessary to handle complex wounds in a systematic and logical way with excellent illustrations and videos. Welcome to an exciting approach to complex wounds.

Christopher E. Attinger, MD
Professor, Plastic Surgery
Georgetown University
Washington, DC, USA

Contents

Contributors

Dean J. Arnaoutakis, MD, MBA Division of Vascular and Endovascular Surgery, Brigham and Women's Hospital, Boston, MA, USA

Lauren R. Bayer, PA-C Wound Care Center, Department of Surgery, Division of Plastic Surgery, Brigham and Women's Hospital – Harvard Medical School, Boston, MA, USA

Charles L. Castiglione, MD, FACS Department of Surgery, Hartford Hospital, Connecticut Children's Medical Center, Hartford, CT, USA

Christopher P. Chiodo, MD Foot and Ankle Division, Brigham Foot and Ankle Center, Brigham and Women's Hospital, Boston, MA, USA

Ernest S. Chiu, MD, FACS Hansjörg Wyss Department of Plastic Surgery, New York Langone Medical Center, New York, NY, USA

Donghoon Choi, MD Department of Plastic Surgery, Asan Medical Center University of Ulsan, Seoul, South Korea

Joshua A. David, BS Hansjörg Wyss Department of Plastic Surgery, New York Langone Medical Center, New York, NY, USA

Michael V. DeFazio, MD Department of Plastic Surgery, Center for Wound Healing, Medstar Georgetown University Hospital, Washington, DC, USA

Tammer Elmarsafi, DPM, MBBCh Department of Plastic Surgery, MedStar Georgetown University Hospital, Washington, DC, USA

Karen Kim Evans, MD Department of Plastic Surgery, Center for Wound Healing, Medstar Georgetown University Hospital, Washington, DC, USA

Chieh-Min Fan, MD Interventional Radiology, Beverly Hospital, Beverly, MA, USA

Jillian L. Fortier, MD Department of Plastic Surgery, Lahey Hospital & Medical Center, Burlington, MA, USA

Robert D. Galiano, MD Division of Plastic and Reconstructive Surgery, Northwestern University Feinberg School of Medicine, Chicago, IL, USA

Division of Plastic Surgery, Northwestern Memorial Hospital, Chicago, IL, USA

Edwin C. Gravereaux, MD Division of Vascular and Endovascular Surgery, Brigham and Women's Hospital, Boston, MA, USA

Lifei Guo, MD, PhD, FACS Department of Plastic Surgery, Lahey Hospital & Medical Center, Burlington, MA, USA

Douglas L. Helm, MD, FACS Division of Plastic and Reconstructive Surgery, Harvard Medical School, Boston, MA, USA

Harvard Medical School, Boston, MA, USA

Joon Pio (Jp) Hong, MD, PhD, MMM Department of Plastic Surgery, Asan Medical Center University of Ulsan, Seoul, South Korea

Sumanas W. Jordan, MD, PhD Division of Plastic and Reconstructive Surgery, Northwestern University Feinberg School of Medicine, Chicago, IL, USA

Paul J. Kim, DPM, MS Georgetown University School of Medicine, Washington, DC, USA

Division of Wound Healing and Hyperbaric Medicine, Department of Plastic Surgery, MedStar Georgetown University Hospital, Washington, DC, USA

Daniel Kwan, MD Department of Plastic and Reconstructive Surgery, Rhode Island Hospital, The Warren Alpert Medical School of Brown University, Providence, RI, USA

Paul Y. Liu, MD, FACS Department of Plastic and Reconstructive Surgery, Rhode Island Hospital, The Warren Alpert Medical School of Brown University, Providence, RI, USA

Alec A. Macaulay, MD Department of Orthopedic Surgery, Brigham and Women's Hospital, Harvard Medical School, Boston, MA, USA

Raman Mehrzad, MD, MHL Department of Plastic and Reconstructive Surgery, Rhode Island Hospital, The Warren Alpert Medical School of Brown University, Providence, RI, USA

Benjamin J. Mitchell, BS Department of Plastic Surgery, Center for Wound Healing, Medstar Georgetown University Hospital, Washington, DC, USA

Dennis P. Orgill, MD, PhD Division of Plastic Surgery, Brigham and Women's Hospital Harvard Medical School, Boston, MA, USA

Joseph Park, DPM Division of Podiatric Surgery, MedStar Washington Hospital Center, Washington, DC, USA

Scott Schmidt, MD Department of Plastic and Reconstructive Surgery, Rhode Island Hospital, The Warren Alpert Medical School of Brown University, Providence, RI, USA

Samir K. Shah, MD Division of Vascular and Endovascular Surgery, Brigham and Women's Hospital, Boston, MA, USA

Indranil Sinha, MD Division of Plastic and Reconstructive Surgery, Harvard Medical School, Boston, MA, USA

Harvard Medical School, Boston, MA, USA

Jessica D. Smith, BA Division of Plastic and Reconstructive Surgery, Harvard Medical School, Boston, MA, USA

Jeremy T. Smith, MD Department of Orthopedic Surgery, Brigham and Women's Hospital, Harvard Medical School, Boston, MA, USA

John S. Steinberg, DPM, FACFAS Department of Plastic Surgery, MedStar Georgetown University Hospital, Washington, DC, USA

Department of Plastic Surgery, Center for Wound Healing and Hyperbaric Medicine, MedStar Georgetown University Hospital, Washington, DC, USA

Hyunsuk (Peter) Suh, MD, PhD Department of Plastic Surgery, Asan Medical Center University of Ulsan, Seoul, South Korea

Kaspar Trocha, MD Division of Vascular and Endovascular Surgery, Brigham and Women's Hospital, Boston, MA, USA

Sergey Y. Turin, MD Division of Plastic and Reconstructive Surgery, Northwestern University Feinberg School of Medicine, Chicago, IL, USA

Eric Robert Zielinski, MD Division of Plastic and Reconstructive Surgery, Northwestern University Feinberg School of Medicine, Chicago, IL, USA

Part I
Surgical Methods and Techniques

Chapter 1
Surgical Debridement

Joshua A. David and Ernest S. Chiu

Introduction

Wound debridement is defined as the removal of devitalized or necrotic tissue, foreign bodies, and microorganisms from a wound bed in order to facilitate or expedite wound healing. Varying types of wound debridement techniques exist, but surgical – or sharp – debridement remains the gold standard in both acute and chronic wound management. First formally described by the eighteenth century French surgeon Pierre Joseph Desault, surgical debridement has evolved into a fundamental technique for restoring the appropriate biochemical conditions required for optimal wound healing. In addition to removing the various types of debris that impair wound healing, surgical debridement offers adjunctive benefits, such as the opportunity to culture the wound, collect biopsies, and perform a comprehensive inspection of the wound bed and local tissues for surgical or therapeutic planning. As we continue to discover more about the biology and physiology of wounds, we are increasingly aware of the significance of surgical debridement in preparing the wound bed, minimizing infection, and stimulating a microenvironment that favors successful wound healing.

Electronic Supplementary Material: The online version of this chapter (https://doi.org/10.1007/978-3-319-66990-8_1) contains supplementary material, which is available to authorized users.

J.A. David, BS • E.S. Chiu, MD FACS (✉)
Hansjörg Wyss Department of Plastic Surgery, New York Langone Medical Center, New York, NY, USA
e-mail: Josh.Adam.David@gmail.com; Ernest.Chiu@nyumc.org

D.P. Orgill (ed.), *Interventional Treatment of Wounds*,
https://doi.org/10.1007/978-3-319-66990-8_1

Wound Healing

Decades of scientific research have redefined the ways in which we evaluate and treat wounds. A more concrete understanding of the molecular and cellular components that facilitate physiologic healing – and propagate impaired healing – has expedited advancements in wound healing modalities such as synthetic and biologic dressings, skin substitutes, and exogenous growth factors. It has also helped us understand how surgical debridement functions to improve wound healing. Normal wound healing consists of four well-described and predictable stages, namely, hemostasis, inflammation, proliferation, and, lastly, remodeling of the extracellular matrix (ECM) [1].

In non-healing wounds, there is failure of regenerating tissue to successfully progress through the normal stages of wound healing. While these wounds remain a topic of intense research, we now know that non-healing wounds do not simply represent deviations of the normal tissue repair process but rather possess irreversible alterations in the timing and mechanisms of normal healing physiology [2]. Factors known to contribute to impaired wound healing include underlying metabolic abnormalities, bacterial contamination, and inadequate tissue perfusion. Irrespective of etiology, it is hypothesized that recurrent injury and ischemia in the wound bed results in overexpression of inflammatory cytokines such as tumor necrosis factor alpha (TNF-a) and interleukin-1 (IL-1), as well as impairments in growth factor action and normal cell migration. Consequently, there are reductions in fibroblast proliferation and connective tissue deposition, and disruptions in regulation of critical proteases, such as metalloproteinase (MMP), which normally function in ECM degradation and deposition [3]. Bacterial infiltration and the ensuing inflammatory response are also an important contributor to non-healing wounds. Surgical debridement is a critical tool for inhibiting this constant state of inflammation and promoting the proliferative phase of wound healing by removing foreign bodies, devitalized tissue, bacteria, and senescent cells at the wound edge and by encouraging platelet activation and the release of endogenous growth factors.

Wound Bed Preparation

The concept of wound bed preparation has emerged as a standard paradigm that encompasses all of the critical components of wound healing, such as debridement, bacterial balance, management of exudate, and the status of the patient. The ultimate goal of this approach is the formation of high-quality granulation tissue that will promote wound closure and either avoid or facilitate advanced healing practices such as skin grafting. The "TIME" (tissue, infection/inflammation, moisture balance, edge of wound) sequence for achieving optimal wound bed preparation was developed by group of international wound care experts in order to create a rational and systematic approach for wound management that would unite expertise and communication within the field of wound management (Table 1.1) [4].

Table 1.1 TIME sequence of wound bed preparation

Clinical observation	Proposed pathophysiology	Intervention	Effects on wound bed preparation
Tissue nonviable or deficient	Nonviable or biologically deficient tissue prevents wound, matrix formation impairs wound healing	Continuous or episodic debridement (surgical, mechanical, autolytic, etc.)	Removal of necrotic or devitalized tissue restores normal wound physiology: ↑ platelet activation, growth factor release, granulation tissue formation, vascularity
Infection/inflammation	Bacterial release of toxins, autolytic enzymes, and biofilm results in a constant inflammatory wound profile	Debridement, topical/systemic antibiotics, nutritional/metabolic optimization of patient	Reduction in bacterial load, and niduses and nutrients for bacterial overgrowth: ↓ inflammatory microenvironment, inhibitory proteases, adherent biofilm
Moisture imbalance	Edema and exudate results in wound desiccation that can impair epithelial cell migration. Excessive fluid causes maceration of wound margin	Mechanical fluid removal (e.g., vacuum) or specialized dressings	Restored moisture balance: ↑ epithelial cell migration and reepithelialization
Edge of wound, non-advancing or undermined	Physical aspects of wound that impair matrix formation and maturation. Includes non-migrating keratinocytes, senescent fibroblasts, and other ECM abnormalities	Debridement, surgical reconstruction (e.g., skin grafts) and adjunctive wound therapies	Advancement of epidermal margin: ↓ wound stage, depth

Debridement Classification

Multiple classification schemes have been developed in order to provide clinicians with objective metrics in order to describe wounds and wound care and for guiding treatment [5]. In general, a wound can be divided into three distinct zones: a zone of necrosis, a marginal zone, and a normal zone. Wounds can also be classified by depth of involved tissue; from superficial to deep, they can include skin, subcutaneous connective tissues, muscle, fascia, and bone. Wound debridement can be classified as one of five numerical categories: a non-debrided wound (0) or an incomplete (1), marginal (2), complete (3), or radical (4) debridement (Fig. 1.1). A non-debrided wound has not yet evolved through the "TIME" sequence of wound bed preparation. An incomplete wound debridement retains nonviable or necrotic tissue despite adequate wound bed preparation, predisposing it to wound complications. If nonviable tissue has been completely excised, but residual areas of tissue are compromised, it is termed marginal debridement. These surrounding tissues may in fact be viable or potentially viable, and thus local and systemic supportive care becomes critical in these cases. Complete debridement entails debridement of both nonviable and potentially viable tissues and usually occurs following multiple debridements. Last, a radical debridement includes excision of a surrounding margin of normal tissue. By using these wound classification systems alone, or in combination with other schemas that describe patient or injury factors – such as those developed by Cierny and Gustilo for host factors and open fractures, respectively – wound practitioners can more accurately describe the unique characteristics and qualities of a particular wound within a patient [6, 7].

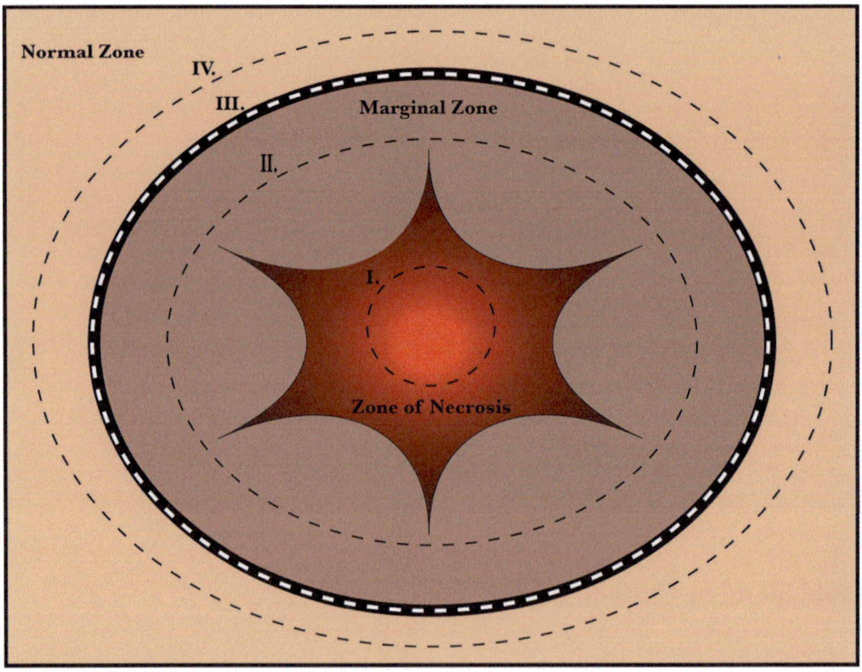

Fig. 1.1 Debridement classification system. The three zones of a wound, overlaid by debridement classifications I (incomplete), II (marginal), III (complete), and IV (radical). (Stage 0 is a non-debrided wound)

Types of Debridement

A variety of alternative debridement types (Table 1.2) exist, and these can be employed either alone, or more commonly, as adjunctive therapies to traditional surgical debridement. These include mechanical, autolytic, enzymatic, and biological debridement. Mechanical debridement forms the basis of techniques such as "wet-to-dry" dressings, which employ force to remove wound debris. Hydrotherapy, a form of mechanical debridement, has become an increasingly popular debridement technique and employs fluid irrigation at varying pressures to eject debris from a wound. Although the efficacy of this option still faces controversy, a novel ultra-high-pressure jet system based on the Venturi effect has shown promising results in studies [8]. Autolytic debridement involves maintaining a moist wound environment in order to accelerate the body's innate mechanisms of devitalized tissue proteolysis. Enzymatic debridement employs exogenous or endogenous enzymes, such as collagenase or papain, to break down necrotic tissue. Biological debridement utilizes maggot larvae, which preferentially digest and eliminate dead tissue. The quantity of necrotic tissue in the wound bed, size and depth of the wound, patient physiological status and comorbidities, and practitioner experience, will dictate the debridement approach. Surgical debridement should be undertaken as a conservative approach when there is an extensive area of tissue loss and large necrotic burden or if there is exposed tendon or bone.

Surgical Debridement: Indications, Instruments, Technique, and Complications

Indications for wound debridement include the presence of devitalized, necrotic tissue in an extensive ulcer, or wound edema or erythema, fluctuance, or discharge. Removal of an adherent eschar may also require debridement, although a stable, healing ulcer with a dry eschar can likely be left alone. In general, patient nutritional and metabolic status should be stabilized prior to any procedure, but in certain situations, such as sepsis or cellulitis, an urgent debridement may be required.

Styles and technique of surgical debridement vary across the world and even within centers. Podiatrists perform the vast majority of surgical debridements, but other practitioners include general, vascular, and plastic surgeons, family and internal medicine physicians, as well as nurse practitioners and physician assistants in some states [9]. Similarly, surgical debridement can occur in a variety of settings. While most occur in the office, they are also commonly performed in outpatient settings or nursing facilities when the extent of the region necessitates general anesthesia, or if there is risk of hemorrhage. Local anesthesia is often satisfactory, but general anesthesia may be necessary for complicated cases, or if adjunctive procedures, such as a bone biopsy for suspected osteomyelitis, are expected. In addition

Table 1.2 Types of debridement

Debridement type	Method	Physiologic effects	Advantages	Disadvantages
Surgical	Direct removal of devitalized tissue, foreign bodies, and microorganisms with sharp surgical instruments	Converts a chronic wound into an acute wound through a reduction in wound bio-burden, decrease in inhibitory load, and excision of senescent rim	• Fast • Comprehensive wound assessment • Wound cultures, biopsies, etc. • Preparation for surgical or nonsurgical wound closure	• May require experienced specialist, anesthesia, sterile surgical setting • Bleeding may occur
Mechanical	Utilizes force to remove debris (e.g., wet-to-dry dressings, vacuum-assisted closure)	Removes necrotic tissue, fibrin slough, and contaminants	• Easy to perform • Cost-effective	• Labor intensive • Nondiscriminatory • Can be painful • Moisture may macerate surrounding tissue
Fluid irrigation	Low (1–15 psi) or high (35–70 psi) pressure systems (pulsatile lavage, hydrosurgery, FluidJet)	Irrigation of foreign material, particulate matter, and contaminants	• Can include use of antimicrobial • Can simultaneously irrigate and debride	• Evidence is controversial • May promote wound contamination • High pressure can damage tissue
Autolytic	Occlusive or hydrocolloid, hydrogel dressings	Re-establishes wound moisture-balance by utilizing endogenous enzymes and stimulating macrophages	• Easy to perform • Capitalizes on endogenous healing mechanisms	• Slow, less aggressive, • Constant dressing changes • Contraindicated in infected wound
Enzymatic	Endogenous or exogenous enzymes (collagenase, elastase, papain/urea)	Proteolytic degradation of collagen or fibrinous tissue	• Works synergistically with endogenous enzymes	• Application may be painful, frequent enzyme changing
Biologic	Maggots of green bottle fly (*Lucilia sericata)*	Enzymatic debridement, decreases bacterial counts, motion stimulation of wound bed	• Minimal pain • Good alternative for non-operable candidate or poorly vascularized tissue	• Patient reluctance

to a sterile environment, essential tools for surgical debridement may include forceps, scalpels, gouge, scissors, curettes, rongeurs, burrs, rasps, saws, saline wash, and syringes, as well as electrocoagulation devices for ensuring hemostasis and clean wound dressings (Fig. 1.2).

Once the patient is properly positioned, and any preoperative markings are drawn (if necessary), the wound and surrounding skin are sterilized with a povidone-iodine solution (Video 1.1). At this point, some practitioners will apply topical methylene blue to the wound, which stains nonviable tissue in order to facilitate a precise, guided debridement. Once the surgical site has been prepared, debridement of devitalized tissue with a sharp instrument such as a scalpel or scissors can proceed (Fig. 1.3). Starting from an area of obvious necrosis, which appears black, and working toward healthier tissue is a reasonable strategy, and tissue appearance and the presence of bleeding can guide the distinction between nonviable and viable tissue. Fibrin tissue, which can be white, yellow, or green, should be debrided as well, while granulation tissue has a pink appearance and should be preserved. Any accumulated exudate should be drained. If the extent of necrosis is ambiguous, a second stage of debridement may be prudent, particularly in deeper tissue layers. In these cases, the short-term use of dilute antiseptics such as acetic acid, povidone-iodine,

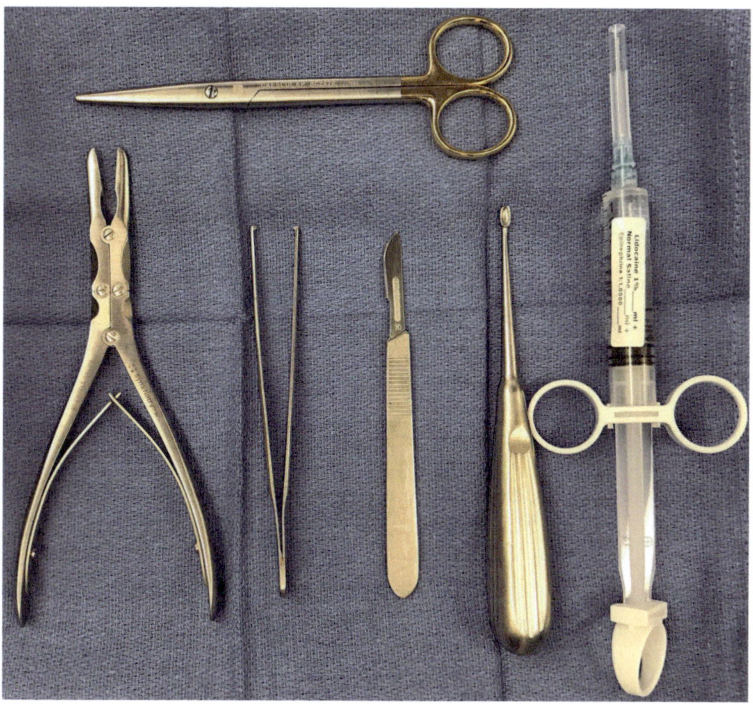

Fig. 1.2 Typical instruments of surgical debridement. Includes a rongeur, forceps, scalpel, curette, and local anesthesia (from *left* to *right*), and surgical scissors (*above*)

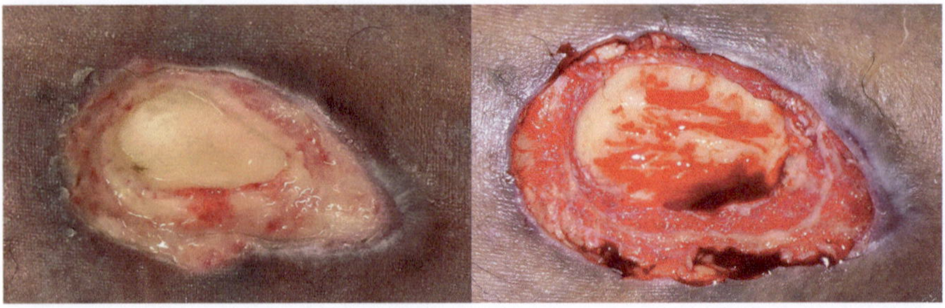

Fig. 1.3 Wound debridement. Wound before (*left*) and after (*right*) debridement. This is a full-thickness wound in the right leg of a 50-year-old man with Type II diabetes mellitus. Note the bone visible at the base of the wound. The bleeding and healthier granulation tissue in the right image indicates the presence of viable tissue and an adequate debridement

or silver dressings can be employed for wound protection. Following debridement, clean, dry dressings should be applied for 8–24 h, after which wet-to-moist or wet-to-dry dressings can be restarted.

There is always a possibility that surgical debridement may not result in proper wound bed preparation or sufficiently eliminate nonviable tissue. Certain medical conditions, particularly those in which vascular integrity is impaired, exhibit a notoriously poor response to surgical debridement. Additionally, surgical debridement carries inherent risks, the most common of which is bleeding. Direct pressure, or the application of topical hemostatic agents such as epinephrine, is usually sufficient to control minor bleeds. For larger pulsatile bleeds however, an instrument clamp, ligation with a suture, or electrocoagulation may be necessary. In chronic wounds, the tissue can be quite lax, and identifying the source of bleeding during debridement may be more difficult.

Infection

Infected wounds pose a difficult challenge for the wound care provider, and local wound care must be delicately balanced with optimization of the patient's immunologic, hemodynamic, and metabolic status. Surgical debridement is considered a prerequisite for successful treatment of bone, joint, and soft-tissue infections, regardless of whether this includes antibiotics, negative-pressure wound therapy, arthroplasty, or open wound therapy [10]. In general, a bacterial count of greater than 10^5 organisms per gram of tissue in a wound is considered an invasive infection and is sufficient to impair healing [11]. The mechanisms by which infection undermines wound healing are multifaceted and involve both bacterial production of toxins and fibrinolytic enzymes, as well as an endogenous inflammatory, cellular, and oxidative response [12]. It is therefore critical that practitioners utilize clinical signs in conjunction with appropriate microbiological assays, such as quantitative or semiquantitative cultures, swab cultures, or needle aspiration, for early recognition of infection and to guide therapeutic intervention. This is particularly important in burns and necrotizing fasciitis, both of which employ surgical debridement as a mainstay of treatment and require early diagnosis and intervention, as well as aggressive empirical antibiotics and septic control for optimal results. Debridement is essential not only for removal of bacteria and the devitalized tissue that provides them with nutrients but also in order to eradicate wound biofilm [13]. Biofilm is composed of bacterial glycocalyx secretions and functions in adherence of microorganisms to the wound, particularly if foreign material such as implants or prostheses is present. These carbohydrate matrices are found in 60–80% of chronic wounds, and render microcolonies resistant to antimicrobials and other debridement techniques such as pulse lavage. Thus, surgical debridement also plays an essential role in the treatment of infected orthopedic prostheses and will require either a single- or two-stage debridement depending on the chronicity of infection, virulence of the organism, and patient factors before reimplantation is attempted.

Acute Traumatic Wounds

Etiologies of acute traumatic wounds can include avulsion, high-powered, and crush injuries. Standard procedures for management of these injuries include prophylactic antibiotic administration, meticulous debridement, irrigation, stabilization, and early soft-tissue coverage. However, due to the high kinetic forces associated with these injuries, the extent of injury often extends well beyond the gross margins of the wound, causing extensive destruction to the surrounding bone and soft tissues. These wounds are also prone to contamination and deep infections, particularly if a foreign object caused the injury.

Open fractures of long bones represent a unique challenge. As a rule of thumb, prompt surgical treatment remains the gold standard. However, the timing of surgical debridement for open fractures remains a point of contention. Historically, infectious concerns support early surgical debridement (<6 h following injury) for open fractures, despite conflicting evidence as to whether delayed treatment (>24 h) augments the risk of infection. Of note, a formal debridement should be avoided upon presentation of a known or suspected open fracture in the emergency room, as nosocomial pathogens can actually facilitate infection in these cases.

In most centers, plastic and orthopedic surgeons will work in conjunction on these cases. Upon inspection, it should be noted that soft-tissue damage will likely expand beyond the margins of the gross wound, and surgeons should expect that extension of the wound will be required in order to perform an adequate debridement, as well as to obtain access for skeletal stabilization, excision of nonviable deep tissue, and removal of necrotic cortical bone. Experience is key for surgeons to accurately assess the viability of fascia, tendons, and muscle, as the decision whether to leave or excise any of these deep structures is challenging and can have profound effects on future form and function. Proper wound irrigation is vital for deeper decontamination, and there are many options with regard to fluid type, volume, and delivery system, each possessing benefits and drawbacks. Notably, tangential high-pressure fluidic debridement has emerged as an effective method of simultaneous debridement and irrigation and is gaining traction for use in open fractures.

Burns

Burn injuries are complicated by sepsis, excessive blood loss, and disfigurement from scarring. It has long been known that early debridement and skin grafting result in enhanced patient survival, healing time, and hospital stay [14, 15]. Consequently, debridement techniques have adapted in order to address the particular challenges of full thickness (third degree) and deep dermal burns. In what is termed tangential excision, the burn eschar is shaved off in thin layers with an angled debridement knife until viable dermis is reached, thus maximizing tissue preservation and, ultimately, esthetic and functional outcomes. In large burns however, sizeable amounts of tissue require debridement, and practitioners will alternatively opt for fascial excision, in which all tissue is removed down to the fascia. This technique, while minimizing blood loss, can eliminate supportive structures, potentially resulting in increased cosmetic deformity and scarring in these patients. Newer techniques for burn debridement include dermabrasion, hydrosurgery, and CO2 lasers, which – unlike tangential and fascial excision – can preserve the maximal amount of dermis. However, these techniques are currently slower than traditional debridement techniques and remain limited by availability.

Chronic Wounds

Chronic wounds are technically defined as wounds that have not healed after 6 weeks, but this term can be broadly applied to most progressive or non-healing wounds. Despite advances in wound care treatments, chronic wounds remain the leading causes of lower extremity amputation in the USA [16]. They tend to occur in the setting of metabolic diseases and vascular insufficiency but are also associated with nutritional deficiencies, pharmacological agents such as steroids, and cutaneous cancers.

Diabetic, arterial, venous, and pressure ulcers constitute the majority of chronic wounds requiring surgical debridement. The role of surgical debridement in this setting is essentially to utilize principles of wound bed preparation in order to convert a chronic wound into an acute one, thus initiating the healing process. While acute wounds generally do not require more than one debridement, chronic non-healing wounds require more frequent debridements, as they continue to generate a necrotic burden, accumulate abnormal cells that impair the healing response, and provide a nidus, nutrients, and an anaerobic environment for bacterial overgrowth. While the management of all chronic wounds adheres to the TIME principles of wound bed preparation, there are certain considerations to keep in mind when treating particular types of chronic wounds.

Diabetic Ulcers

In 2004, more than half of all Medicare claims or surgical debridement were for patients with a diagnosis of diabetes [9]. Chronic hyperglycemia and nerve damage are fundamental pathologies involved in the formation of these ulcers, and surgical debridement has been validated as a vital component of treatment for these wounds, resulting in accelerated healing times and a lower recurrence rate [17]. The unique characteristics of these wounds include a hyperkeratotic callus surrounding the rim of the ulcer, absence of pain due to a neuropathic etiology, and development over an area subject to heavy loads, which may require an exostectomy. A vascular assessment should be performed prior to surgery to rule out arterial occlusive disease, in addition to a thorough assessment of the wound and a patient history that includes the course of the lesion and previous treatment attempts. Particular attention should be paid to the presence of infection, abscess, and/or gangrene. Prevention is the key of diabetic ulcer management, and the patient should be counseled on how to properly and regularly conduct self-assessments of their feet.

Decubitus Ulcers

Decubitus ulcers, also referred to as pressure sores, affect an estimated 1.3–3 million people in the USA alone [18]. Decubitus ulcers occur when the skin overlying bony prominences, particularly the sacrum or heels, are subjected to extended bouts of pressure. They are more likely to occur in terminally ill or elderly patients, particularly when paralysis, hip fractures, or spinal cord injuries necessitate long periods of confinement to a bed or wheelchair.

Comprehensive patient assessment and proper staging of the decubitus ulcer according to the National Pressure Ulcer Advisory Committee (NPUAC) are important factors in guiding wound management strategies in these patients. In general, stage III and IV decubitus ulcers, which possess full-thickness skin loss, should be considered for surgical debridement. Decubitus ulcers should always raise concern for underlying osteomyelitis, and radiographic and imaging studies such as radiolabeled leukocyte scintigraphy and magnetic resonance imaging (MRI) are useful tools for monitoring the periosteal surfaces and bone marrow for signs of infection.

Post-debridement Wound Management

The management of a wound following surgical debridement is equally important to proper wound healing as the debridement itself, and failure to appreciate or recognize the appropriate postsurgical requirements can result in devastating consequences. A clean, but unhealed, postoperative soft-tissue matrix will likely require a combination of additional debridements – surgical or other – before ultimate wound closure. Wound closure techniques range from simple skin approximation to grafts and complex tissue rearrangements such as flaps but possess the common goal of reestablishing arterial, venous, and lymphatic flow in order to restore nutrient delivery and metabolic waste elimination, as well as maximizing esthetic and functional outcomes.

Regardless of ultimate wound closure modality, the importance of postsurgical wound monitoring cannot be overstated. This affords the clinician additional opportunities to comprehensively survey the wound for the appearance, quality, and quantity of drainage and also, if necessary, excise wound margins or remove hypertrophic granulation tissue. Proper dressings and physiologic optimization are also key requirements for proper wound healing. Additionally, infection control, either through topical or systemic antibiotics, is paramount and should be monitored and treated appropriately in order to minimize inflammation, particularly in patients who have immune or vascular compromise. Maintaining a delicate moisture balance is cited, but often neglected; excessive moisture causes maceration of the wound margin, while desiccation results in impaired epithelial cell migration. Additionally, newer therapeutic modalities such as vacuum-assisted closure (VAC) devices and supra-atmospheric hyperbaric oxygen chambers are increasingly utilized as adjunctive wound healing measures by optimizing local hygiene and oxygen delivery.

Conclusion

Wound management remains an essential component of holistic patient care, particularly as we face challenges such as an aging population and an increase in the prevalence in diabetes. Even with the advent of novel debridement strategies, such as the use of ultrasound, radiofrequency ablation, or erbium:YAG lasers, traditional surgical debridement remains a fundamental aspect of acute and chronic wound care treatment. Although the basis of surgical debridement – the removal of nonviable tissue and foreign bodies – may seem relatively straightforward at first glance, variations in wound mechanism of injury and anatomical location, underlying patient medical morbidities, timing of surgery and adjunctive debridement techniques, and the variety of wound closure options complicate this critical component of wound management. An experienced practitioner who is well versed in the molecular, physiological, and technical aspects of surgical debridement is critical for successful wound management.

References

1. Schilling JA. Wound healing. Surg Clin North Am. 1976;56(4):859–74.
2. Panuncialman J, Falanga V. The science of wound bed preparation. Surg Clin North Am. 2009;89(3):611–26.

3. Eming SA, Krieg T, Davidson JM. Inflammation in wound repair: molecular and cellular mechanisms. J Investig Dermatol. 2007;127(3):514–25.
4. Schultz GS, Sibbald RG, Falanga V, Ayello EA, Dowsett C, Harding K, et al. Wound bed preparation: a systematic approach to wound management. Wound Repair and Rregen. 2003;11(Suppl 1):S1–28.
5. Granick MS, Gamelli RL. Surgical wound healing and management. New York: Informa Healthcare; 2007.
6. Cierny G. 3rd. Chronic osteomyelitis: results of treatment. Instr Course Lect. 1990;39:495–508.
7. Gustilo RB, Gruninger RP, Davis T. Classification of type III (severe) open fractures relative to treatment and results. Orthopedics. 1987;10(12):1781–8.
8. Webb LX, Smith TL, Morykwas MJ. Wound debridement: a comparison of two techniques for particle clearance. HydroCision Doc. No. 1000–1161, Rev. A09/03. www.wounds.Smith-Nephew.com
9. Department of Health and Human Services. Medicare Payments for surgical debridement services in 2004. 2007. OEI-02-05-00390.
10. Lew DP, Waldvogel FA. Osteomyelitis. Lancet. 2004;364(9431):369–79.
11. Robson MC, Heggers JP. Quantitative bacteriology and inflammatory mediators in soft tissue. Soft and hard tissue repair. New York: Praeger; 1984. p. 484–507.
12. Penhallow K. A review of studies that examine the impact of infection on the normal wound-healing process. J Wound Care. 2005;14(3):123–6.
13. Black CE, Costerton JW. Current concepts regarding the effect of wound microbial ecology and biofilms on wound healing. Surg Clin North Am. 2010;90(6):1147–60.
14. Cope O, Langohr JL, et al. Expeditious care of full-thickness burn wounds by surgical excision and grafting. Ann Surg. 1947;125(1):1–22.
15. Burke JF, Bondoc CC, Quinby WC. Primary burn excision and immediate grafting: a method shortening illness. J Trauma. 1974;14(5):389–95.
16. American Diabetes Association. Economic costs of diabetes in the U.S. in 2012. Diabetes Care. 2013;36:1033–46.
17. Piaggesi A, Schipani E, Campi F, Romanelli M, Baccetti F, Arvia C, et al. Conservative surgical approach versus non-surgical management for diabetic neuropathic foot ulcers: a randomized trial. Diabet Med. 1998;15(5):412–7.
18. Panel for the Prediction and Prevention of Pressure Ulcers in Adults. Pressure ulcers in adults: prediction and prevention. Clinical practice guideline, 3. Rockville: Agency for Healthcare Policy and Research, Public Health Service, US Department of Health and Human Services, 1992 May: HCPR Publication No. 92–0047.

Chapter 2
Bacterial Control

Jessica D. Smith, Indranil Sinha, and Douglas L. Helm

Introduction

Bacterial skin and soft tissue infections (SSTIs) have become increasingly common and, left untreated, can progress to sepsis. SSTIs are caused by microbes, which invade the skin, subcutaneous tissue, fascia, and muscle. SSTI severity ranges from localized to rapidly progressing and systemic infections. These bacterial infections vary greatly in their clinical presentation and recommended interventions [1]. Accurate diagnosis and management with a comprehensive treatment plan that takes into account the patient's overall health, comorbidities, and severity and location of the infection are critical to proper SSTI management. Comprehensive SSTI treatment may require multimodal therapy, including oral and intravenous antibiotics, topical agents, antibacterial dressings, and surgical debridement.

The financial burden of SSTIs is not well understood, but preliminary studies suggest surgical intervention can result in substantial cost and vary widely. One study suggests that direct costs of treatment ranges from $400 per patient to $30,000 per patient [2], depending on the intervention required. Following orthopedic and cardiac surgery procedures, complicated by SSTI, the medical costs can be upwards of an additional $40,000 per case [3]. Meanwhile, surgical intervention to address a breast tissue-expander infection costs between $18,500 and $28,000 more per

---

Electronic Supplementary Material: The online version of this chapter (https://doi.org/10.1007/978-3-319-66990-8_2) contains supplementary material, which is available to authorized users.

J.D. Smith, BA
Division of Plastic and Reconstructive Surgery, Harvard Medical School, Boston, MA, USA

I. Sinha, MD • D.L. Helm, MD, FACS (✉)
Division of Plastic and Reconstructive Surgery, Harvard Medical School, Boston, MA, USA

Harvard Medical School, Boston, MA, USA
e-mail: dhelm@partners.org

D.P. Orgill (ed.), *Interventional Treatment of Wounds*,
https://doi.org/10.1007/978-3-319-66990-8_2

patient [4]. Although there are no statistics that describe the overall cost of SSTIs and surgical intervention, it is evident that the additional financial burden is enormous. As a result, the World Health Organization has established numerous recommendations for preoperative, intraoperative, and postoperative measures to prevent surgical site infections [5, 6]. If, however, an infection does occur, prompt and effective treatment is paramount. This chapter will discuss the various treatment regimens and, in particular, the timing, frequency, and extent of surgical debridement that is required to eradicate an infection as well as ancillary approaches to SSTI treatment.

At Risk Patient Populations

Although SSTIs may affect anyone, several distinct patient populations are at an elevated risk of developing soft tissue infections. People who suffer from diabetes mellitus, burns, radiation, paraplegia, obesity, immune disorders, and addiction to tobacco products have a higher risk of SSTIs.

Diabetes Mellitus

Diabetes mellitus (DM) is a risk factor for SSTIs and infection-related mortality [7, 8]. The elevated risk of infection results from impaired immune function, uncontrolled glucose levels, nerve and microvascular damage, and insufficient blood flow. Though not immunocompromised, diabetic patients display altered immune function due to impaired cell-mediated immunity and humoral immunity [7, 9, 10]. Neutrophils and macrophages exhibit poor chemotaxis and impaired function in diabetic patients [10, 11]. In addition, hyperglycemia impairs neutrophil bactericidal efficacy [7, 12]. Consequently, diabetic patients inadequately respond to acute bacterial infections. Furthermore, hyperglycemia interferes with wound healing, which can lead to the development of chronic wounds with bacterial colonization [13].

DM also frequently causes nerve damage and, subsequently, autonomic and peripheral neuropathy. Autonomic neuropathy can lead to abnormal sweating, dry skin, impaired tissue perfusion, and eventually cracking and fissuring of the skin, which creates an entryway for bacteria [14, 15]. Peripheral neuropathy decreases an individual's sensitivity to stimuli, as well as muscle tone, which predisposes to altered pressure distributions and deformation of the feet [11, 16]. Altered pressure distribution in conjunction with autonomic neuropathy may cause diabetic patients to develop skin breakdown through which bacteria can enter [7]. Patients that suffer from diabetic peripheral neuropathy are seven times more likely to develop a foot ulcer than those without peripheral neuropathy [14, 17].

Diabetic patients commonly suffer from vascular compromise of both large and small vessels, referred to as peripheral arterial disease (PAD). Secondary to local tissue hypoxia and reduced circulation, anaerobic bacteria can thrive, while immune cells and antibiotic access to the infected areas are reduced [11, 18, 19]. Patients with diabetes and concomitant PAD are not only more likely to develop an infection, they are three times more likely to experience infection-associated mortality [7, 8].

Patients with DM have an increased risk of developing multiple types of SSTIs, including skin infection, surgical site infections, periprosthetic joint infections, and chronically infected pressure injuries [7, 20]. Lenz et al. demonstrated that diabetics HBA1c, a measure of glucose control, correlates with a 9% increase in risk of sternal wound infection [21]. Jamsen et al. found that diabetes increases a patient's risk of periprosthetic joint infection by 2.3 times [22], and Kunutsor et al. report that the relative risk of wound infection following total joint arthroplasty was 2.57 for patients with DM [23]. A diabetic patient's risk ratio for hospitalization or physician claim secondary to infection is 1.21 compared to a nondiabetic patient [7, 24]. SSTI treatment in this patient population must be accordingly aggressive to prevent further sequelae.

Burn Injuries

The skin serves as a critical barrier for first line defense to pathogens. Thermal or chemical burn injury breaks down this barrier. The skin is comprised of several layers, the outermost formed by keratinocytes covering a well-vascularized dermal layer, which is home to a rich supply of lymphocytes, blood vessels, and glandular tissues. When damaged by a burn injury, this defensive structure becomes a rich media for attacking microorganisms. Utilizing the protein exudate, microbes colonize the wound in the first 48 h and can rapidly lead to serious, even life-threatening, infections [25–27]. Burn infections can be severe, and approximately 75% of deaths in patients who suffered over 40% total body surface area (TBSA) burns were from sepsis due to burn wound infections or infection complications [25].

In addition to damaging the human body's physical barrier to infection, burn injury impairs the immune system and its natural response to injury. The mechanism by which burns cause immunosuppression is not fully understood, but studies have suggested that the production of granulocytes and monocytes/macrophages decreases following burn injury and that there are other biochemical changes that affect the immune system by way of impacting the endocrine system, arachidonic acid cascade, and cytokine network [25, 28]. As a result, burn patients are susceptible to infection and infection-related mortality [29, 30].

Radiation

Radiation therapy, a common cancer treatment, disrupts the DNA replication process. In doing so, radiation destroys rapidly dividing neoplastic cells but with unwanted damage to healthy surrounding tissue as well. Long-term effects of radiation include loss of tissue elasticity, scarring, fragility of blood vessels,

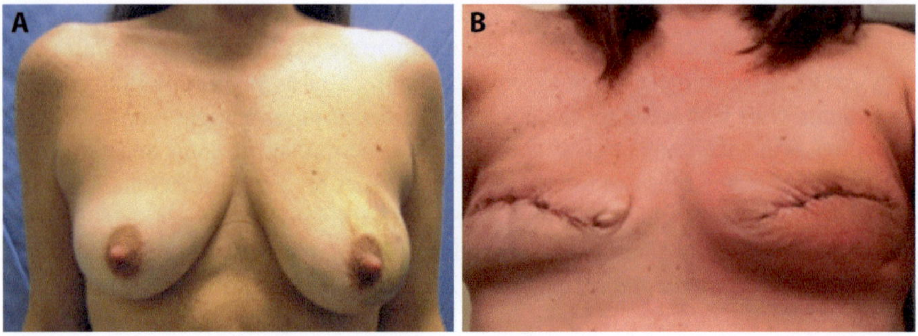

Fig. 2.1 A patient with unilateral, left breast cancer presented prior to bilateral mastectomy and implant-based reconstruction (**a**). She received preoperative, unilateral radiation. Following bilateral mastectomy and tissue-expander placement, she developed an acute infection of her left breast prosthesis (**b**). The erythema and induration are indicative of cellulitis, which is a common clinical sign of an infectious process and likely infection of the implant. Treatment for early infections includes antibiotics, but infections that are prolonged or in an irradiated field, as in this patient's case, often require removal of the implant, debridement and washout, closure, and eventually delayed breast reconstruction

arteriosclerosis, erythema, swelling, and as a result, impaired wound healing [31]. Operative intervention in radiated sites may also increase the rates of surgical site infections (SSIs).

Following breast reconstruction with a silicone or saline prosthesis, numerous studies have shown that patients who receive radiation therapy have a higher risk of developing an infection, such as cellulitis, in the irradiated field (Fig. 2.1). Patients having undergone radiation therapy are five times more likely to develop an implant infection than those who did not receive radiation [32]. Other studies have described similar outcomes, and some have shown that patients who receive postoperative radiation also have an increased risk of developing later infections (greater than 90 days postoperative), but limited research exists regarding the mechanism of SSTIs following radiation therapy [33–38].

Risk for infection following radiation to other areas of the body has not been well described. Sutton et al. suggest that rectal cancer patients who received radiation therapy prior to elective rectal cancer resection had a greater risk of developing a delayed superficial infection [39]. Concurrent chemotherapy and corticosteroid treatment, both of which are immunosuppressive, further puts patients at greater risk for infection [40, 41]. A depiction of SSTI in a patient following surgical resection of sarcoma within a radiated field is shown in Fig. 2.2.

Paraplegia

Paraplegia, independent of etiology, increases an individual's risk for infection. Paraplegics are frequently wheel chair bound and, given their immobility, are highly susceptible to pressure injuries. Loss of sensation below the level of injury leads to

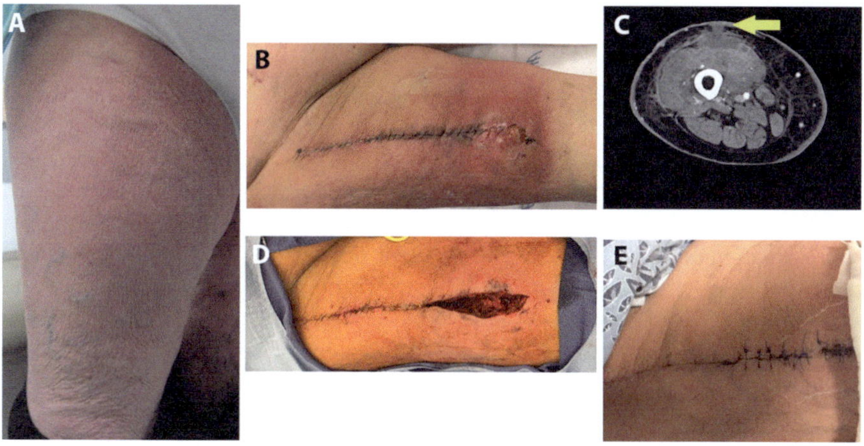

Fig. 2.2 Although the risk of infection following radiation to areas of the body other than the breasts is not well described, our center has experienced a greater number of infections following surgery in an irradiated field. This patient presented with a previously irradiated muscle sarcoma of her right anterior thigh (**a**). Three month status post radiation, the sarcoma was resected. Approximately 1 month later she developed a fluid collection with surrounding erythema and induration (**b**). A CT scan confirmed the presence of a fluid collection (**c**). The patient was taken back to the operating room, and the area was irrigated and debrided (I&D). The surrounding erythema immediately resolved following washout (**d**). One month after I&D, there were no signs of infection, and the area was healing well (**e**)

increased pressure in recumbent areas and moisture buildup, ultimately causing skin maceration and eventual ulceration [42]. Studies have shown that the prevalence of pressure injuries in spinal cord injury (SCI) patients ranges from 13% to 69% during their initial hospitalization [43, 44]. Other paraplegics are susceptible to skin break down as well because they have limited ability to reposition themselves. Once there is a break in the skin, microorganisms can move into, colonize, and lead to infection in the area.

Research has examined the overall effect of paraplegia on the immune system. Paralysis, especially from high-level SCIs, has been shown to impair the immune system, especially early on, and further increase a paraplegic's susceptibility to infection. According to Cruse et al., both the natural and adaptive immune responses are affected by SCI; natural-killer cell function and T-cell function and activation decrease acutely in individuals who suffer SCIs [45]. Additionally, Rubin-Asher et al. report that macrophage phagocytosis and cellular adhesion molecules are negatively affected by paralysis [45–48]. Cruse et al. also describe that SCI patients who undergo rehabilitation typically regain the majority of both natural and adaptive immune functions, although natural-killer cell function only reaches the lower end of the normal range; when patients stopped active rehabilitation, natural-killer cell function decreased once again [45]. Given the initial decline in immune function, it is important to recognize the elevated risk of infection for SCI patients in the early months following their injury and to be cognizant that all paraplegics have an increased risk of infection compared to their uninjured counterparts.

Obesity

Obesity, defined as a body mass index (BMI) greater than 30 kg/m^2, elevates the risk of infection. In patients with obesity, adipose tissue has decreased vascularity and, as a result, suffers from hypoxia. Infected wounds in the adipose tissue can, therefore, rapidly progress secondary to decreased exposure to neutrophils, macrophages, and antibiotics [30, 31, 35, 49]. Obesity further causes patients to consistently be in a pro-inflammatory state due to the constant degradation of adipose tissue and increased production of adipokines [50], which possibly restrains T-lymphocyte function [51–53]. Additionally, studies have indicated that obesity may independently impair T-cell, B-cell, macrophage, and dendritic cell activity [51–54]. As a result, obese patients are significantly more susceptible to infection. Balachandran et al. reported an odds ratio of 2.59 for sternal infection in an obese patient population [49]. Marmor et al. state that the infection risk for total knee arthroplasty is 6.7 times greater for severely obese patients (BMI > 35), while it is 4.2 times great for severely obese patients undergoing total hip arthroplasty [46, 55]. Waisbren et al. describe a fivefold increase in SSI in an obese population [56].

Tobacco

Many studies have shown that tobacco smoke is reported to delay primary wound healing and lead to subsequent infection. Tobacco smoke contains nicotine, carbon monoxide, and hydrogen cyanide, all of which contribute to tissue hypoxia [57]. Nicotine stimulates the sympathetic nervous system, which then releases epinephrine, causes vasoconstriction, and leads to tissue ischemia. Simultaneously carbon monoxide increases tissue hypoxia by binding to hemoglobin in place of oxygen thereby decreasing tissue oxygen availability. Hydrogen cyanide furthers this problem of tissue hypoxia by inhibiting cellular oxygen metabolism and further diminishing the effectiveness of the delivered oxygen [57, 58]. The resulting hypoxic environment causes surgical sites and wounds to remain open for longer periods of time and allows for microorganism colonization [59].

Research has also demonstrated the negative effects of tobacco on the immune system though the exact mechanism is still not fully understood. Studies have suggested both cell-mediated and humoral-mediated immunity are impacted by smoking, including decreased levels of circulating immunoglobulins, CD4$^+$ lymphocytes, and pro-inflammatory cytokines. Additionally, smoking may increase CD8$^+$ lymphocyte counts and impair phagocyte activity [60, 61]. These effects may be temporary and reversible following cessation [60, 62, 63]. To obtain optimal healing following surgery, research has indicated that patients should quit smoking at least 30 days before their procedure [59]. Otherwise, many studies have shown that current smokers have an increased risk of SSIs, especially following breast cancer surgery, cardiac surgery, and spinal surgery [35, 64–66].

Immunocompromise

Impairment of the central immune system has several causes including neutrophil defects, HIV, immunosuppressive medications required after a transplant, corticosteroid use, and chemotherapy treatment [67, 68]. A thorough discussion of various immunocompromised states is beyond the scope of this chapter, but, collectively, these patients are at high risk for SSTIs and must be monitored vigilantly. These patients may not present with normal clinical manifestations of infection, and they have a higher risk of hematogenous dissemination of infection [67]. Furthermore, infections can progress and become life threatening more rapidly in a compromised host. Lastly, immunocompromised patients have a greater susceptibility to infection from unusual microorganisms, which makes diagnosis and treatment of SSTIs in this patient population particularly difficult and yet paramount [69]. Aggressive treatment is warranted and required for SSTIs in this patient population to limit further morbidity and mortality.

Categories of Bacterial Infection

Given the broad range of bacterial SSTIs, the Infectious Diseases Society of America developed a classification system for skin and soft tissue infections based on skin extension, rate of progression, and tissue necrosis [68, 70]. Skin extension is divided into uncomplicated infections, such as impetigo and cellulitis, and complicated infections, which normally involve deeper tissues. Rate of progression is further divided into acute wound infections and chronic wound infections. Acute infections include traumas and postoperative infections, while diabetic foot infections and pressure injuries are chronic wound infections. Lastly, the SSTIs are classified as necrotizing and non-necrotizing infections [70]. It is important to determine which categories an infection falls into so that the necessary and proper treatment or treatments can be utilized. Further complicating bacterial infections is antibiotic resistance, which is an increasing problem secondary to improper use of antibiotic therapy.

Wound Colonization

Wound colonization refers to the presence of microorganisms without a host response [71–75]. Given the presence of pathogens, a colonized wound may experience delayed wound healing without clinical manifestations of infection [71]. However, bacterial colonization, especially high perioperative bacterial load, is often a precursor to infection [72].

Acute Infections

Acute bacterial infections occur when microorganisms invade an area following a breach in the integumentary barrier, frequently resulting from surgery or trauma [76]. Immediately following injury, planktonic bacteria, which are single, independent, bacterial cells, will colonize the area and adhere to host cells in low numbers [77]. If the bacterial load increases, evades the host defenses, and begins to cause tissue damage, an SSTI develops, and the body mounts an inflammatory reaction in response to the bacterial toxins. On clinical examination, patients may exhibit varying symptoms, but common clinical presentations include erythema, edema, warmth, pain, and tenderness. More severe infections may cause fever, hypotension, tachycardia, altered mental status, and pain. Prompt diagnosis and targeted treatment of an acute SSTI are important [78]. *Staphylococcus aureus (S. aureus)*, Alpha-hemolytic streptococci, *Pseudomonas aeruginosa (P. aeruginosa)*, and *Escherichia coli (E. coli)* are the most common pathogens responsible for acute bacterial infections [76].

Chronic Infections

Chronic infections are characterized by prolonged inflammatory responses, which damage tissues and prevent collagen synthesis and epithelialization [79, 80]. Chronic infections tend to progress more slowly than acute infections but also tend to have higher rates of morbidity and mortality [77, 80]. Rather than solely being caused by planktonic bacteria, these infections are frequently caused by a combination of planktonic bacteria and biofilms, which are polymicrobial colonies of bacteria encased in an extracellular polymeric matrix. The protective biofilm matrix provides the microorganisms with enhanced protection from the surrounding environment [81], as well as the ability to adhere to both inert and living surfaces [80]. As a result, biofilms are difficult to eradicate and often do not respond to antibiotic treatment. Additionally, biofilms are frequently found in chronic wounds, such as diabetic foot ulcers and pressure injuries, as well as on the surface of foreign bodies, such as prosthetic implants [77]. Similar to acute infections, *Staphylococcus aureus* and *Pseudomonas aeruginosa* are two of the most common bacteria present in biofilms, though their mechanisms of infection and chronicity differ [81].

Common SSTIs and Their Treatment

SSTIs have become an increasingly common reason for ambulatory visits, emergency care, and hospitalization. Further complicating this clinical problem is the increased prevalence of drug-resistant infections, which lead to a dramatic increase in the cost of caring for SSTIs [70]. For example, treatment of *Staphylococcus aureus* SSTIs in 2008 alone cost $4.84 billion, which was a 44% increase in cost from 2001 [82]. Although the general treatment of SSTIs are the same, certain types of SSTIs require special considerations for treatment including diabetic foot infections, sternal wound infections, lower extremity periprosthetic joint infections, infected burns, previously irradiated implant-based breast reconstruction infections, and infected pressure injuries.

Diabetic Foot Infections

Diabetic foot infections (DFIs) are a common consequence of diabetic foot ulcers (DFUs), which are full-thickness wounds in diabetics distal to the ankle [14, 83]. A diabetic patient has approximately a 25% lifetime risk of developing a DFU [14, 84]. Once the skin has ulcerated, bacteria and other pathogens can easily enter into and colonize the area. Staphylococcus, especially *S. aureus*, and streptococci are the most common causes of bacterial infections, though DFIs are frequently caused by a combination of microbes [14]. DFUs and DFIs are difficult to heal due to the patient's altered immune function, insufficient circulation, and neural damage. In patients that also suffer from PAD, the risk of developing a DFI is even higher because PAD prevents wound healing by further limiting the blood supply to the area. With a diminished blood supply, a DFU does not receive sufficient oxygen or nutrition, thus causing DFUs to become chronic and easily infected by both planktonic bacteria and biofilms [14].

DFIs must be treated promptly and effectively otherwise they can rapidly develop into a limb-threatening condition, requiring amputation, or even death [14, 85]. DFIs are the leading cause of non-traumatic lower extremity amputations with about 66,000 DFI-related amputations in the United States annually. Overall, DFIs are associated with a public health cost of approximately $174 billion each year in the United States [86, 87].

Treatment of DFIs often requires surgical intervention because they do not usually respond well to antibiotic therapy alone. This is largely due to the insufficient circulation that diabetics, and especially those with PAD, suffer from [24]. As a result, sharp debridement is usually required. In order to ensure adequate debridement, all nonviable tissue should be excised systematically, working from the outer edges in, and until healthy, bleeding tissue is attained [88]. All infected tissue, bone, bursa, and cicatrix must be removed; if any infection remains, the ulcer will persist and require further debridement [19].

Additionally, studies have recommended placing the patient on antibiotics for at least 2 weeks after surgery; although the antibiotics will not directly target the DFI, they are meant to sterilize the surrounding soft tissues [19]. Following debridement, the wound should be dressed with a sterile, nonadhesive dressing that maintains a moist environment around the wound and absorbs exudates. To improve healing the wound should be off-loaded with a custom splint or orthotic [14]. In cases where tissue hypoxia and chronic ischemia are present, hyperbaric oxygen therapy (HBOT) is an additional treatment that should be considered [19].

HBOT has been shown to increase healing rates of DFUs, but studies are still being conducted on the use of HBOT as an adjuvant therapy and on its use alone versus in conjunction with surgical debridement [14, 89]. Lastly, researchers are investigating alternative methods of treatment, especially those that target biofilms, including the use of calcium sulfate beads with local application of antibiotics [90], silver dressings, honey-impregnated dressings [14], dispersal enzymes [91], tryptophan dressings [92], and the use of copper-containing nanofibers [93].

Burn Infections

Patients suffering from burn injuries are at an elevated risk of infection following loss of the skin barrier [29]. Given the risk of infection that burn patients suffer from, it is of utmost importance to control infections as rapidly as possible. Early excision of burned tissue and closure is recommended and has been shown to decrease infection-related morbidity and mortality [29, 94].

Burn wound cellulitis is an infection that spreads into surrounding healthy tissue and causes pain, erythema, and edema around the burn (Fig. 2.3a–d) [29]. *S. aureus* is the most common pathogen responsible for burn wound cellulitis, though *P. aeruginosa* is another common cause [29, 95].

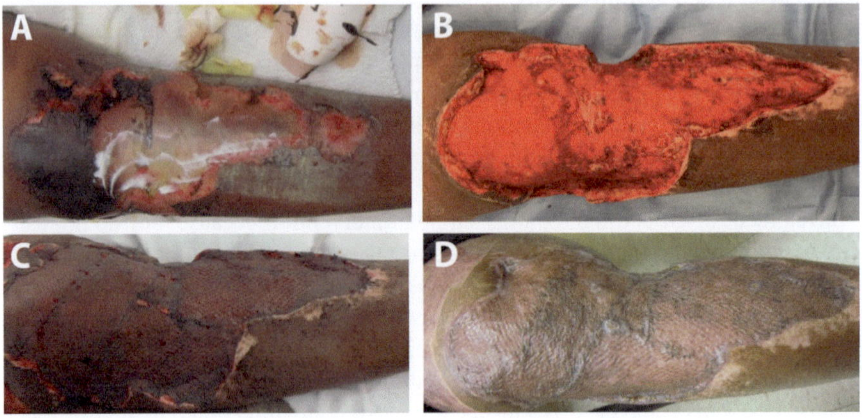

Fig. 2.3 A patient with a right, anterior leg burn was transferred from an outside hospital and presented with fevers, chills, and mild erythema around the edges of the burn (**a**). Given the clinical signs of infection, she was taken to the operating room for debridement and washout. She was found to have cellulitis and an infected hematoma, which required a more extensive debridement, placement of a VAC dressing, and a subsequent debridement and washout 3 days later (**b**). After the second debridement, multiple skin grafts were placed (**c**) and a VAC dressing was used as a bolster. Due to adequate debridement and bacterial control, the skin grafts were well healed 1 month later (**d**)

Invasive burn infections arise from unexcised burn eschars and rapidly convert partial-thickness burns into full-thickness injuries. *P. aeruginosa* is often the cause of invasive burn infection, but any bacterium can be present in and responsible for these infections. Timely surgical excision of all affected tissue followed by administration of broad-spectrum antibiotics is required to treat invasive burn infections [29]. After surgery, a topical antimicrobial agent, usually silver sulfadiazine or mafenide acetate cream, should be applied to further reduce the wound's microbial load [29, 96].

Impetigo encompasses infections that cause loss of epithelium from a previously epithelialized surface. Impetigo is commonly caused by gram-positive skin flora, specifically staphylococci. To efficaciously treat impetigo, all abscesses must be opened, the area should be cleansed twice a day with a surgical detergent disinfectant, and a topical antimicrobial, such as mupirocin, should be applied twice a day [29].

As an adjunct for small, infected areas, certain dressings that are easily applicable, are absorbent, have broad-spectrum antibiotic properties, and do not cause adverse reactions may be used to treat topical infections [97, 98]. Silver dressings, specifically silver-containing soft-silicone foam dressings, are an ideal choice because wound secretions ionize the silver into an active form that can bind to cell membranes and proteins. The activated silver impairs the function of respiratory enzymes of bacteria and binds to bacterial DNA bases, which prevents bacterial replication [97].

Breast Prosthesis Infection

Prosthetic breast reconstruction is the most common form of postmastectomy reconstruction [99]. The insertion of prosthetic material into a field with incumbent and required cancer treatment, including chemotherapy and potential radiation, increases the potential for SSTIs. The risk is further elevated with an increasing numbers of comorbidities, such as radiation, obesity, and/or diabetes [99–101]. Breast implant infections vary in severity and can be classified as mild or superficial, requiring solely treatment by oral antibiotics, chronic due to the presence of a biofilm on the implant, or severe and life threatening requiring immediate surgical intervention [99].

Patients who present with normal signs of infection, such as erythema, induration, and increased localized pain, should be placed on a broad-spectrum antimicrobial regimen covering the common pathogens responsible for prosthesis infection at your hospital, as well as those that can form biofilms [4]. For example, rifampin and tetracycline, daptomycin, or minocycline are antimicrobial regimens designed to target methicillin-resistant staphylococci [4, 102]. Wound cultures should be taken and microbiologically analyzed for bacterial speciation and antibiotic sensitivities and resistance [102]. *Pseudomonas* infections and gross infections of the periprosthetic fluid do not respond to antimicrobial treatment alone and require operative washout and removal of prosthesis [4, 103]. Staphylococci may also form biofilm on prosthetics and must be similarly treated with operative washout and removal of the prosthetic device [4, 103, 104]. The initial stage of a periprosthetic infection is depicted in Fig. 2.1.

Surgical intervention is also indicated if the infection persists longer than 14 days regardless of antimicrobial treatment or if prosthesis becomes exposed [4]. In these cases, the prosthesis should be explanted, and the capsule with the surrounding infected tissue should be thoroughly debrided and irrigated. If there are no overwhelming signs of infection and there is enough tissue to cover a prosthesis, the surgeon may consider placing a new prosthesis at that time, otherwise the site should be closed primarily and allowed to heal [105]. After the area has healed sufficiently, patients can elect to undergo subsequent reconstructive procedures.

Infections of Pressure Injuries

Pressure injuries are localized areas of tissue necrosis that develop when soft tissue is compressed between a bony prominence and an external surface for an extended length of time. These commonly arise in paraplegics and quadriplegics, as these individuals have decreased mobility and sensation. Common locations for pressure injuries include the ischium, sacrum, and greater trochanter, although pressure injuries can develop anywhere [69]. Pressure injuries are a common site of SSTIs (Fig. 2.4a, b). Given the severity of the ulcer, infection may cause cellulitis, abscess formation, osteomyelitis, infection of the joint or bursa, and sepsis [43, 106]. Prompt and effective treatment is critical. Pressure injury infections are usually polymicrobial and include gram-positive and gram-negative facultative aerobes, as well as anaerobic organisms. Broad-spectrum antibiotics must be used to treat these infections in conjunction with excisional debridement of the necrotic tissue and bone as needed (Fig. 2.4c) [43, 69, 106].

The goal of surgery is to excise the unhealthy tissue to reduce the bacterial load on healthy tissue (Fig. 2.4d). Video 2.1 demonstrates debridement of a pressure injury, which is outlined in methylene blue to ensure complete resection of infected tissue (Video 2.1). Following debridement, the wound may need to be left open to ensure that all of the infection has been eradicated and that the wound bed is healthy. Temporary use of negative-pressure wound therapy may be useful in these cases, as it has been shown to remove fluid, regulate inflammation, stimulate the wound-healing pathways, and prevent the formation of biofilms (Fig. 2.4e) [107]. When there are no longer local signs of infection or drainage, and the area is well vascularized, the wound can be closed. If the defect is large enough and/or the ulcer includes the muscle, bone, bursa, or joint, a myocutaneous flap may be needed to restore soft tissue coverage to the area. Following the flap procedure, directed antibiotic therapy should be continued to prevent infection [43].

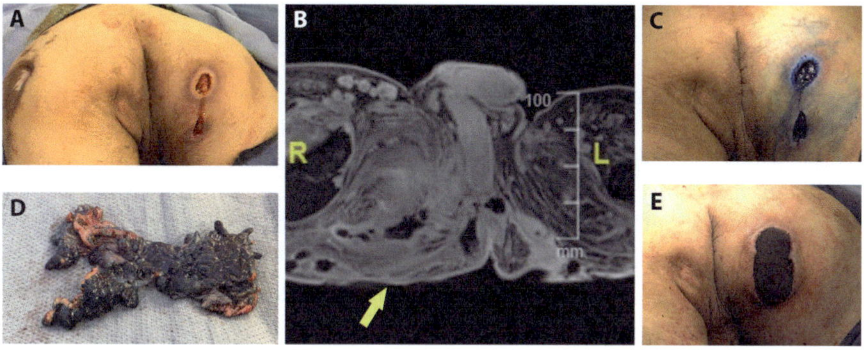

Fig. 2.4 An elderly paraplegic with a history of pressure injuries presented with fever, chills, and localized pain in his right buttock. Based on clinical presentation, he was diagnosed with a *right* buttock pressure injury and possible infection (**a**). An MRI confirmed the presence of a fluid collection deep to the ulcer (**b**). It was determined that treatment of the infected ulcer would require surgical debridement. *Methylene blue* was used to mark the ulcer so as to ensure that all affected tissue was excised (**c**). The ulcer was resected in its entirety as shown by the resected specimen (**d**). Given the patient's history of infection, the area was left open, and a VAC sponge dressing was placed (**e**)

Sternal Wound Infections

Sternal wound infections (SWIs), a complication in patients who undergo cardiac surgery, are more common in diabetic and obese patients [21]. The reported overall risk of developing a SWI is 0.5–3%, while the in-hospital mortality rate for SWIs is 8–28% [108–110]. Patients suffering from a deep SWI may present with increased chest pain, sternal instability, fever, and/or purulent discharge from the mediastinum. Blood, fluid, or tissue cultures should be obtained to confirm the diagnosis of deep SWIs. As soon as a deep SWI is diagnosed, early surgical debridement is paramount as antibiotic treatment alone cannot cure a deep SWI [111]. Debridement should occur urgently following SWI diagnosis. Delayed treatment is associated with increased hospital readmissions and stay [112].

As with other SSTIs, operative debridement should remove all infected and necrotic tissue from the sternum. If purulence tracks through from the retrosternal area, closed suction drains should be placed before closure is performed [108]. A pectoralis, omental, or rectus abdominis flap may be necessary to close the resulting defect and obliterate space where microbes can colonize and lead to further infection [112]. Following debridement, patients should receive antibiotics specific to the culture results. Infectious disease specialists may be useful in determining the proper antimicrobial regimen and necessary length of antimicrobial treatment [108].

Periprosthetic Joint Infection

Periprosthetic joint infections (PJIs) are a devastating complication following total joint arthroplasty. Unlike most local infections, PJIs do not usually respond to antibiotics alone and frequently require surgical intervention, possibly due to the presence of biofilms that form on the metal surfaces of the implant. Effectively treating the PJI requires eliminating the biofilm and any other surrounding organisms [113, 114].

Several surgical approaches have been described for PJIs including debridement with retention of the joint prosthesis, debridement with removal of the implant, debridement with replacement of the joint prosthesis, and debridement with removal of the implant followed by replacement of the prosthesis at a later date (two-stage replacement) [115]. Current literature suggests that patients who suffer from a chronic PJI, which normally present months after the original operation and cause persistent symptoms of infection, should receive a two-stage surgical treatment [115–117]. First, the infected implant should be completely removed and replaced with a temporary antimicrobial spacer. The patient should then be placed on a 6-week course of antibiotics. Following completion of the antibiotic course, the patient can undergo the subsequent surgery, in which a new joint prosthesis is placed [115].

There is less of a consensus regarding the appropriate treatment of acute PJIs, although the Infectious Diseases Society of America recommends debridement and prosthesis retention if infection occurs within 30 days of total joint arthroplasty or if treatment occurs within 3 weeks of onset of signs of infections [118, 119]. Some studies suggest that biofilm-active antibiotic treatment in conjunction with irrigation and radical debridement with retention of the joint prosthesis is sufficient to treat early PJIs [113, 116, 120, 121]; however, these studies clarify that this approach should not be used in elderly patients, immunocompromised patients, patients with Staphylococcal SSTIs, or those that have significant medical comorbidities [113, 116, 118]. Other studies suggest that irrigation and debridement with component retention do not have a high success rate and should be used cautiously [122–125].

Given the variety of treatment options, PJIs require an individualized treatment plan that is based on the clinical presentation of infection and organisms involved. Early detection and understanding of the complexity of these infections due to the presence of biofilms are important and will lead to improved overall prosthesis survival and patient outcomes.

Conclusion

Skin and soft tissue infections continue to be an enormous problem for patients everywhere. Certain patient populations are at an increased risk for SSTIs, and caregivers need to be aware of these high-risk patient populations to ensure that they receive prompt and effective treatment at the first signs of infection. Fastidious monitoring of these patients while they undergo treatment is also necessary as they can rapidly decline and have an increased risk of mortality due to SSTIs. A comprehensive plan to treat SSTIs begins with an accurate diagnosis of the type of SSTI as well as an understanding of the associated comorbidities. The plan of care for the SSTI should include antibiotic therapy and judicious use of adjuvant therapy including surgical debridement to remove the bio-burden of infection. Although all SSTIs are different, the principles of treatment can be applied to all skin and soft tissue infections to improve global health.

References

1. Sukumaran V, Senanayake S. Bacterial skin and soft tissue infections. Aust Prescr. 2016;39:159–63.
2. Gillespie BM, Chaboyer W, Erichsen-Andersson A, Hettiarachchi RM, Kularatna S. Economic case for intraoperative interventions to prevent surgical-site infection. Br J Surg. 2017;104(2):e55–64.
3. Saadatian-Elahi M, Teyssou R, Vanhems P. *Staphylococcus aureus*, the major pathogen in orthopaedic and cardiac surgical site infections: a literature review. Int J Surg. 2008 Jun;6(3):238–45.
4. Viola GM, Selber JC, Crosby M, Raad II, Butler CE, Villa MT, Kronowitz SJ, Clemens MW, Garvey P, Yang W, Baumann DP. Salvaging the infected breast tissue expander: a standardized multidisciplinary approach. Plast Reconstr Surg Glob Open. 2016 Jun;4(6):e732–43.
5. Allegranzi B, Bischoff P, de Jonge S, Kubilay NZ, Zayed B, Gomes SM, Abbas M, Atema JJ, Gans S, van Rijen M, Boermeester MA, Egger M, Kluytmans J, Pittet D, Solomkin JS. New WHO recommendations on preoperative measures for surgical site infection prevention: an evidence-based global perspective. Lancet Infect Dis. 2016;16(12):e276–87.
6. Allegranzi B, Zayed B, Bischoff P, Kubilay NZ, de Jonge S, de Vries F, Gomes SM, Gans S, Wallert ED, Wu X, Abbas M, Boermeester MA, Dellinger EP, Egger M, Gastmeier P, Guirao X, Ren J, Pittet D, Solomkin JS. New WHO recommendations on intraoperative and postoperative measures for surgical site infection prevention: an evidence-based global perspective. Lancet Infect Dis. 2016;16(12):e288–303.
7. Dryden M, Baguneid M, Eckmann C, Corman S, Stephens J, Solem C, Li J, Charbonneau C, Baillon-Plot N, Haider S. Pathophysiology and burden of infection in patients with diabetes mellitus and peripheral vascular disease: focus on skin and soft-tissue infections. Clin Microbiol Infect. 2015;21:527–32.
8. Bertoni AG, Saydah S, Brancati FL. Diabetes and the risk of infection-related mortality in the U.S. Diabetes Care. 2001;24(6):1044–9.
9. Rajagopalan S. Serious infections in elderly patients with diabetes mellitus. Clin Infect Dis. 2005;40:990–6.
10. Geerlings SE, Hoepelman AI. Immune dysfunction in patients with diabetes mellitus (DM). FEMS Immunol Med Microbiol. 1999;26:259–65.
11. Pozzilli P, Leslie RD. Infections and diabetes: mechanisms and prospects for prevention. Diabet Med. 1994;11:935–41.
12. Gallacher SJ, Thomson G, Fraser WD, Fisher BM, Gemmell CG, MacCuish AC. Neutrophil bactericidal function in diabetes mellitus: evidence for association with blood glucose control. Diabet Med. 1995;12:916–20.
13. Kok TW, Agrawal N, Sathappan SS, Chen WK. Risk factors for early implant-related surgical site infection. J Orthop Surg (Hong Kong). 2016;24(1):72–6.

14. Amin N, Doupis J. Diabetic foot disease: from the evaluation of the "foot at risk" to the novel diabetic ulcer treatment modalities. World J Diabetes. 2016;7(7):153–64.
15. Young MJ, Boulton AJ, MacLeod AF, Williams DR, Sonksen PH. A multicenter study of the prevalence of diabetic peripheral neuropathy in the United Kingdom hospital clinic population. Diabetologia. 1993;36:150–4.
16. Boulton AJM. The importance of abnormal foot pressures and gait in causation of foot ulcers. In: Connor H, Boulton AJM, Ward JD, editors. The foot in diabetes. Chichester: Wiley; 1987. p. 11–26.
17. Shaw JE, Boulton AJ. The pathogenesis of diabetic foot problems: an overview. Diabetes. 1997;46(Suppl 2):S58–61.
18. Wheat LJ, Allen SD, Henry M, Kernek CB, Siders JA, Keubler T, Fineberg N, Norton J. Diabetic foot infections. Arch Intern Med. 1986;146:1935–40.
19. Strauss MB, Moon H, La S, Craig A, Ponce J, Miller S. The incidence of confounding factors in patients with diabetes mellitus hospitalized for diabetic foot ulcers. Wounds. 2016;28(8):287–94.
20. National Pressure Ulcer Advisory Panel. NPUAP pressure injury stages [Internet]. 2016 April [cited 11 May 2017]. Available from: http://www.npuap.org/resources/educational-and-clinical-resources/npuap-pressure-injury-stages/
21. Lenz K, Brandt M, Fraund-Cremer S, Cremer J. Coronary artery bypass surgery in diabetic patients – risk factors for sternal wound infections. GMS Interdiscip Plast Reconstr Surg DGPW. 2016;5:Doc 18.
22. Jamsen E, Nevalainen P, Eskelinen A, Huotari K, Kalliovalkama J, Moilanen T. Obesity, diabetes, and preoperative hyperglycemia as predictors of periprosthetic joint infection. J Bone Joint Surg Am. 2012;94:e101(1–9).
23. Kunutsor SK, Whitehouse MR, Blom AW, Beswick AD, INFORM Team. Patient-related risk factors for periprosthetic joint infection after total joint arthroplasty: a systematic review and meta-analysis. PLoS One. 2016;11(3):e0150866.
24. Shah BR, Hux JE. Quanitifying the risk of infectious diseases for people with diabetes. Diabetes Care. 2003;26(2):510–3.
25. Church D, Elsayed S, Reid O, Winston B, Lindsay R. Burn wound infections. Clin Microbiol Rev. 2006;19(2):403–34.
26. Erol S, Altoparlak U, Akcay MN, Celebi F, Parlak M. Changes of microbial flora and wound colonization in burned patients. Burns. 2004 Jun;30(4):357–61.
27. Sheridan RL. Evaluating and managing burn wounds. Dermatol Nurs. 2000; 12(1):17–8, 21–8.
28. Gamelli RL, He LK, Liu H. Marrow granulocyte-macrophage progenitor cell response to burn injury as modified by endotoxin and indomethacin. J Trauma. 1994;37(3):339–46.
29. Coban YK. Infection control in severely burned patients. World J Crit Care Med. 2012;1(4):94–101.
30. Tancheva D, Hadjiiski O. Effect of early nutritional support on clinical course and septic complications in patients with severe burns. Ann Burns Fire Disasters. 2005;18:74–8.
31. Anderson K, Hamm RL. Factors that impair wound healing. J Am Coll Clin Wound Spec. 2012;4(4):84–91.
32. Nahabedian MY, Tsangaris T, Momen B, Manson PN. Infectious complications following breast reconstruction with expanders and implants. Plast Reconstr Surg. 2003;112(2):467–76.
33. Cordeiro PG, Albornoz CR, McCormick B, Hu Q, Van Zee K. The impact of postmastectomy radiotherapy on two-stage implant breast reconstruction: an ananlysis of long-term surgical outcomes, aesthetic results, and satisfaction over 13 years. Plast Reconstr Surg. 2014;134:588–95.
34. Kearney AM, Brown MS, Soltanian HT. Timing of radiation and outcomes in implant-based breast reconstruction. J Plast Reconstr Aesthet Surg. 2015;68:1719–26.
35. Olsen MA, Lefta M, Dietz JR, Brandt KE, Aft R, Matthews R, Mayfield J, Fraser VJ. Risk factors for surgical site infection following major breast surgery. J Am Coll Surg. 2008;207(3):326–35.

36. Reish RG, Damjanovic B, Austen WG Jr, Winograd J, Liao EC, Cetrulo CL, Balkin DM, Colwell AS. Infection following implant-based reconstruction in 1952 consecutive breast reconstructions. Plast Reconstr Surg. 2013;131(6):1223–30.
37. Francis SH, Ruberg RL, Stevenson KB, Beck CE, Ruppert AS, Harper JT, Boehmler JH 4th, Miller MJ. Independent risk factors for infection in tissue expander breast reconstruction. Plast Reconstr Surg. 2009;124(6):1790–6.
38. Viola GM, Baumann DP, Mohan K, Selber J, Garvey P, Reece G, Raad II, Rolston KV, Crosby MA. Improving antimicrobial regiments for the treatment of breast tissue expander-related infections. Plast Reconstr Surg Glob Open. 2016 May;4(5):e704–14.
39. Sutton E, Miyagaki H, Bellini G, Shantha Kumara HM, Yan X, Howe B, Feigel A, Whelan RL. Risk factors for superficial surgical site infection after elective rectal cancer resection: a multivariate analysis of 8880 patients from the American College of Surgeons National Surgical Quality Improvement Program database. J Surg Res. 2017;207:205–14.
40. Hughes MA, Parisi M, Grossman S, Kleinberg L. Primary brain tumors treated with steroids and radiotherapy: low CD4 counts and risk of infection. Int J Radiat Oncol Biol Phys. 2005;62(5):1423–6.
41. Panghal M, Kaushal V, Kadayan S, Yadav JP. Incidence and risk factors for infection in oral cancer patients undergoing different treatments protocols. BMC Oral Health. 2012;12:22.
42. National Institute for Health and Care Excellence. The prevention and management of pressure ulcers in primary and secondary care [Internet]. 2014 April [cited 24 December 2016]. Available from: https://www.ncbi.nlm.nih.gov/pubmedhealth/PMH0068960/
43. Montgomerie JZ. Infections in patients with spinal cord injuries. Clin Infect Dis. 1997;25:1285–92.
44. Richardson RR, Meyer PR Jr. Prevalence and incidence of pressure sores in acute spinal cord injuries. Paraplegia. 1981;19:235–47.
45. Cruse JM, Lewis RE, Roe DL, Dilioglou S, Blaine MC, Wallace WF, Chen RS. Facilitation of immune function, healing of pressure ulcers, and nutritional status in spinal cord injury patients. Exp Mol Pathol. 2000;68:38–54.
46. Rubin-Asher D, Zeilig G, Klieger M, Adunsky A, Weingarden H. Dermatological findings following acute traumatic spinal cord injury. Spinal Cord. 2005;43:175–8.
47. Dahl MV. Dermatophytosis and the immune response. J Am Acad Dermatol. 1994;31(3 part 2):S34–41.
48. Nash MS. Known and plausible modulators of depressed immune functions following spinal cord injuries. J Spinal Cord Med. 2000;23:111–20.
49. Balachandran S, Lee A, Denehy L, Lin KY, Royse A, Royse C, El-Ansary D. Risk factors for sternal complications after cardiac operations: a systematic review. Ann Thorac Surg. 2016;102:2109–17.
50. Marmor S, Kerroumi Y. Patient-specific risk factors for infection in arthroplasty procedure. Orthop Traumatol Surg Res. 2016;102:S113–9.
51. Hainer V, Zamrazilova H, Kunesova M, Bendlova B, Aldhoon-Hainerova I. Obesity and infection: reciprocal causality. Physiol Res. 2015;64(Suppl 2):S105–19.
52. Tanaka S, Inoue S, Isoda F, Waseda M, Ishihara M, Yamakawa T, Sugiyama A, Takamura Y, Okuda K. Impaired immunity in obesity: suppressed but reversible lymphocytes responsiveness. Int J Obes Relat Metab Disord. 1993;17:631–6.
53. Tanaka S, Isoda F, Ishihara Y, Kimura M, Yamakawa T. T lymphopaenia in relation to body mass index and TNF-alpha in human obesity: adequate weight reduction can be corrective. Clin Endocrinol. 2001;54:347–54.
54. Nieman DC, Hanson DA, Nehlsen-Cannarella SL, Ekkens M, Utter AC, Butterworth DE, Fagoaga OR. Influence of obesity on immune function. J Am Diet Assoc. 1999;99:294–9.
55. Namba RS, Paxton L, Fithian DC, Stone ML. Obesity and perioperative morbidity in total hip and total knee arthroplasty patients. J Arthroplast. 2005;20(7 Suppl. 3):46–50.
56. Waisbren E, Rosen H, Bader AM, Lipsitz SR, Rogers SO Jr, Eriksson E. Percent body fat and prediction of surgical site infection. J Am Coll Surg. 2010;210(4):381–9.

57. Guo S, DiPietro LA. Factors affecting wound healing. J Dent Res. 2010;89(3):219–29.
58. Ahn C, Mulligan P, Salcido RS. Smoking-the bane of wound healing: biomedical interventions and social influences. Adv Skin Wound Care. 2008;21(5):227–36.
59. Mangram AJ, Horan TC, Pearson ML, Silver LC, Jarvis WR. Guideline for prevention of surgical site infection 1999. Infect Control Hosp Epidemiol. 1999;20:250–78.
60. Arcavi L, Benowitz NL. Cigarette smoking and infection. Arch Intern Med. 2004;164:2206–16.
61. Sopori ML, Kozak W, Savage SM, Geng Y, Soszynski D, Kluger MJ, Perryman EK, Snow GE. Effect of nicotine on the immune system: possible regulation of immune responses by central and peripheral mechanisms. Psychoneuroendocrinology. 1998;23:189–204.
62. Mili F, Flanders WD, Boring JR, Annest JL, Destefano F. The associations of race, cigarette smoking, and smoking cessation to measures of the immune system in middle-aged men. Clin Immunol Immunopathol. 1991;59:187–200.
63. Hersey P, Prendergast D, Edwards A. Effects of cigarette smoking on the immune system: follow-up studies in normal subjects after cessation of smoking. Med J Aust. 1983;2:425–9.
64. Edwards BL, Stukenborg GJ, Brenin DR, Schroen AT. Use of prophylactic postoperative antibiotics during surgical drain presence following mastectomy. Ann Surg Oncol. 2014;21(10):3249–55.
65. Nagachinta T, Stephens M, Reitz B, Polk BF. Risk factors for surgical wound infection following cardiac surgery. J Infect Dis. 1987;156:967–73.
66. Kong L, Liu Z, Meng F, Shen Y. Smoking and risk of surgical site infection after spinal surgery: a systematic review and meta-analysis. Surg Infect. 2016;(2):206–14.
67. Moffarah AS, Al Mohajer M, Hurwitz BL, Armstrong DG. Skin and soft tissue infections. Microbiol Spectr. 2016 Aug;4(4): DMIH2-0014–2015.
68. Stevens DL, Bisno AL, Chambers HF, Dellinger EP, Goldstein EJC, Gorbach L, Hirschmann JV, Kaplan SL, Montoya JG, Wade JC. Practice guidelines for the diagnosis and management of skin and soft tissue infections: 2014 update by the infectious diseases society of America. Clin Infect Dis. 2014;59:147–59.
69. Sartelli M, Malangoni MA, May AK, Viale P, Kao LS, Catena F, Ansaloni L, Moore EE, Moore FA, Peitzman AB, Coimbra R, Leppaniemi A, Kluger Y, Biffl W, Koike K, Girardis M, Ordonez CA, Tavola M, Cainzos M, Di Saverio S, Fraga GP, Gerych I, Kelly MD, Taviloglu K, Wani I, Marwah S, Bala M, Ghnnam W, Shaikh N, Chiara O, Faro MP, Pereira GA, Gomes CA, Coccolini F, Trana C, Corbella D, Brambillasca P, Cui Y, Lohse HAS, Khokha V, Kok KYY, Hong S-K, Yuan K-C. World Society of Emergency Surgery (WSES) guidelines for management of skin and soft tissue infections. World J Emerg Surg. 2014;9(57):1–18.
70. Esposito S, Noviello S, Leone S. Epidemiology and microbiology of skin and soft tissue infections. Curr Opin Infect Dis. 2016;29:109–15.
71. White RJ, Cutting KF. Critical colonization – the concept under scrutiny. Ostomy Wound Manage. 2006;52(11):50–6.
72. Turtiainen J, Hakala T, Hakkarainen T, Karhukorpi J. The impact of surgical wound bacterial colonization on the incidence of surgical site infection after lower limb vascular surgery: a prospective observational study. Eur J Vasc Endovasc Surg. 2014;47(4):411–7.
73. Yu Y, Tan M, Chen H, Wu Z, Xu L, Li J, Cao J, Yang Y, Xiao X, Lian X, Lu X, Tu Y. Non-thermal plasma suppresses bacterial colonization on skin wound and promotes wound healing in mice. J Huazhong Univ Sci Technolog Med Sci. 2011;31(3):390–4.
74. Saleh K, Sonesson A, Persson B, Riesbeck K, Schmidtchen A. A descriptive study of bacterial load of full-thickness surgical wounds in dermatologic surgery. Dermatol Surg. 2011;37(7):1014–22.
75. Lineaweaver WC, Jacob S, Yan H, Zhang F. Wound cultures as predictors of complications in reconstructive flap procedures. Ann Plast Surg. 2011;66(5):572–4.
76. Cardona AF, Wilson SE. Skin and soft-tissue infections: a critical review and the role of telavancin in their treatment. Clin Infect Dis. 2015;61(Suppl 2):S69–78.
77. Bjarnsholt T. The role of bacterial biofilms in chronic infections. APMIS Suppl. 2013; 136:1–51.

78. Ki V, Rotstein C. Bacterial skin and soft tissue infections in adults: a review of their epidemiology, pathogenesis, diagnosis, treatment and site of care. Can J Infect Dis Med Microbiol. 2008;19(2):173–84.
79. Rondas AA, Schols JM, Stobberingh EE, Halfens RJ. Prevalence of chronic wounds and structural quality indicators of chronic wound care in Dutch nursing homes. Int Wound J. 2015;12(6):630–5.
80. Clinton A, Carter T. Chronic wound biofilms: pathogenesis and potential therapies. Lab Med. 2015;46(4):277–84.
81. Jeffery Marano R, Jane Wallace H, Wijeratne D, William Fear M, San Wong H, O'Handley R. Secreted biofilm factors adversely affect cellular wound healing responses *in vitro*. Sci Rep. 2015;5:13296–306.
82. Suaya JA, Mera RM, Cassidy A, O'Hara P, Amrine-Madsen H, Burstin S, Miller LG. Incidence and cost of hospitalizations associated with *Staphylococcus aureus* skin and soft tissue infections in the United States from 2001 through 2009. BMC Infect Dis. 2014;14:296–303.
83. Reiber GE, Ledoux WR. Epidemiology of diabetic foot ulcers and amputations: evidence for prevention. In: Williams R, Herman W, Kinmonth AL, Wareham NJ, editors. The evidence base for diabetes care. Chichester/Hoboken: Wiley; 2003. p. 641–65.
84. Lavery LA, Armstrong DG, Wunderlich RP, Mohler MJ, Wendel CS, Lipsky BA. Risk factors for foot infections in individuals with diabetes. Diabetes Care. 2006;29:1288–93.
85. Veves A, Giurini J, LoGerfo F. The diabetic foot: medical and surgical management. Totowa: Humana Press; 2006.
86. Reveles KR, Duhon BM, Moore RJ, Hand EO, Howell CK. Epidemiology of methicillin-resistant *Staphylococcus aureus* diabetic foot infections in a large academic hospital: implications for antimicrobial stewardship. PLoS One. 2016;11(8):1–8.
87. Centers for Disease Control and Prevention. 2014 National diabetes statistics report [Internet]. 2015 May 15 [cited 31 December 2016]. Available from: https://www.cdc.gov/diabetes/pubs/statsreport14/national-diabetes-report-web.pdf
88. Wei C, Granick MS. Surgical management of chronic wounds. Wounds. 2008;20(3):62–6.
89. Strauss MB. Hyperbaric oxygen as an intervention for managing wound hypoxia: its role and usefulness in diabetic foot wounds. Foot Ankle Int. 2005;26:15–8.
90. Price BL, Lovering AM, Bowling FL, Dobson CB. Development of a novel collagen wound model to stimulate the activity and distribution of antimicrobials in soft tissue during diabetic foot infection. Antimicrob Agents Chemother. 2016;60(11):6880–9.
91. Watters CM, Burton T, Kirui DK, Millenbaugh NJ. Enzymatic degradation of in vitro *Staphylococcus aureus* biofilms supplemented with human plasma. Infect Drug Resist. 2016;9:71–8.
92. Brandenburg KS, Calderon DF, Kierski PR, Brown AL, Shah NM, Abbott NL, Schurr MJ, Murphy CJ, McAnulty JF, Czuprynski CJ. Inhibition of *Pseudomonas aeruginosa* biofilm formation on wound dressings. Wound Repair Regen. 2015;23(6):842–54.
93. Ahire JJ, Hattingh M, Neveling DP, Dicks LM. Copper-containing anti-biofilm nanofiber scaffolds as a wound dressing material. PLoS One. 2016;11(3):1–12.
94. Barret JP, Herndon DN. Modulation of inflammatory and catabolic responses in severely burned children by early burn wound excision in the first 24 hours. Arch Surg. 2003;138(2):127–32.
95. Altoparlak U, Erol S, Akcay MN, Celebi F, Kadanali A. The time-related changes of antimicrobial resistance patterns and predominant bacterial profiles of burn wounds and body flora of burned patients. Burns. 2004;30:660–4.
96. Heggers, JP, Hawkins, H, Edgar, P, Villarreal, C, Herndon, D.N. Treatment of infections in burns. Herndon DN, Burn care. 2 London: W.B. Saunders/Bailliere Tindall; 2001. 120–169.
97. Yang B, Wang X, Li Z, Qu Q, Qiu Y. Beneficial effects of silver foam dressing on healing of wounds with ulcers and infection control of burn patients. Pak J Med Sci. 2015;31(6):1334–9.
98. Selig HF, Lumenta DB, Giretzlehner M, Jeschke MG, Upton D, Kamolz LP. The properties of an "ideal" burn wound dressing – what do we need in daily clinical practice? Results of a worldwide online survey among burn care specialists. Burns. 2012;38(7):960–6.

99. Ooi AS, Song DH. Reducing infection risk in implant-based breast-reconstruction surgery: challenges and solutions. Breast Cancer (Dove Med Press). 2016;8:161–72.
100. McCarthy CM, Mehrara BJ, Riedel E. Predicting complications following expander/implant breast reconstruction: an outcomes analysis based on preoperative clinical risk. Plast Reconstr Surg. 2008;121(6):1886–92.
101. Kato H, Nakagami G, Iwahira Y, Otani R, Nagase T, Iizaka S, Tamai N, Matsuyama Y, Sanada H. Risk factors and risk scoring tool for infection during tissue expansion in tissue expander and implant breast reconstruction. Breast J. 2013;19(6):618–26.
102. Phillips BT, Wang ED, Mirrer J, Lanier ST, Khan SU, Dagum AB, Bui DT. Current practice among plastic surgeons of antibiotic prophylaxis and closed-suction drains in breast reconstruction: experience, evidence, and implications for postoperative care. Ann Plast Surg. 2011;66:460–5.
103. Reish RG, Damjanovic B, Austen WG Jr, Winograd J, Liao EC, Cetrulo CL, Balkin DM, Colwell AS. Infection following implant-based reconstruction in 1952 consecutive breast reconstructions: salvage rates and predictors of success. Plast Reconstr Surg. 2013;131:1223–30.
104. Spear SL, Seruya M. Management of the infected or exposed breast prosthesis: a single surgeon's 15 year experience with 69 patients. Plast Reconstr Surg. 2010;125:1074–84.
105. Spear SL, Howard MA, Boehmler JH, Ducic I, Low M, Abbruzzesse MR. The infected or exposed breast implant: management and treatment strategies. Plast Reconstr Surg. 2004;113(6):1634–44.
106. Schiffman J, Golinko MS, Yan A, Flattau A, Tomic-Canic M, Brem H. Operative debridement of pressure ulcers. World J Surg. 2009;33:1396–402.
107. Li T, Zhang L, Han L, Wang G, Yin P, Li Z, Zhang L, Guo Q, Liu D, Tang P. Early application of negative pressure wound therapy to acute wounds contaminated by *Staphylococcus aureus*: an effective approach to prevention biofilm formation. Exp Ther Med. 2016;11(3):769–76.
108. Dubert M, Pourbaix A, Alkhoder S, Mabileau G, Lescure FX, Ghodhbane W, Belorgey S, Rioux C, Armand-Lefevre L, Wolff M, Raffoul R, Nataf P, Yazdanpanah Y, Lucet JC. Sternal wound infection after cardiac surgery: management and outcome. PLoS One. 2015;10(9):1–11.
109. Milano CA, Kesler K, Archibald N, Sexton DJ, Jones RH. Mediastinitis after coronary artery bypass graft surgery. Risk factors and long-term survival. Circulation. 1995;92(8):2245–51.
110. Vos RJ, van Putte BP, Sonker U, Kloppenburg GTL. Primary closure using Redon drains for the treatment of post-sternotomy mediastinitis. Interact Cardiovasc Thorac Surg. 2014;18(1):33–7.
111. De Feo M, Gregorio R, Della Corte A, Marra C, Amarelli C, Renzulli A, Utili R, Cotrufo M. Deep sternal wound infection: the role of early debridement surgery. Eur J Cardiothorac Surg. 2001;19(6):811–6.
112. Wu L, Chung KC, Waljee JF, Momoch AO, Zhong L, Sears ED. A national study of the impact of initial debridement timing on outcomes for patients with deep sternal wound infection. Plast Reconstr Surg. 2016;137(2):414e–23e.
113. Kim JH, Chun SK, Yoon YC, Lakhotia D, Shon WY. Efficacy of debridement for early periprosthetic joint infection after hip arthroplasty. Hip Pelvis. 2014;26(4):227–34.
114. Song Z, Borgwardt L, Hoiby N, Wu H, Sorensen TS, Borgwardt A. Prosthesis infections after orthopedic joint replacement: the possible role of bacterial biofilms. Orthop Rev (Pavia). 2013;5:65–71.
115. Darouiche RO. Treatment of infections associated with surgical implants. N Engl J Med. 2004;350:1422–9.
116. Koyonos L, Zmistowski B, Della Valle CJ, Parvizi J. Infection control rate of irrigation and debridement for periprosthetic join infection. Clin Orthop Relat Res. 2011;469:3043–8.
117. Diermengian C, Greenbaum J, Lotke PA, Boothe RE Jr, Lonner JH. Limited success with open debridement and retention of components in the treatment of acute *Staphylococcus aureus* infections after total knee arthroplasty. J Arthoplasty. 2003;18:22–6.

118. Holmberg A, Thorhallsdottir VG, Robertsson O, W-Dahl A, Stefansdottir A. 75% success rate after open debridement, exchange of tibial insert, and antibiotics in knee prosthetic joint infections. Acta Orthop. 2015;86(4):457–62.
119. Osmon DR, Berbari EF, Berendt AR, Lew D, Zimmerli W, Steckelberg JM, Rao N, Hanssen A, Wilson WR. Diagnosis and management of prosthetic join infection: clinical practice guidelines by the Infectious Diseases Society of America. Clin Infect Dis. 2013;56(1):1–25.
120. Mont MA, Waldman B, Banerjee C, Pacheco IH, Hungerfor DS. Multiple irrigation, debridement, and retention of components in infected total knee arthroplasty. J Arthroplast. 1997;12:426–33.
121. Tsukayama DT, Estrada R, Gustilo RB. Infection after total hip arthroplasty: a study of the treatment of one hundred and six infections. J Bone Joint Surg Am. 1996;78:512–23.
122. Bradbury T, Fehring TK, Taunton M, Hanssen A, Azzam K, Parvizi J, Odum SM. The fate of acute methicillin-resistant *Staphylococcus aureus* periprosthetic knee infections treated by open debridement and retention of components. J Arthroplast. 2009;(Suppl 6):101–4.
123. Zmistowski BM, Manrique J, Patel R, Chen AF. Recurrent periprosthetic joint infection after irrigation and debridement with component retention is most often due to identical organisms. J Arthroplast. 2016;31:S148–51.
124. Fehring TK, Odum SM, Berend KR, Jiranek WA, Parvizi J, Bozic KJ, Della Valle CJ, Gioe TJ. Failure of irrigation and debridement for early postoperative periprosthetic infection. Clin Orthop Relat Res. 2013;471(1):250–7.
125. Odum SM, Fehring TK, Lombardi AV, Zmistowski BM, Brown NM, Luna JT, Fehring KA, Hansen EN. Irrigation and debridement for periprosthetic infections: does the organism matter? J Arthroplast. 2011;26(Suppl 6):114–8.

Chapter 3
Amputations of the Lower Extremity

Joseph Park, Tammer Elmarsafi, and John S. Steinberg

Introduction

According to Banks the term amputation was first used in English medical literature in 1597 by Peter Lowe in his treatise *A Discourse in the Whole Art of Chirurgerie*. Lower extremity amputations are commonly performed procedures [1]. Moxey et al. report that most common indications for amputation of the lower extremity are trauma, infection, and ischemia [2]. Less common reasons for amputation include thermal injury, malignancy, congenital deformity, and, in rare instances, intractable pain.

Despite being one of the oldest surgical procedures, surgeons continue to develop and refine their surgical techniques. Additionally, many innovations related to endovascular interventions and wound healing therapies have improved patient outcomes before and after amputations. Other improvements relate to patient quality of life. Novel techniques such as nerve coaptation as described by Economides et al. have

Electronic Supplementary Material: The online version of this chapter (https://doi.org/10.1007/978-3-319-66990-8_3) contains supplementary material, which is available to authorized users.

J. Park, DPM
Division of Podiatric Surgery, MedStar Washington Hospital Center,
110 Irving Street NW, Washington, DC 20010, USA

T. Elmarsafi, DPM, MBBCh
Department of Plastic Surgery, MedStar Georgetown University Hospital,
3800 Reservoir Road NW, Washington, DC 20007, USA

J.S. Steinberg, DPM, FACFAS (✉)
Department of Plastic Surgery, MedStar Georgetown University Hospital,
3800 Reservoir Road NW, Washington, DC 20007, USA

Department of Plastic Surgery, Center for Wound Healing and Hyperbaric Medicine, MedStar Georgetown University Hospital, 3800 Reservoir Road NW, Washington, DC 2007, USA
e-mail: Jss5@gunet.georgetown.edu

D.P. Orgill (ed.), *Interventional Treatment of Wounds*,
https://doi.org/10.1007/978-3-319-66990-8_3

the potential to reduce postoperative phantom pain in those who require below-knee amputations [3]. Perhaps the greatest recent advancement, however, has been the emphasis on the multidisciplinary approach to lower extremity amputations. The collaborate efforts of podiatric surgery, vascular surgery, plastic surgery, orthopedic surgery, infectious disease, psychiatry, and orthotists/prosthetics have transformed the paradigm of amputation from admission of defeat to the commencement of rehabilitation.

Attinger and Brown state that the guiding principle in any lower extremity amputation is to improve the patient's functional status and quality of life [4]. Clinicians must not sacrifice biomechanical stability in exchange for maximizing length, and it is of utmost importance that the surgeon properly conveys this message to the patient. The surgeon must consider the following factors when performing an amputation: level of amputation, resultant biomechanical function, perioperative management, and rehabilitation including proper orthoses and prostheses.

Indications for Amputation

The ultimate purpose of any amputation is to excise tissues which impart greater patient harm if not removed. In most cases the underlying etiology can be broken down into two main primary pathologies: ischemia and infection. As noted by Weledji and Fokam, in the limb which presents with pure ischemia, vascular optimization and prevention of superimposed infection may result in favorable outcomes [5]. The degree of tissue loss, however, is highly dependent on the time of discovery and time to vascular intervention to the success of management. The anatomic distribution (proximal disease versus distal disease) and degree of the vascular insult (severity of stenosis or occlusion) are all important parameters which can influence the level of amputation. Amputations can range from partial digital amputation to hip disarticulation. Nather and Wong describe that the ankle joint traditionally delineates a minor from major amputation [6].

Patients who have any open skin lesions are predisposed to lower extremity infection, particularly in the immunocompromised and diabetic patient population. Infections can be either acute or chronic and include soft tissue and bone infections. As shown by Altemeier and Fullen, fulminant infections such as necrotizing infections, gas gangrene, and infections that cause hemodynamic instability all require emergent debridement [7]. In such cases, the postoperative soft tissue deficit and the predicted functional outcome often dictate the level of final amputation. In her review, Price demonstrated that chronic infections have a dramatic impact on patient quality of life, increase the risk of osteomyelitis, and have major implications on amputation risk [8].

Deformity alone is not typically a primary indication for amputation. However, in patients with failed osseous reconstructions or those who are high risk for complex surgical correction of lower extremity deformities, such as those seen in

Charcot neuroarthropathy, amputation should be considered if functional status and quality of life can be improved. Acquired skeletal deformities predispose the neuropathic patient to ulcer development and increased fall risk. Raspovic et al. demonstrated that when ulcers develop secondary to biomechanical causes, healing the ulcer without addressing the underlying osseous structure will inevitably lead to re-ulceration, increased amputation risk, and a decrease in quality of life [9].

Most patients have a combination of the aforementioned cardinal pathologies. They present with a biomechanically induced ulcer, have peripheral neuropathy, have some degree of ischemia, and are typically infected. Beaulieu et al. reported that these patients often have multiple conditions and comorbidities which increase the risks for amputation [10] and challenge limb salvage efforts. Furthermore, Hobizal and Wukich illustrated that host factors such as the patient's overall comorbidities, nutritional status, glycemic control, adherence to medical regimens, and socioeconomic status clearly have an impact on patient outcomes [11], but they can be difficult to quantify. Without question, the complicated host presents clinical and socioeconomic complexity to the discussion of lower extremity amputations.

Amputations must be understood as a part of a process within a continuum in a patient's disease state. Each patient has a subset of known medical conditions each of which may or may not be well controlled, have associated risks, and each have a particular pattern of progression. Though each patient presents with unique and distinct challenges, the overall sequence of events can be somewhat predictable if risks are properly elucidated, stratified, and mitigated in a timely and continuous fashion.

Yazdanpanah et al. demonstrated how optimization of disease-modifiable factors such as glycemic control, blood pressure, and vascular insufficiency may allow patients to have more favorable long-term health outcomes [12]. However, once ulceration, deformity, neuropathy, or infection occurs, the risk for amputation remains undeniably high. Every effort must be taken to slow the rate of progression and prevent the onset of disease-related complications. Fernandez et al. report how healthcare disparities, food insecurity, and cultural, ethnic, and language barriers all carry socioeconomic implications which impact the overall quality of care in the at-risk population [13]. Ultimately, amputations are cumulatively based on patient-specific risks and may be unavoidable.

The surgical indications for amputations must not be made in isolation of the patient's ambulatory status and must include a realistic assessment of the patient underlying cardiopulmonary capacity to walk after amputation. The level of amputation must be carefully taken into account during surgical planning and must be inclusive of the patient's wishes and expectations. Regardless of the level of amputation, disease progression, advancing age, and worsening vascular integrity almost guarantee additional surgery, revisions, and more proximal amputations. Furthermore, Glaser et al. elucidated how the contralateral extremity becomes a high-risk limb due to the increased load subsequent to an amputation and peripheral arterial disease [14]. Bilateral foot pathologies leading to amputations are common.

Risk Factors for Amputations

Diabetic Foot Ulcer (Figure 3.1)

According to Boulton, up to 50% of patients with diabetes as part of the disease natural history develop symmetrical peripheral polyneuropathy [15]. Singh et al. documented that the lifetime incidence of a patient with diabetes developing a foot ulcer is up to 25% [16]. The loss of protective sensation disarms the patient's ability to identify pain from traumatic injury, ischemic necrosis, or infection and can delay the recognition of the active pathologic process. The lag in time from clinical onset to the time the patient seeks medical attention can lead to an initial presentation which requires urgent or emergent medical and surgical management. When wounds fester, particularly in the presence of uncontrolled diabetes, the lower extremity becomes at risk for increased tissue loss and the patient at increased risk for systemic complications including sepsis and shock. Soft tissue infections can result in a non-salvageable limb if they are not promptly and effectively managed. In certain cases, complex soft tissue reconstruction techniques such as free tissue transfer may be an option for those who are surgical candidates after the underlying infection and/or ischemia have been fully addressed.

Acute ulcers can result from a direct trauma such as stepping on a sharp object, a retained foreign body, open fractures, or any condition which results in skin breakdown. Sheer forces can also exert trauma to the foot resulting in open wounds such as those that occur from ill-fitting shoe gear worn for extended periods of time in feet with underlying skeletal deformities such as hammertoes. These acute traumatic wounds can be preceded with early warning signs such as erythema or blistering or may present with frank ulceration. Once the acute trauma occurs, the

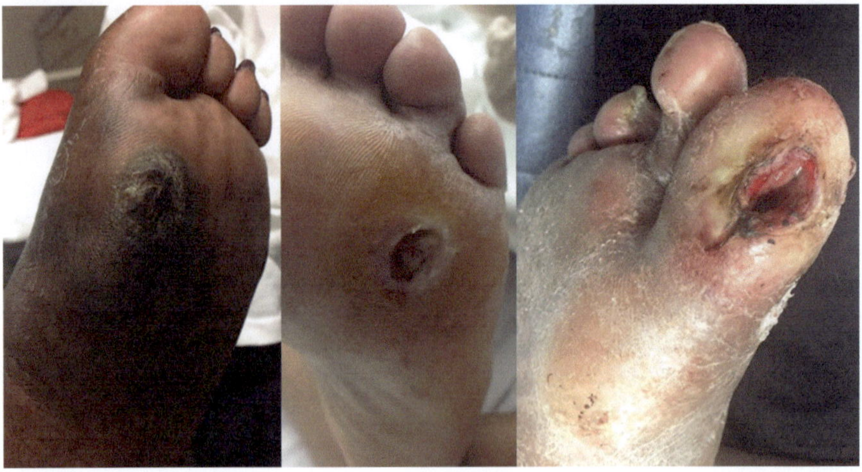

Fig. 3.1 Diabetic foot ulcer

immune-competent patient will launch the normal cascade of events of acute inflammatory and tissue healing. However, Muller et al. described immunocompromised patients such as diabetics have a blunted and faulty cascade resulting in an unchecked rapid bacterial diabetic infection [17].

Many patients develop superficial chronic ulcerations typically to the plantar, medial, and lateral foot and to the distal and dorsal toes. Caselli et al. reported that these ulcers often are a result of biomechanically induced areas of high pressure and sheer forces which are typically preceded by hyperkeratotic lesions [18]. Irrespective of location, chronic ulcers increase risk for cellulitis, deep tissue abscess, sepsis, osteomyelitis, and ultimately amputation. Frequently, chronic ulcers require multiple and frequent interventions including outpatient and inpatient management and require an excessively high utilization of medical resources and cost. Apelqvist et al. state that the total cost is $16,100 for primary healed patients without critical ischemia, $26,700 for primary healed patients with critical ischemia, $43,100 for a healed minor amputation, and $63,100 after a healed major amputation [19]. Diabetic foot ulcerations are associated with frequent hospital readmissions and a high morbidity and mortality rates. A complete patient-centered treatment plan via a multidisciplinary team can help decrease these burdens. These chronic wounds are often classified as non-healing or are recalcitrant to standard wound care modalities, particularly if the underlying biomechanics are not addressed. Chronicity and ulcer recurrence in the foot predispose to osteomyelitis, a strong independent risk factor for amputation. It should be noted that long-standing ulcers which may be primarily addressed with an amputation may be an appropriate management consideration.

Neuropathy

Polyneuropathy can be caused by a wide variety of processes. Although understanding the etiology is important, once neuropathy occurs, it is often irreversible. The degree of clinical symptoms and the rate of progression can vary from patient to patient and is largely dependent on the underlying cause. Mold et al. discuss that the most common causes of peripheral polyneuropathy are diabetes, chronic alcohol abuse, and HIV medications [20]. The side effects of certain medications include neuropathy, and in some cases once discontinued, normal sensation is restored. Other medications exhibit a dose- or duration-dependent causation.

In the diabetic population, the onset is insidious and begins with loss of temperature and vibratory sensation and further develops into loss of light touch and eventually a dense neuropathy. Partanen et al. described the slow progression and reported that it often takes about 10 years from the time diabetes is identified [21]. Patients with such sensory loss do not respond appropriately to noxious stimuli such as those that result in injury to the skin. Frequently, they only become aware of the injury if they are cued by other senses such as seeing blood or drainage on socks or becoming aware of malodor. Often, however, as a result of diabetic retinopathy, and same neuropathic changes that occur peripherally, the sense of smell can also be diminished; thus, the only cues of these patients are others which tend to their care. Diabetes-induced peripheral neuropathy is a spectrum of disease, with some patients exhibiting diminished sensation, while others becoming profoundly numb. Still others develop an array of neural disturbances which manifest as paresthesias most often described by the patient as a burning, tingling, or pin and needle sensation. Painful diabetic peripheral neuropathy can be problematic for patients. Marchettini et al. note that these symptoms are often difficult to treat and the medications available do not come without side effects [22]. It is, however, important to note that patients with this type of neuropathic condition often attribute pain secondary to a real and dangerous pathologic process, to the expected waxing and waning episodes of painful diabetic neuropathy.

Neuropathy is and must be understood as a principal independent risk factor for diabetic foot ulceration. The downstream consequences of ulcer formation in a patient with diabetes with sensory loss are cyclical and often result in amputations. Lavery et al. discovered that patients with neuropathy have a 1.7 times greater risk of ulceration than patients without neuropathy [23]. Both type I and type II diabetic patients develop loss of protective sensations with differing rates of progression. Additionally, both classifications of diabetes are prone to symptomatic painful neuropathy.

Aside from sensory loss, there are other forms of neuropathy that occur simultaneously which may have an impact on amputation risk. Autonomic neuropathy is multisystem conglomerate of symptoms that include cardiovascular, gastrointestinal, genitourinary, endocrine, and sudomotor dysfunction. Duby et al. state that the symptoms most commonly manifest as resting tachycardia, orthostatic hypotension, gastroparesis, constipation, diarrhea, fecal incontinence, erectile dysfunction, neurogenic bladder, hypoglycemia unawareness, and changes in skin quality with either increased or decreased sweating [24]. All autonomic neuropathies must be viewed as important surrogate markers for overall health outcomes and amputation risk stratification. Patients with cardiovascular autonomic neuropathy have a significantly higher risk for fall-related injuries, including those of the lower extremity. Patients with gastroparesis have decreased absorption of important vitamins such as vitamin B12 which accelerates progression and exacerbates peripheral sensory loss. In addition, those on oral medications may have suboptimal pharmacodynamics and thus decreased therapeutics effects resulting in increased risk profiles for this cohort of patients. Semel and Goldin discuss how increased sweating of the feet amplifies risk for interdigital maceration, increases risk for bacterial and fungal colonization, and leads to a greater propensity for skin breakdown [25]. Autonomic dysfunction resulting in dry skin of the feet is equally problematic. Dry skin decreases skin turgor and pliability, becomes prone to micro-abrasions and overt fissures, and in the partially sensate patient increases itching which can lead to secondary lesions such as excoriations. These micro-abrasions become portals of entry which can lead to skin and soft tissue infection. All forms of neuropathy have important implications on amputation risk.

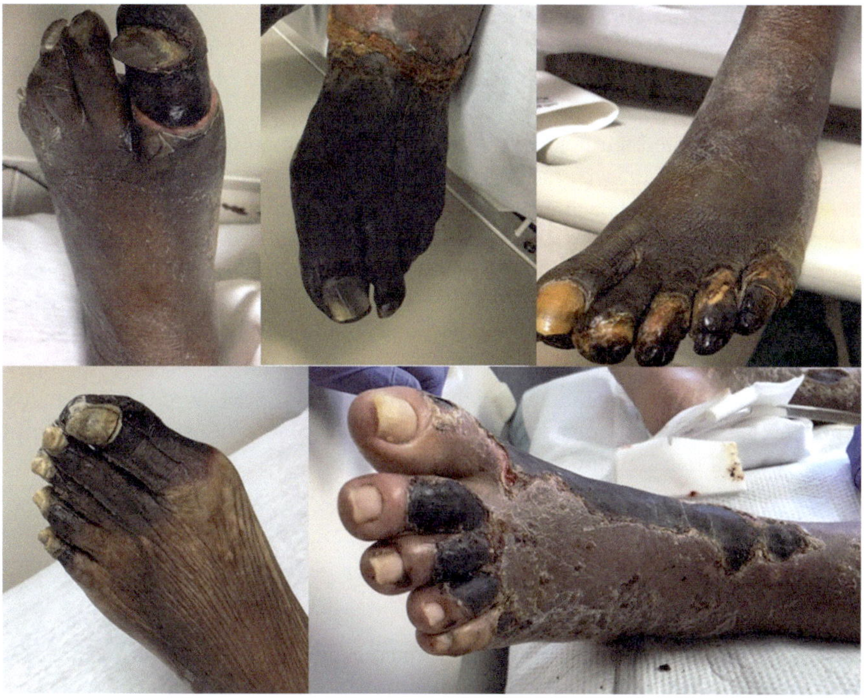

Fig. 3.2 Ischemia

Ischemia (Figure 3.2)

Peripheral vascular disease can occur as a consequence of multiple host factors. Shammas found that the most important independent risk factors for peripheral arterial disease include advanced age, diabetes, smoking, hypertension, and dyslipidemia [26]. A strong family history of vascular disease is important to ask about in all patients with diabetes. Patients with a history coronary artery disease and/or cerebrovascular accidents are also at high risk for peripheral arterial disease. These indicate that the patient has some predisposition toward macrovascular compromise which should prompt early screening for peripheral arterial disease. Claudication is an important symptom which, when present, easily identifies patients with clinically significant vasculopathy. Patients with diabetes are susceptible to both macrovascular and microvascular compromise.

Microvascular insufficiency has a major influence on lower extremity ulcer morbidity and amputation risk. Patients with diabetes with retinopathy, nephropathy, and/or neuropathy are likely to also have impaired tissue perfusion in lower extremity which predispose to ulcer non-healing and suboptimal results after revascularization. Fowler states that although macrovascular disease can be corrected, there are currently no direct treatments for microvascular disease of the lower extremity

[27]. The distribution of microvascular disease is similar to that of peripheral neuropathy. The most distal tissue of the foot is most affected and improves proximally. The level and quality of microvascular disease however are often elusive and difficult to objectively quantify.

Both medical and surgical interventions play an important role in improving long-term outcomes in ischemic patients. The patient history, vascular examination, and clinical impression each provide valuable information that can direct management of peripheral arterial disease. The presence of any type of ulcer or ischemic necrosis (dry gangrene) should prompt early endovascular angiography. A clinical algorithm is outlined in Fig. 3.3. Although CT and MR angiograms are alternative methods to assess the macrovascular anatomy, endovascular angiograms offer the advantage of intervention. Vascular reconstruction should be reserved for those patients in whom the benefits outweigh the risks. Taylor et al. argued that primary amputations should be considered in the non-salvageable limb and for those in whom medical risk contraindicates revascularization [28].

Skin and Soft Tissue Infection (Figure 3.4)

Ulcerations of the lower extremity remain the most important risk factor in patients with diabetes for foot and major lower extremity amputations. Chronic ulcers predispose to cellulitis and deep tissue abscess and can lead to acute infection and potential sepsis. All infections in patients with diabetes must be treated promptly and must not be underestimated. Rapid bacterial growth, spread within the fascial and tendinous planes of the foot, and close proximity to the joints and bones make the diabetic foot especially at risk for irreparable damage [7]. Because of the inherent immune-compromised state, patients may become bacteremic, develop systemic inflammatory response syndrome, or become frankly septic. Often systemic manifestations of infection such as fevers, leukocytosis, tachycardia, and hypotension are late presentations. In many patients, only mild constitutional symptoms such as lethargy and loss of appetite guide clinical suspicion of a severe systemic infection. An unusual spike from the patient's baseline plasma glucose levels is a clinical clue to an ensuing infection.

Bacterial infections of the diabetic foot can be isolated to the skin only and present as cellulitis. However, in most cases, deep tissues are also infected, and a delay in treatment can cause tissue death. The mainstay of treatment is to establish extent of involvement, decompression, and debridement of all infected and devitalized tissue and to provide empiric intravenous antibiotics until they can be tailored to intraoperative deep tissue cultures [7]. The initial surgical intervention must be aggressive enough to stabilize the medically compromised patient. Attinger et al. believe that multiple serial debridements should be undertaken before primary closure or soft tissue coverage is attempted [29]. The postsurgical soft tissue deficits left as a consequence of infection are a major factor in the determination of the final level of amputation.

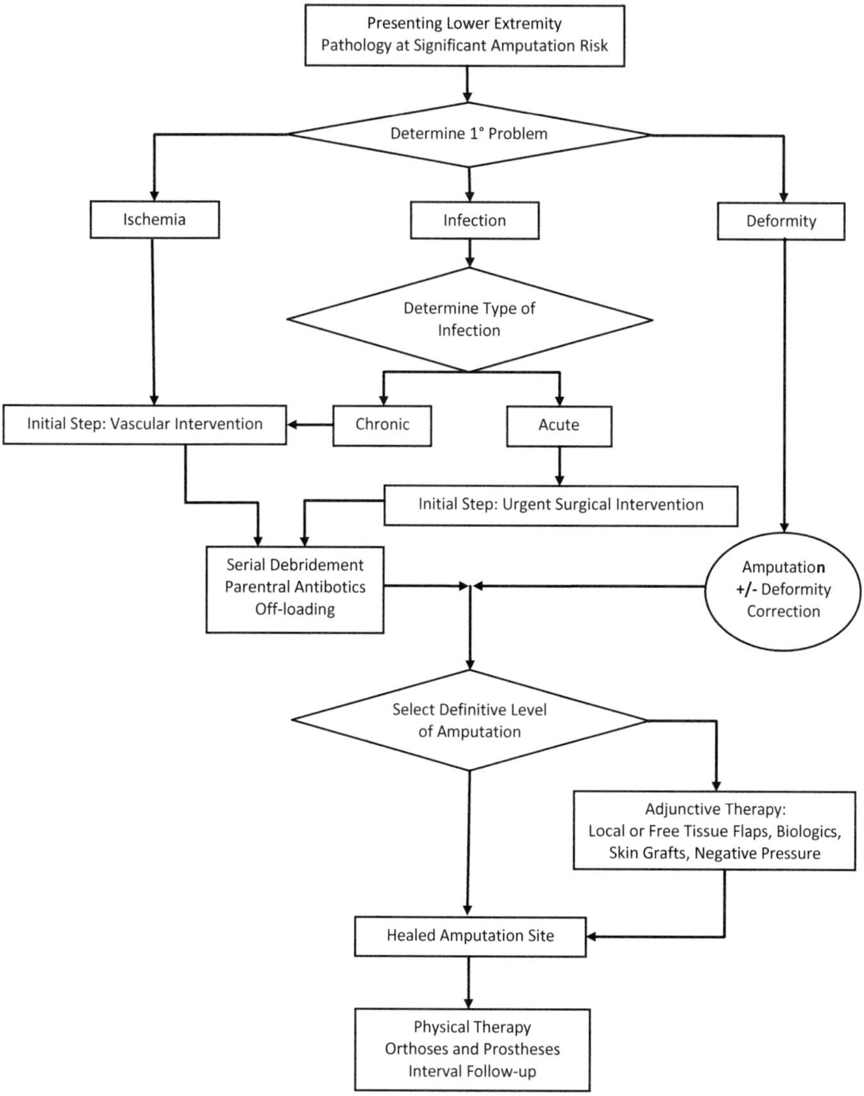

Fig. 3.3 Treatment algorithm for the ischemic and/or infected lower extremity

All patients with a foot infection must receive plain radiographs. X-ray imaging is widely available and is a simple screening test to rule out soft tissue emphysema and overt osteomyelitis. Both the extent and level of gas on radiographs so long as the radiographs are taken to the next proximal major joint can give an indication for inclusion of amputation within the treatment differential.

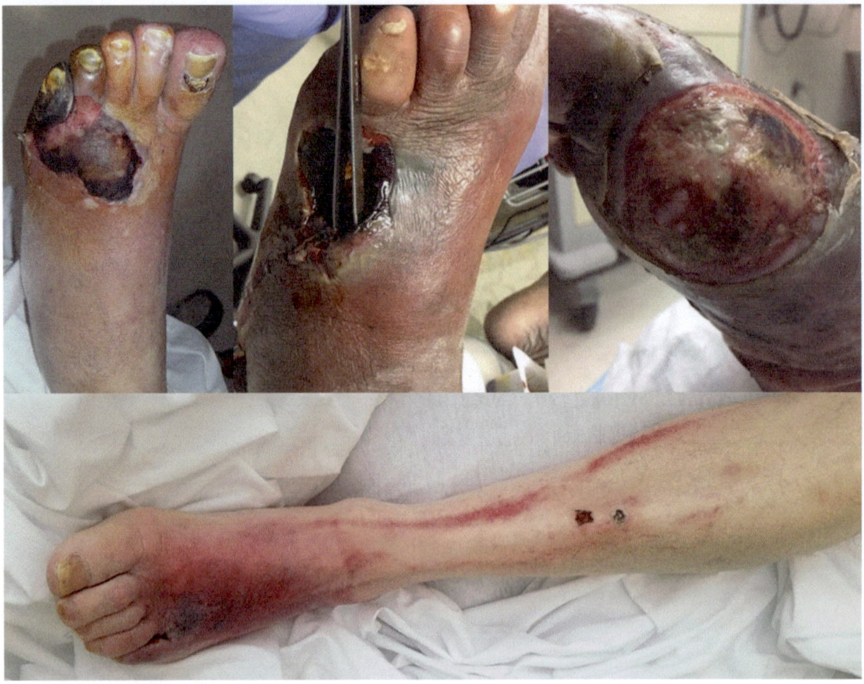

Fig. 3.4 Skin and soft tissue infection

Osteomyelitis

When infection of the bone is present, resection offers a definitive cure; however, this often results in some type of amputation. The soft tissue envelope of the foot and distal lower extremity are within millimeters of the skeletal structure. Diabetic foot infections whether acute or chronic expose the tissues to bacteria which may seed the underlying bone. According to Lam et al. [30], exposed bone and the bone that can be probed should be considered positive for osteomyelitis until proven otherwise. In those scenarios, clinical suspicion may be more important than diagnostic testing. Delay in treatment in the diabetic population consistently results in unfavorable outcomes. Early resection of grossly infected bone can prevent more proximal resection. Resection of an infected osseous structure essentially means an amputation of a portion of the infected foot. Lazaro-Martinez et al. have shown that the alternative to surgical resection is to give patients long courses of multiple intravenous antibiotics, usually for a minimum of 6 weeks, but that it may only be successful in patients without ischemia or necrotizing soft tissue infections [31]. Because the microvascular system is only marginally improved with macrovascular revascularization, delivery of effective plasma-level antibiotics with sufficient bone penetration is too uncertain to objectively define for each patient. Thus, the only definitive and objective standard is surgical removal with culture-endorsed clean margins.

Progression and severity of microvascular disease can be predicted by the presence of retinopathy and/or nephropathy in those with diabetes.

It must be noted that the surgical treatment of osteomyelitis must incorporate the anatomic location and the biomechanical effect of surgical resection. In some cases, only partial bone resection may be adequate, while in other cases, an entire bone or multiple bones may require removal. Faglia et al. have shown that calcaneal osteomyelitis has poorer outcomes and higher rates of transtibial amputations compared to forefoot or midfoot osteomyelitis [32]. Thus, the location of the bone can have an important effect on postsurgical patient outcomes. In patients with adequate circulation, and a low degree of bony involvement, a case-by-case evaluation of surgical management must include discussion with infectious disease. The consequences of unresolved osteomyelitis include wound non-healing, ulcer recurrence, systemic illness, and an increased risk for major lower extremity amputation.

Jeffcoate and Lipsky have demonstrated that a combination of clinical signs supplemented by laboratory results, imaging modalities, and bone biopsies all play an important role in the comprehensive evaluation of osteomyelitis [33]. No single test, including tissue-based diagnostics, should drive treatment decisions. When the clinical impression suggests osteomyelitis, while other diagnostic tests are conflicting or equivocal, the emphasis should err on the side of treatment. The intraoperative clinical evaluation of the bone by the surgeon may help determine the definitive treatment plan.

Deformity

The foot serves a unique and complex musculoskeletal purpose. The foot and its associated bones and joints collectively work to efficiently disperse immense loads during gait. Disturbances in lower extremity biomechanics ultimately result in changes in gait and load distribution which can lead to degenerative processes. In patients with normal sensation, changes in anatomic structure progress slowly but lead to pain and manifest in clinical syndromes which are easy to identify. Deformities of the forefoot are common and can occur in all age groups. Digital hammering and hallux abductovalgus are examples of common digital pathologies, which can present with a wide range of clinical symptoms. Hindfoot and midfoot pathologies are often more complex and may require major reconstruction to fix. As Faglia et al. described, perhaps the most difficult pathology to treat in the lower extremity is plantar heel ulceration secondary to calcaneal gait [32]. Major lower extremity amputations may be required.

Types of Lower Extremity Amputation

When the clinical indications are met, the extent of the amputation must be evaluated from a risk benefit perspective. Risk assessment depends on level of acuity and hemodynamic stability and must take into account laboratory parameters that might

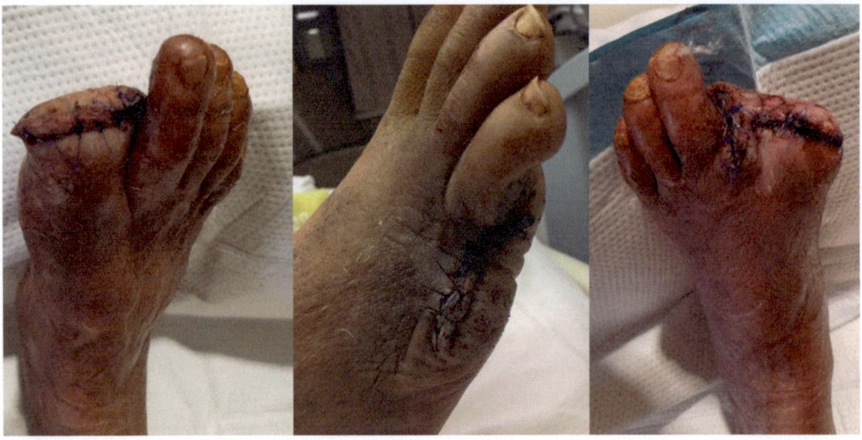

Fig. 3.5 Toe amputations

require medical optimization for each patient prior to undergoing amputation. As Roukis et al. have shown, preservation of lower extremity length is important, but the resultant biomechanical function must take precedence [34]. There are several levels of amputations and variations that are commonly performed.

Minor Amputations of the Foot

Toe Amputations (Figure 3.5)

Toe amputations are those in which an entire digit is removed at the metatarsophalangeal joint. For the lesser digits 2–4, the biomechanical implications are more forgiving than the amputation of the hallux. Although a disarticulation amputation of the hallux and the fifth toe can be performed, soft tissue closure may require the excision of the fifth metatarsal head. From a functional perspective, little sequelae occur when the digit is removed without the need for resection of the respective metatarsal head. When the metatarsal parabola is changed, the weight distribution during the gait cycle and in stance is greatly disturbed. Typically the weight is directed to the unaffected metatarsal adjacent to the one resected. A transfer lesion results in a new area of high pressure. Sage explained how this predisposes the patient to the same cycle of ulceration and risk of osteomyelitis and amputation [35]. When the lateral column of the foot has freedom of movement, this risk is lessened. When the lateral ray range of motion is limited, increased transfer ulcerations and complications undoubtedly occur. Rinonapoli et al. state that the greatest complication encountered with a second toe amputation is the occurrence of a hallux valgus deformity [36]. In the insensate patient, this type of deformity can predispose to ulcerations at the medial aspect of the first metatarsophalangeal joint.

When the base of the proximal phalanx can be preserved, the stump can provide a buttress that has the potential to decrease the development of hallux valgus. The third toe is part of the immobile central column, and thus, the implications of a total third toe disarticulation bear minimal consequence for amputation.

When only a part of the toe requires amputation, the partial toe amputation is simple to perform. Generally, disarticulation at the interphalangeal joints is acceptable. Although the length of the toe does not have an impact on overall outcomes, it is more important to create an amputation with soft tissue closure in mind. All toe amputations should be designed with primary or delayed primary closure in mind. The soft tissue envelop of the digit often dictates the level of amputation. Most digital ulcerations occur either at the distal toe or over the dorsal proximal interphalangeal joint. In the case of the distal ulceration, excision of the ulcer and the nail plate and extirpation of the distal phalanx can provide a plantar flap that can provide a durable closure. When ulceration occurs over the dorsal proximal interphalangeal joint, an excisional arthroplasty is an option. However, if too much bone is required to be removed secondary to underlying osteomyelitis, a partial toe amputation transecting the proximal phalanx is a practical amputation.

When the hallux is involved, the biomechanics of the foot is greatly influenced by the level of amputation. A partial hallux amputation preserves both length and the attachment of the flexor hallucis brevis tendon at the base of the proximal phalanx, which is an important stabilizer. Typically, closure of this type of amputation requires the resection of the head of the proximal phalanx. Oliver et al. discussed the importance of evaluating the presence of hallux rigidus, as partial hallux amputations should be avoided to prevent re-ulceration [37]. Disarticulation at the level of the first metatarsophalangeal joint maintains the metatarsal parabola and thus mitigates the risk of transfer ulceration. Evaluation of the first metatarsophalangeal joint range of motion is important to delineate type of hallucal amputation. Because most ulcerations occur plantar or medial to the first metatarsophalangeal joint, partial hallux and disarticulation amputations may not provide adequate soft tissue coverage. Although there are hallux-sparing procedures, often the only viable option is a partial first ray amputation, where the head of the first metatarsal is resected. The removal of the head of the metatarsal, where osteomyelitis is most likely to occur, addresses the infection while allowing soft tissue coverage. Quebedeaux et al. explain that because the hallux is an integral component during the push-off phase of gait, its removal imparts dramatic biomechanical consequences, which can result in progressive ulcerations laterally [38]. The loss of length and disturbance of the normal parabola predispose to transfer ulcerations which have the potential to lead to further amputations. Elmarsafi et al. reported that the use of permanent cement spacers after resection of the metatarsal head in these cases can result in improved rates of hallux salvage and decreases risk of transfer ulcerations [39].

In the case of ischemic necrosis, without infection, and in the setting of a patient who is not a surgical candidate, auto-amputation of the digit can be an acceptable option. Patients in whom vascular interventions are not possible, so long as infection has not developed to the afflicted foot, auto-amputation is a safe and noninvasive method. Topical drying and antiseptic agents must be used, however, with

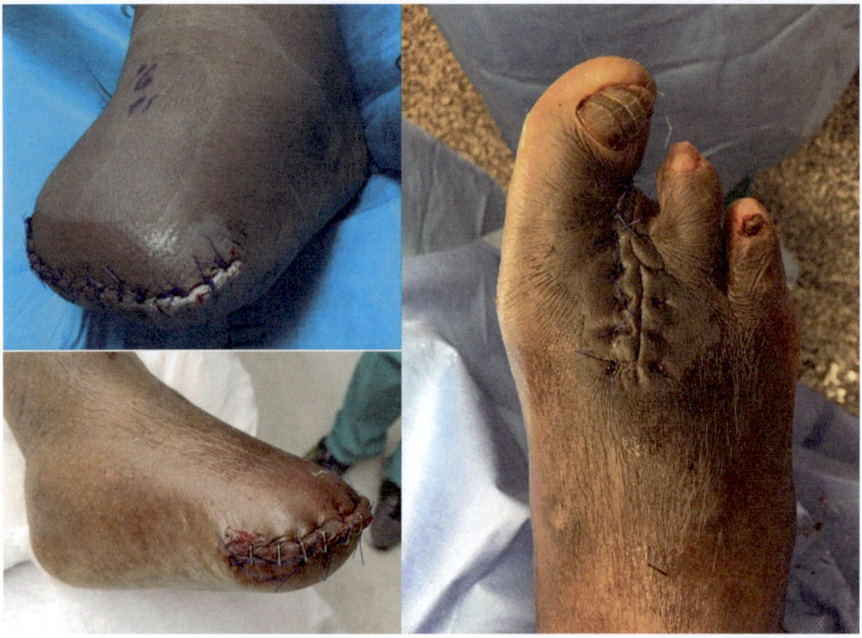

Fig. 3.6 Partial ray and transmetatarsal amputations

frequent inspection for the occurrence of early signs of infection. Once infection occurs, surgical amputation must be considered. Furthermore, when large areas undergo ischemic necrosis, such as an entire foot or leg, evidence of systemic toxicity other than infection can be an indication for amputation. In these cases, when vascular correction of the ischemic limb is not possible, amputation should not be delayed. The risks and benefits or all interventions must be reviewed in light of each patient's wishes, expectations, and functional status.

Partial Ray Amputations and Transmetatarsal Amputations (Figure 3.6)

Partial ray amputations and transmetatarsal amputations (TMA) are commonly performed procedures, both as primary and salvage procedures for forefoot infection and ischemia. According to Landry et al., in a series of 62 TMAs performed in 57 patients, healing occurred in 53%, 22 ended up with below-knee amputations, and 11% died without healing [40]. A meta-analysis performed by Thorud et al. revealed that the reoperation rate was 24%; reamputation rate was 28%; and 30% required major amputations following initial TMA [41]. These poor results have caused surgeons to evaluate their surgical technique and consider adjunct procedures. Garwood and Steinberg investigated procedures such as Achilles lengthening, anterior tibial tendon lengthening, or anterior tibial tendon transfer and found that they may play a role in decreasing postoperative complication rates [42]. Furthermore, Boffeli et al. reported a 75% radiographic incidence of heterotopic ossification (HO) following partial ray resection with 18% exhibiting HO-related ulceration [43]. These findings suggest that risk stratification and prophylaxis against heterotopic ossification may be warranted in certain patients.

Surgical technique: Partial ray amputation incisions are made longitudinally over the operative metatarsal. The TMA incision is designed to create a long, thick myocutaneous plantar flap. A slightly curved dorsal transverse incision is made at the level of the mid-to-proximal metatarsal shafts. The apices of the incision on the medial and lateral sides are made slightly proximally at the level of the glabrous junction. The plantar incision is made as distally as possible as any excess tissue can later be trimmed. The plantar flap is reflected plantarly and the metatarsals are exposed. It is critical to maintain the metatarsal parabola during the osseous cuts. For both partial ray resections and transmetatarsal amputations, more bone should be removed from the plantar than dorsal aspect for all five metatarsals. The first and fifth metatarsals should also have slightly more bone resected on the medial and lateral aspects, respectively. The exposed flexor and extensor tendons should be sharply excised. The plantar tissue is then flapped dorsally to be primarily closed with the dorsal skin. Closure is performed in multiple anatomic layers, and the authors prefer to close the skin with vertical mattresses without tension.

Postoperative course: The patient should be non-weight bearing for 2–4 weeks or until the incision has completely healed. At this point the sutures are removed. The patient may require a special ankle-foot orthosis, a rigid rocker-bottom shoe, or a toe filler. After the patient has fully healed, regular follow-ups should be performed every 6 months to check for signs of irritation, soft tissue breakdown, or infection.

Major Amputations

Below-Knee Amputations (Figure 3.7)

Transtibial or below-knee amputation is the most common major lower extremity amputation performed. BKAs are performed when it is deemed that the foot and ankle are non-salvageable. It can also be performed for intractable pain such as that from untreatable critical limb ischemia. Despite being a commonly performed procedure, BKAs have relatively poor outcomes. Aulivola et al. report that the 30-day mortality rate for below-knee amputation is 5.7%. In their study of 704 BKAs, 18.4% required subsequent operation, and 9.4% required conversion to above-knee amputation [44]. The overall survival rates at 1 and 5 years were 69.7% and 34.7%, respectively.

The tibia can be transected at different lengths, but at least 8 cm of tibia distal to the knee joint is required for optimal fitting of a prosthesis. A short transtibial amputation is when less than 20% of original length is preserved, a standard amputation is between 20% and 50%, and a long transtibial amputation is when greater than 50% is preserved. Waters et al. report that the energy expenditure above baseline is

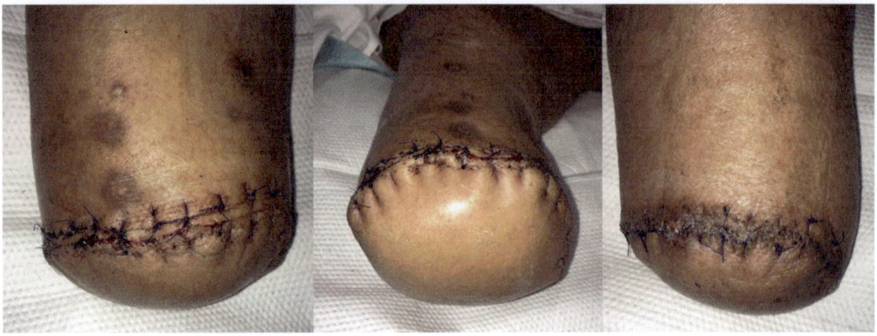

Fig. 3.7 Below-knee amputations

40% for short BKA, 25% for an average BKA, and 10% for a long BKA [45]. This increased energy requirement is because of the shorter moment arm making knee extension and therefore ambulation more difficult. Despite a long BKA requiring less energy expenditure, it is usually not advised in the diabetic patient with peripheral arterial disease because the likelihood of wound healing complications increases dramatically.

Surgical technique: A transverse anterior incision is made approximately 15 cm distal to the knee joint or 10 cm distal to the tibial tuberosity. It extends approximately two-thirds of the total circumference of the leg. The posterior incision is made as far distally as possible to create a long flap that can later be trimmed as needed for proper closure. The anterior tibial neurovascular structures are identified, clamped, and ligated. The tibial cut is made 2–3 cm proximal to the anterior skin flap, with the fibula transected 1–2 cm proximal to the tibial cut at 45° on the coronal plane. The anterior portion of the tibia is beveled and rasped to make it smooth. At this point, an Ertl procedure, which consists of a distal tibiofibular synostosis, can be performed. According to Bosse et al., the Ertl may provide a better prosthetic fit, increase the weight bearing surface, and improve function especially among high-performing individuals [46]. However, it is more technically challenging, requires a longer operative time, has a longer healing time, and possibly has a higher complication rate. Once the osseous cuts have been made, the posterior vessels are identified, clamped, and ligated. The common peroneal and tibial nerves are either sharply transected under tension or an end-to-end neurodesis is performed to prevent phantom limb pain. At the authors' institution, the nerves are injected with liposomal bupivacaine before closure. The deep posterior muscles and soleus are isolated and transected just distal to the level of the tibia. The peroneal muscles and gastrocnemius are myodesed to the distal tibia to provide a stable and cushioned distal stump. Closure is performed in multiple anatomic layers, and the authors prefer to close the skin with alternating vertical mattresses and staples. A closed suction drain is usually placed and removed once the drainage decreases to less than 20 ml over 24 h for 2 consecutive days.

Transgenicular, also known as through-knee or knee disarticulation amputation, is another option for patients with infrapopliteal vascular disease. The benefits of this procedure include relative technical ease, short procedure time, and less traumatic dissection. It offers weight bearing over a large surface area and a biomechanically advantageous long lever arm. It also preserves all muscle groups which help prevent muscle imbalances and contractures. Historically, the greatest problem has been fitting standard prosthesis with the double condylar, bulbous end. Morse et al. published a series of 50 patients [47]. They reported a 6% mortality rate and 81% uncomplicated healing rate. The survival probabilities at 3 and 5 years were 0.60 and 0.44, respectively. The disadvantages of this type of amputation mostly relate to fit of prostheses and patient comfort in a prosthetic.

Surgical technique: A fishmouth incision with equal anterior and posterior flaps is created. The flap should extend past the tibial tuberosity. The patellar tendon is detached from the tibia. A circumferential knee capsulotomy is performed, along with a transection of the cruciate ligaments. Care should be taken to preserve the superior genicular artery when dissecting the gastrocnemius. The popliteal artery is identified, clamped, and ligated. The common peroneal and tibial nerves are either sharply transected under tension or an end-to-end neurodesis is performed to prevent phantom limb pain. At the authors' institution, the nerves are injected with liposomal bupivacaine before closure. The hamstring tendons are myodesed to the knee capsule to prevent flexion contracture. The iliotibial band is anastomosed to the knee capsule to preserve abductor function. The patellar tendon is attached to the cruciate ligaments with the hip in extension to prevent flexion contracture. There is some debate whether to excise the patella or to perform a patellofemoral arthrodesis, with good results reported in the literature for both techniques. The protruding surfaces of the distal femoral condyles are resected, and a conical stump is formed. Closure is performed in multiple anatomic layers, and the authors prefer to close the skin with alternating vertical mattresses and staples. A closed suction drain is usually placed and is removed once the drainage decreases to less than 20 ml over 24 h for 2 consecutive days.

Patients who require a BKA and who were previously ambulatory are more likely to function well with a prosthetic. Patients who were minimally able to ambulate independently prior to a BKA are less likely to function well with a prosthetic. The decision process however should not change; the indications for a BKA should be well delineated. If a patient is a good candidate for a BKA and is offered diligent and comprehensive physical rehabilitation, outcomes may prove favorable, particularly if cardiopulmonary reserve is adequate to support exertion. It is important to note that in patients who are bedridden, and for those with contractures of the lower extremity, an above-knee amputation is a better choice to prevent distal stump necrosis and pressure-induced ulcerations for BKA's with subsequent flexion contracture at the knee. A well-performed BKA is a versatile amputation that affords patients with a robust soft tissue closure, at a level with more tissue perfusion, and amenable to fitting and ambulation in a prosthetic (Video 3.1).

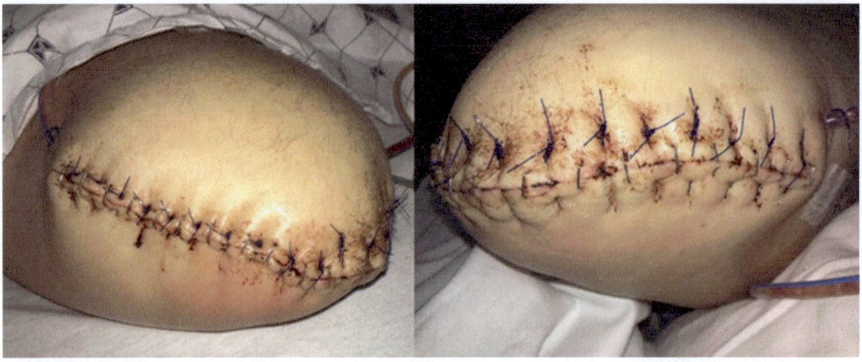

Fig. 3.8 Above-knee amputations

Above-Knee Amputation (Figure 3.8)

Transfemoral or above-knee amputation (AKA) is the procedure of choice when a patient has severe peripheral vascular disease at the popliteal or infrapopliteal level without revascularization options or when the patient has extensive soft tissue loss or infection with resultant inadequate tissue coverage to heal a more distal procedure. Alternatively, patients with severe lower extremity contractions which contraindicate endovascular intervention, and are poor candidates for a more distal amputation, are best served with this type of amputation. The proximal nature of the procedure allows for the greatest chance of wound healing. However, AKAs come with greater morbidity and mortality risks compared to BKA. Research conducted by Aulivola et al. shows that the 30-day mortality rate for AKAs was 16.5% and the 1- and 5-year survival rates were 50.6% and 22.5%, respectively [44]. According to Waters et al., the energy expenditure is 65% above baseline for ambulation [45]. This increased effort results in less than one-third of AKA patients successfully rehabilitating with prosthesis.

AKAs can be performed at various levels along the femur. In order to properly fit a prosthetic device, the residual limb must be at least 4–6 inches from the groin and at least 4 inches above the distal aspect of the femur. Long, medium, and short transfemoral amputations occur when greater than 60%, between 35% and 60%, and less than 30% of the original femoral length is preserved, respectively.

Surgical technique: After the level of bone resection has been determined, a fishmouth incision is made distal to that level. The anterior flap should be longer in order to create a posterior scar. The adductors should be preserved and should be myodesed to the distal aspect of the femur at the end of the procedure to prevent an abduction contracture. The femur is transected at the desired level. The major blood vessels should be identified, clamped, and ligated. The sciatic nerve can either be cauterized or end-to-side loop anastomosis may be performed to prevent phantom limb pain. At the authors' institution, the nerve is injected with liposomal bupivacaine before closure. The anterior and posterior muscle groups are transected sharply to retract to the level of bone resection. Quadriceps myodesis is performed with the femur in full extension to prevent hip flexion contracture. Closure is performed in multiple anatomic layers, and the authors prefer to close the skin with alternating vertical mattresses and staples. A closed suction drain is usually placed and is removed once the drainage decreases to less than 20 ml over 24 h for 2 consecutive days.

Postoperative course for major amputations: The patient should be non-weight bearing for 6–9 weeks. The staples are removed at 7–10 days and the sutures are removed at 3–5 weeks. The leg should be compressed with lymphedema wraps. The patient should be fitted for prosthesis at 6–8 weeks in order to create the proper fit. Premature fitting for prosthesis will create one that is too large as the patient's swelling will continue to improve. At approximately 6–9 weeks, patients are allowed to weight bear as tolerated and gradually increase activity. Physical therapy is initiated after delivery of prosthesis and should be continued for 3–4 weeks to increase functional status. After the patient has fully healed, regular follow-ups should be performed every 6 months to check for signs of irritation, soft tissue breakdown, or infection.

Conclusions (Figure 3.9)

Although amputation cases can be challenging, if the basic approach to each patient is comprehensive and complete, successes can be met with amicable frequency. There are several other types of infrequently used amputations which have not been described in this chapter. However, the overwhelming majority of cases can be

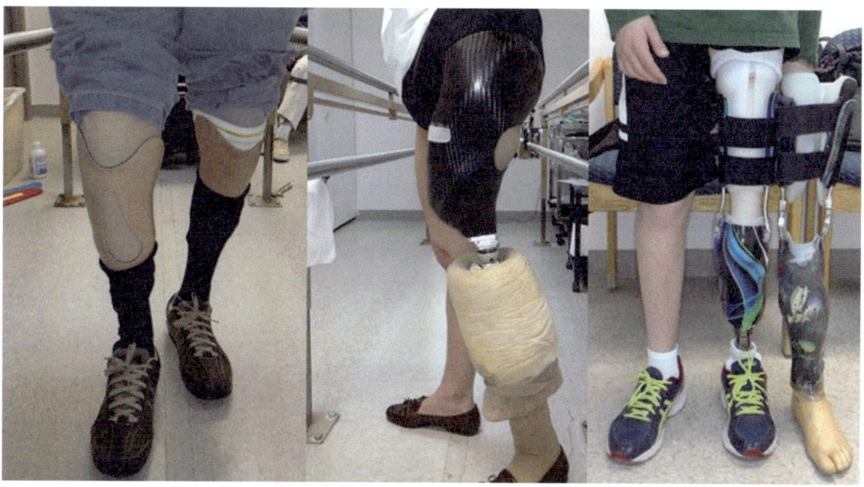

Fig. 3.9 Prosthetic limbs

successfully addressed in keeping within the context of the information provided herein.

Traumatic amputations though not discussed in detail should follow the general principles and guidelines of any amputation. For all levels of amputation of the lower extremity, acute and post-traumatic causes can be executed as a staged or in a single operation. Postoperative complications and long-term outcomes are dramatically different in the typically young healthy amputee, versus amputations in the complex host. Traumatic amputations in the diabetic patient should be exercised with the same precautions outlined in this chapter.

There are many conditions which can contribute to the need for a lower extremity amputation. Understanding the underlying etiology, mitigating risk factors which lead to poor postoperative outcomes and performing the proper type of amputation are important surgical considerations. Knowing patient expectations and performing amputations which preserve function provide the foundation for proper salvage. Once a patient undergoes an amputation at any level, continued interval surveillance for the detection of other risk factors which may lead to additional amputations must be established. The contralateral limb must always be evaluated for the same risks. Optimizing glycemic control, nutritional status, and other modifiable parameters can prove beneficial. When a major lower extremity amputation is required, the advancements in prosthetics and the materials they are made from have made functional outcomes possible even in the most challenging cases. Physical rehabilitation is always an appropriate part of recovery.

Authorship Role, Participation, and Acknowledgments 1. Joseph Park: Provided substantial contributions to conception and design; acquisition of data, analysis, and interpretation of findings; drafting the article and revising it critically for important intellectual content; and final approval of the version to be published.

2. Tammer Elmarsafi: Provided substantial contributions to conception and design; acquisition of data, analysis, and interpretation of findings; drafting the article and revising it critically for important intellectual content; and final approval of the version to be published.
3. John S. Steinberg: Provided substantial contributions to conception and design; acquisition of data, analysis, and interpretation of findings; drafting the article and revising it critically for important intellectual content; and final approval of the version to be published.
4. Jocelyn Lu: MS4 Georgetown University School of Medicine – A special thank you for her contribution in clinical photography and video editing.

Financial Disclosures Joseph Park, Tammer Elmarsafi, and John S. Steinberg have no financial disclosures, commercial associations, or any other conditions posing a conflict of interest to report.

References

1. Banks M. The surgeon of old in war. JAMA. 1897 Oct;29(14):665–7.
2. Moxey PW, Gogalniceanu P, Hinchliffe RJ, Loftus IM, Jones KJ, Thompson MM, Holt PJ. Lower extremity amputations – a review of global variability in incidence. Diabet Med. 2011 Oct;28(10):1144–53.
3. Economides JM, DeFazio MV, Attinger CE, Barbour JR. Prevention of painful neuroma and phantom limb pain after transfemoral amputation through concomitant nerve coaptation and collagen nerve wrapping. Neurosurgery. 2016 Sept;79(3):508–13.
4. Attinger CE, Brown BJ. Amputation and ambulation in diabetic patients: function is the goal. Diabetes Metab Rev. 2012 Feb;28(Suppl 1):93–6.
5. Weledji EP, Fokam P. Treatment of the diabetic foot – to amputate or not? BMC Surg. 2014;14:83.
6. Nather A, Wong KL. Distal amputations for the diabetic foot. Diabet Foot Ankle. 2013;4:10.
7. Altemeier WA, Fullen WD. Prevention and treatment of gas gangrene. JAMA. 1971;217(6):806–13.
8. Price P. The diabetic foot: quality of life. Clin Infect Dis. 2004;39(Suppl 2):S129–31.
9. Raspovic KM, Hobizal KB, Rosario BL, Wukich DK. Midfoot charcot neuroarthropathy in patients with diabetes: the impact of foot ulceration on self-reported quality of life. Foot Ankle Spec. 2015 Aug;8(4):255–2559.
10. Beaulieu RJ, Grimm JC, Lyu H, Abularrage CJ, Perler BA. Predictors for readmission and reamputation following minor lower extremity amputation. J Vasc Surg. 2015 Jul;62(1):101–5.
11. Hobizal KB, Wukich DK. Diabetic foot infections: current concept review. Diabet Foot Ankle. 2012 Jan;1;3(1):18409.
12. Yazdanpanah L, Nasiri M, Adarvishi S. Literature review on the management of diabetic foot ulcer. World J Diabetes. 2015 Feb 15;6(1):37–53.
13. Fernandez A, Schillinger D, Warton EM, Adler N, Moffet HH, Schenker Y, Salgado MV, Ahmed A, Karter AJ. Language barriers, physician-patient language concordance, and glycemic control among insured latinos with diabetes: the diabetes study of northern California. J Gen Intern Med. 2011 Feb;26(2):170–6.
14. Glaser JD, Bensley RP, Hurks R, Dahlberg S, Hamdan AD, Wyers MC, Chaikof EL, Schermerhorn ML. Fate of the contralateral limb after lower extremity amputation. J Vasc Surg. 2013 Dec;58(6):1571–7.
15. Boulton AJM. Management of diabetic peripheral neuropathy. Clin Diabetes. 2005 Jan;23(1):9–15.
16. Singh N, Armstrong DG, et al. Preventing foot ulcers in patients with diabetes. JAMA. 2005;293:217–28.
17. Muller LM, Gorter KJ, Hak E, Goudzwaard WL, Schellevis FG, Hoepelman AI, et al. Increased risk of common infections in patients with type 1 and type 2 diabetes mellitus. Clin Infect Dis. 2005;41:281–8.
18. Caselli A, Pham H, Giurini JM, Armstrong DG, Veves A. The forefoot-to-rearfoot plantar pressure ratio is increased in severe diabetic neuropathy and can predict foot ulceration. Diabetes care. 2002 Jun;1;25(6):1066–71.
19. Apelqvist J, Ragnarson-Tennvall G, Larsson J, Persson U. Long-term costs for foot ulcers in diabetic patients in a multidisciplinary setting. Foot Ankle Int. 1995 Jul;16(7):388–94.
20. Mold JW, Vesely SK, Keyl BA, Schenk JB, Roberts M. The prevalence, predictors, and consequences of peripheral sensory neuropathy in older patients. J Am Board Fam Med. 2004 Sep-Oct;17(5):309–18.
21. Partanen J, Niskanen L, Lehtinen J, Mervaala E, Siitonen O, Uusitupa M. Natural history of peripheral neuropathy in patients with non-insulin-dependent diabetes mellitus. N Engl J Med. 1995 Jul 13;333(2):89–94.

22. Marchettini P, Lacerenza M, Mauri E, Marangoni C. Painful peripheral neuropathies. Curr Neuropharmacol. 2006 Jul;4(3):175–81.
23. Lavery LA, Armstrong DG, Vela SA, Quebedeaux TL, Fleischli JG. Practical criteria for screening patients at high risk for diabetic foot ulceration. Arch Intern Med. 1998 Jan 26;158(2):157–62.
24. Duby JJ, Campbell RK, Setter SM, White JR, Rasmussen KA. Diabetic neuropathy: an intensive review. Am J Health Syst Pharm. 2004 Jan 15;61(2):160–73.
25. Semel JD, Goldin H. Association of athlete's foot with cellulitis of the lower extremities: diagnostic value of bacterial cultures of ipsilateral interdigital space samples. Clin Infect Dis. 1996 Nov;23(5):1662–164.
26. Shammas NW. Epidemiology, classification, and modifiable risk factors of peripheral arterial disease. Vasc Health Risk Manag. 2007 Apr;3(2):229–34.
27. Fowler MJ. Microvascular and macrovascular complications of diabetes. Clin Diabetes. 2008 Nov;26(2):77–82.
28. Taylor LM, Hamre D, Dalman RL. Limb salvage vs amputation for critical limb ischemia: the role of vascular surgery. Arch Surg. 1991;126(10):1251–8.
29. Attinger CE, Bulan E, Blume PA. Surgical debridement. The key to successful wound healing and reconstruction. Clin Podiatr Med Sug. 2000;17:599–630.
30. Lam K, van Asten SA, Nguyen T, La Fontaine J, Lavery LA. Diagnostic accuracy of probe to bone to detect osteomyelitis in the diabetic foot: a systematic review. Clin Infect Dis. 2016 Oct 1;63(7):944–8.
31. Lazaro-Martinez JL, Aragon-Sanchez J, Garcia-Morales E. Antibiotics versus conservative surgery for treating diabetic foot osteomyelitis: a randomized comparative trial. Diabetes Care. 2014;37(3):789–95.
32. Faglia E, Clerici G, Caminiti M, Curci V, Somalvico F. Influence of osteomyelitis location in the foot of diabetic patients with transtibial amputation. Foot Ankle Int. 2013 Feb;34(2):222–7.
33. Jeffcoate WJ, Lipsky BA. Controversies in diagnosing and managing osteomyelitis of the foot in diabetics. Clin Infect Dis. 2004;39(Supplement_2):S115–22.
34. Roukis TS, Singh N, Andersen CA. Preserving functional capacity as opposed to tissue preservation in the diabetic patient: a single institution experience. Foot Ankle Spec. 2010 Aug;3(4):177–83.
35. Sage RA. Biomechanics of ambulation after partial foot amputation: prevention and management of reulceration. J Prosthet Orthot. 2007 Jul;19(8):P77–9.
36. Rinonapoli G, Ceccarini P, Altissimi M, Caraffa A. Critical appraisal of foot and ankle amputations in diabetes. Clin Res Foot Ankle. 2014;S3:005.
37. Oliver NG, Attinger CE, Steinberg JS, Evans KK, Vieweger D, Kim PJ. Influence of hallux rigidus on reamputation in patients with diabetes mellitus after partial hallux amputation. J Foot Ankle Surg. 2015;54(6):1076–80.
38. Quebedeaux T, Lavery L, Lavery D. The development of foot deformities and ulcers after great toe amputation in diabetes. Diabetes Care. 1996;19:165–7.
39. Elmarsafi T, Oliver NG, Steinberg JS, Evans KK, Attinger CE, Kim PJ. Long-term outcomes of permanent cement spacers in the infected foot. J Foot Ankle Surg. 2017 Mar;56(2):287–90.
40. Landry GJ, Silverman DA, Liem TK. Predictors of healing and functional outcomes following transmetatarsal amputations. Arch Surg. 2011;146(9):1005–9.
41. Thorud JC, Jupiter DC, Lorenzana J, Nguyen TT, Shibuya N. Reoperation and reamputation after transmetatarsal amputation: a systematic review and meta-analysis. J Foot Ankle Surg. 2016 Sep-Oct;55(5):1007–12.
42. Garwood CS, Steinberg JS. Soft tissue balancing after partial foot amputations. Clin Podiatr Med Surg. 2016 Jan;33(1):99–111.
43. Boffeli TJ, Thompson JC, Waverly BJ, Pfannenstein RR, Mahoney KJ. Incidence of clinical significance of heterotopic ossification after partial ray resection. J Foot Ankle Surg. 2016 Jul-Aug;55(4):714–9.

44. Aulivola B, Hile CN, Hamdan AD, Sheahan MG, Veraldi JR, Skillman JJ, Campbell DR, Scovell SD, LoGerfo FW, Pomposelli FB Jr. Major lower extremity Amputation Outcome of a modern series. Arch Surg. 2004;139(4):395–9.
45. Waters RL, Perry J, Antonelli D, Hislop H. Energy cost of walking of amputees: the influence of level of amputation. J Bone Joint Surg Am. 1976 Jan;58(1):42–6.
46. Bosse MJ, Morshed S, Reider L, Ertl W, Toledano J, Firoozabadi R, Seymour RB, Carroll E, Scharfstein DO, Steverson B, MacKenzie EJ. Transtibial amputation outcomes study (TAOS): comparing transtibial amputation with and without a tibiofibular synostosis (Ertl) procedure. J Orthop Trauma. 2017 Apr;31(Suppl 1):S63–9.
47. Morse BC, Cull DL, Kalbaugh C, Cass AL, Taylor MD. Through-knee amputation in patients with peripheral arterial disease: a review of 50 cases. J Vasc Surg. 2008 Sep;48(3):638–43.

Chapter 4
Gastrocsoleus Lengthening

Christopher P. Chiodo

Background

The gastrocsoleus complex, also known as the triceps surae, is located in the superficial posterior compartment of the leg. It is comprised of the gastrocnemius and soleus muscles, which ultimately join to form the Achilles tendon. The gastrocnemius muscle is larger and superficial to the soleus. It has two heads that originate on the medial and lateral condyles of the distal femur. Distally, it terminates into a broad, fascia-like tendon that then joins with the terminal soleus to form the Achilles tendon. Functionally, the gastrocnemius crosses both the knee and ankle joints. The soleus, meanwhile, is a broad, multipennate structure that originates from the posterior tibia and fibula. Its distal tendon is often lest distinct. Unlike the gastrocnemius, the soleus does not cross the knee.

Concentric contracture of the gastrocsoleus complex is responsible for forward propulsion through active ankle plantarflexion. This occurs during the second half of the stance phase of gait. Meanwhile, eccentric contraction of the gastrocnemius and soleus muscles allows with controlled ankle dorsiflexion during the swing phase of gait. Additionally, isometric contracture of the soleus muscle is instrumental in controlling sway and stabilizing the ankle during normal standing.

A gastrocsoleus contracture can substantially alter the biomechanics of gait and weight-bearing. In the setting of a contracture, the gastrocnemius and soleus muscles are unable to fully elongate during the stance phase of gait. With this, ankle dorsiflexion is restricted, and the leg is unable to fully progress over the planted foot. This results in premature and increased loading of the forefoot, which in turn may contribute to the development of an ulcer. Alternatively, it may inhibit healing or lead to recurrence of preexisting ulcers.

C.P. Chiodo, MD (✉)
Foot and Ankle Division, Brigham Foot and Ankle Center, Brigham and Women's Hospital, Boston, MA, USA
e-mail: cchiodo@partners.org

D.P. Orgill (ed.), *Interventional Treatment of Wounds*,
https://doi.org/10.1007/978-3-319-66990-8_4

It follows that addressing a gastrocsoleus contracture is an important component of treating nonhealing foot ulcers. Nonoperative measures may include home stretching, physical therapy, and the use of a night splint. Surgical lengthening is most often accomplished by either a gastrocnemius recession or an Achilles tendon lengthening. A gastrocnemius recession entails division of the gastrocnemius tendon just distal to the musculotendinous junction [1]. Following an early review in 1950, this operation is often referred to as a "Strayer" procedure [2]. It is indicated for contractures isolated to the gastrocnemius muscle without concomitant involvement of the soleus.

Meanwhile, an Achilles tendon lengthening is used for combined contractures of the gastrocnemius and soleus muscles. While such lengthening may be accomplished with an open Z-plasty, this more extensive procedure is usually not necessary in patients with plantar wounds. Instead, the triple hemisection technique as described by Hoke is a useful alternative [3]. This procedure lengthens the Achilles through three percutaneous incisions and sequential, transverse step cuts that alternate between the medial and lateral halves of the tendon.

In the presence of a contracture, both gastrocnemius recession and Achilles lengthening can reduce the mechanical loads exerted on a plantar foot ulcer. This facilitates healing and prevents recurrence of future ulceration.

Indications

Surgical lengthening of the gastrocnemius or Achilles is indicated for recalcitrant ulcers of the *plantar* forefoot associated with a gastrocsoleus contracture. A Strayer procedure is indicated for contractures isolated to the gastrocnemius muscle. Meanwhile, surgical lengthening of the Achilles tendon is indicated for plantar forefoot wounds associated with combined contractures of the gastrocnemius and soleus muscles.

Distinguishing between an isolated gastrocnemius contracture and a combined contracture of the gastrocnemius and soleus muscles is based on physical examination, in particular the Silfverskiold test. The anatomic basis of this test is the fact that the gastrocnemius muscle crosses both the ankle and knee joints, while the soleus crosses only the ankle joint. As such, knee flexion will relax the gastrocnemius, but not the soleus. The Silfverskiold test assesses passive ankle dorsiflexion first with the knee extended and then flexed to 90° (Fig. 4.1). In the absence of contracture, ankle dorsiflexion will be similar with both knee flexion and extension (approximately 10°–15° in healthy individuals). With an isolated gastrocnemius contracture, there will be decreased ankle dorsiflexion with the knee extended, but not with the knee flexed. With a combined gastrocsoleus contracture, there will be decreased ankle dorsiflexion both with the knee flexed and extended.

In the author's experience, most contractures associated with plantar forefoot ulcers are limited to the gastrocnemius muscle. As such, they can usually be addressed with a Stayer procedure. While a Hoke lengthening may also suffice, it

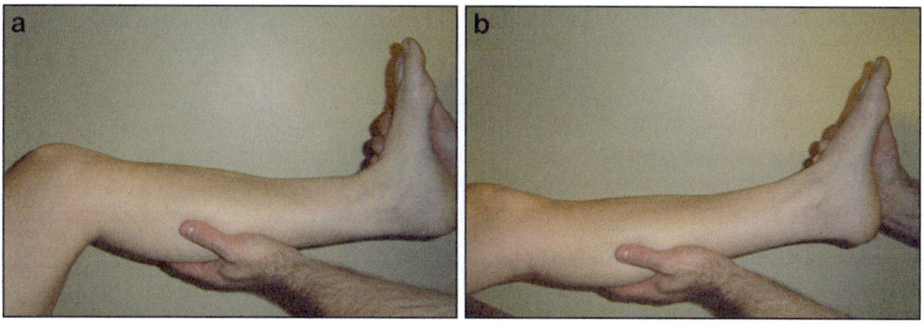

Fig. 4.1 With the Silfverskiold test, an isolated gastrocnemius contracture is characterized by normal ankle dorsiflexion with the knee flexed (**a**) but decreased ankle dorsiflexion with the knee extended (**b**)

can result in excessive lengthening [4]. This, in turn, can lead to the development of heel ulceration.

Contraindications

Gastrocsoleus lengthening may result in increased loading of the heel and is therefore contraindicated for plantar *heel* wounds. It may also be contraindicated in the setting of compromised soft tissues, as seen after extensive trauma or burn injuries. However, in these instances, a percutaneous Achilles lengthening may still be possible.

Active distal infection is not considered a contraindication for surgery. In fact, those wounds for which gastrocsoleus lengthening is indicated are often infected. In these instances, the surgeon has two options. First, the procedure can be staged, and lengthening pursued after local control of the ulcer is obtained. Alternatively, lengthening can be performed simultaneously with ulcer debridement. In this setting, the extremity is prepped and draped as described below.

Pearls and Pitfalls

Preoperative Evaluation

An assessment of the patient's general health status and medical comorbidities is essential. The history should be explored for diabetes, smoking, thromboembolism, social support systems, restrictions in the home living environment, and the ability to adhere to non-weight-bearing restrictions. The physical examination should include the Silfverskiold test, as well as evaluation of the limb alignment, both with and without weight-bearing. The neurovascular status must also be carefully assessed. Manual sensory testing with a 5.07 monofilament nylon wire can be used to assess protective sensation. Peripheral pulses should be manually palpated. If both the dorsalis pedis and posterior tibial pulses are diminished or non-palpable, then vascular testing or consultation with a vascular surgeon is indicated.

Radiographs of the foot and ankle should be obtained and, if possible, performed with the patient standing. These are helpful to assess alignment and as well to rule out ankle impingement or arthritis. The latter can mimic a soft tissue contracture and also manually block any correction afforded by a gastrocsoleus lengthening. Advanced imaging, usually in the form of magnetic resonance or nuclear studies, is performed as needed to assess for infection.

Surgical Prepping

As noted, a gastrocsoleus lengthening frequently performed in the setting of distal infections. In these instances, the foot is immediately isolated with an impermeable stockinette after the extremity has been prepped and draped. The proximal lengthening is then performed. Following a layered closure, the incision is protected with an occlusive dressing. Thereafter, the surgeon proceeds with distal ulcer debridement and other indicated procedures.

Avoiding Sural Nerve Injury

With either a Strayer or Hoke procedure, the sural nerve is at risk for transection. This may result in numbness or a painful neuroma. With a Strayer, the sural nerve is also at risk for stretch injury due overzealous retraction. The sural nerve travels in the midline of the posterior leg proximally and then courses laterally in the distal third of the leg. It exists the crural fascia in the region of the gastrocnemius musculotendinous junction and thus is particularly vulnerable to injury during a Strayer procedure. In one cadaver study, Pinney and colleagues found that in 57.5% of specimens, the nerve was still deep to the crural fascia at the level of a Strayer procedure [5]. Moreover, the nerve was directly applied to the gastrocnemius tendon in 12.5% of specimens and needed to be gently dissected off of the tendon. With a Hoke lengthening, the nerve is on average 7.9 mm from the lateral edge of the tendon, and as such extra care must be taken with the lateral hemisection [6].

Incomplete Correction

Incomplete correction of a contracture following a Strayer procedure is usually due to one of two factors. First, the surgeon may have failed to release the far lateral fibers of the tendon. Alternatively, the surgeon may have failed to identify a combined gastrocsoleus contracture. In the latter scenario, there are two options. One is to release the fascia of the soleus muscle and see if this affords further correction. The other is to proceed with a distal percutaneous Achilles lengthening.

Incomplete correction following a Hoke lengthening is usually due to inadequate release of central or peripheral fibers. In this setting, the surgeon should revisit each cut to make sure that adequate tendon has been resected.

Achilles Rupture

Inelasticity of the tendon fibers can lead to complete rupture of the Achilles when performing a Hoke lengthening. To avoid this, care should be taken not to extend past the midline when performing the hemisections. If a rupture does occur, the author's protocol is to treat this with observation, as the paratenon is still intact and the tendon can heal. To avoid over-lengthening in this situation, however, the ankle should not be allowed to dorsiflex past 0°–5° of dorsiflexion.

Approaches and Techniques

Gastrocnemius Recession (Strayer Procedure)

With a Strayer procedure, the patient can be positioned either prone or supine. This is dependent on surgeon preference and the nature of any other procedures being performed at the time of surgery. In the author's experience, supine positioning is usually adequate. With this, the extremity is allowed to externally rotate at the hip, facilitating access to the medial calf. A thigh tourniquet may be used but generally is not needed.

An 8–10 cm medial longitudinal incision is centered over the musculotendinous junction of the gastrocnemius muscle (Fig. 4.2). The inflection point at the distal aspect of the posterior calf musculature is a helpful landmark to guide incision placement. The subcutaneous tissues are then bluntly dissected. A communicating branch of the lesser saphenous vein is often encountered and is cauterized or gently retracted (Fig. 4.3).

The crural fascia is then incised in line with the skin incision, exposing the distal edge of the gastrocnemius muscle and the medial aspect of the gastrocnemius tendon (Fig. 4.4). The tendon is a broad, flat structure which will distally merge with the soleus tendon to form the Achilles tendon.

Next, the gastrocnemius tendon is carefully isolated. Doing so will protect the soleus muscle (deep) and the sural nerve (superficial). It is particularly helpful to dissect the epitenon layer off of the superficial surface of the tendon and then place a malleable retractor between this layer and the tendon (Fig. 4.5). This helps to ensure that the sural nerve is separated away from the tendon prior to transection.

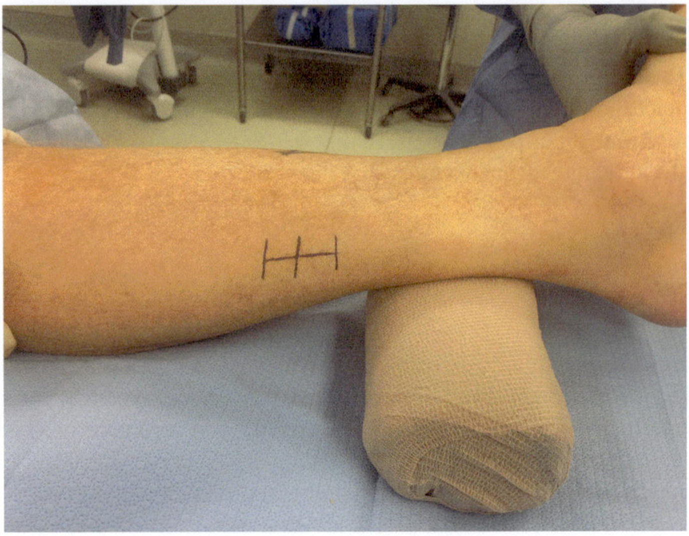

Fig. 4.2 Skin incision for the Strayer procedure

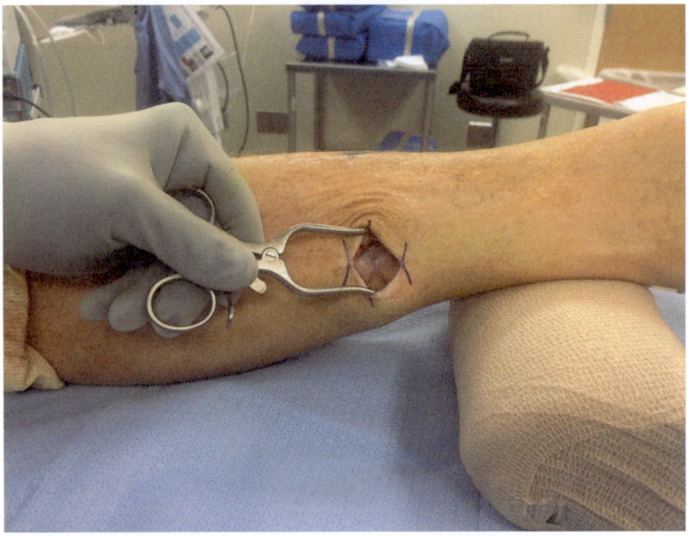

Fig. 4.3 A communicating branch of the lesser saphenous vein is encountered in the subcutaneous dissection

Once the tendon has been isolated, it is transversely transected from medial to lateral using Metzenbaum scissors (Fig. 4.6). Two Kocher clamps are utilized to deliver the central and far lateral portions of the tendon into the medial wound. While the tendon is transected, the ankle is gently dorsiflexed with the knee straight. This puts the tendon under tension and also allows the surgeon to

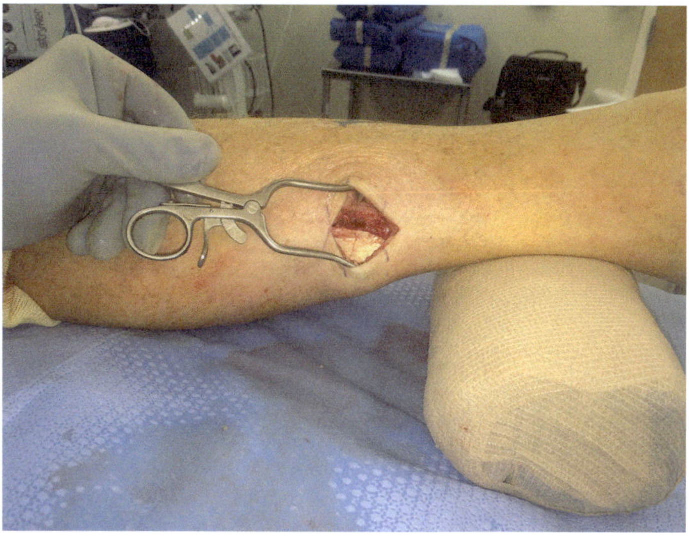

Fig. 4.4 Following division of the crural fascia, the medial edge of the gastrocnemius tendon is identified

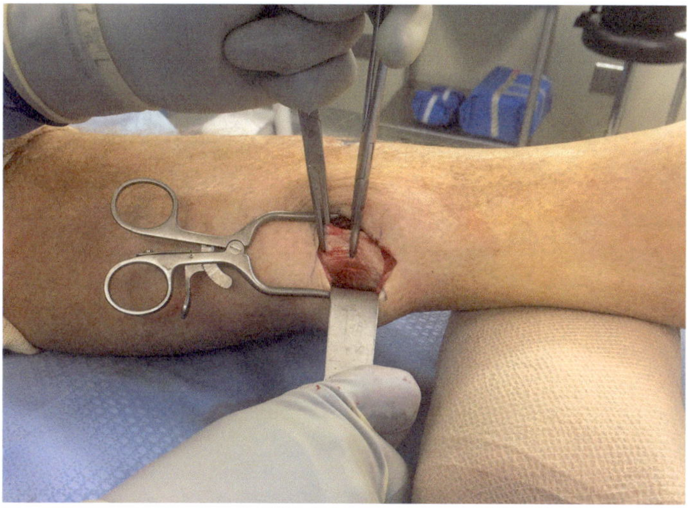

Fig. 4.5 A malleable retractor placed immediately superficial to the gastrocnemius tendon protects the adjacent sural nerve

know when the release is complete. With final release of the lateral tendon fibers, ankle dorsiflexion will suddenly improve, moving well past neutral. A gap in the tendon will be visible, as will the underlying soleal muscle fibers (Fig. 4.7). The latter often elongate as well due to their adherence to the adjacent gastrocnemius tendon.

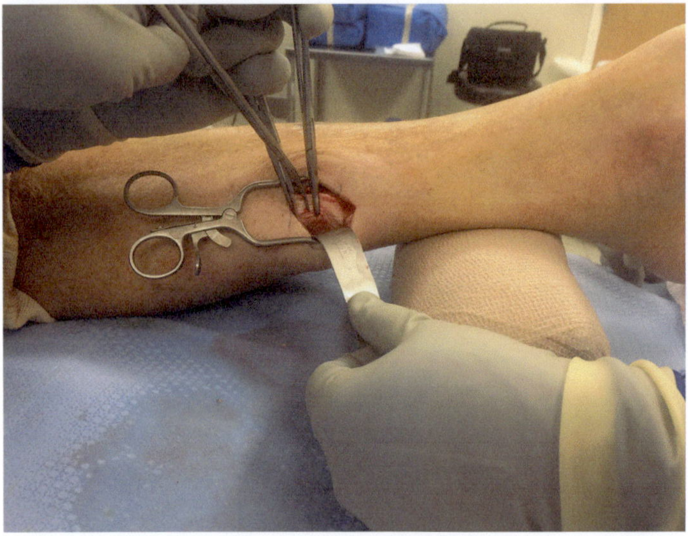

Fig. 4.6 The gastrocnemius tendon is transected with scissors

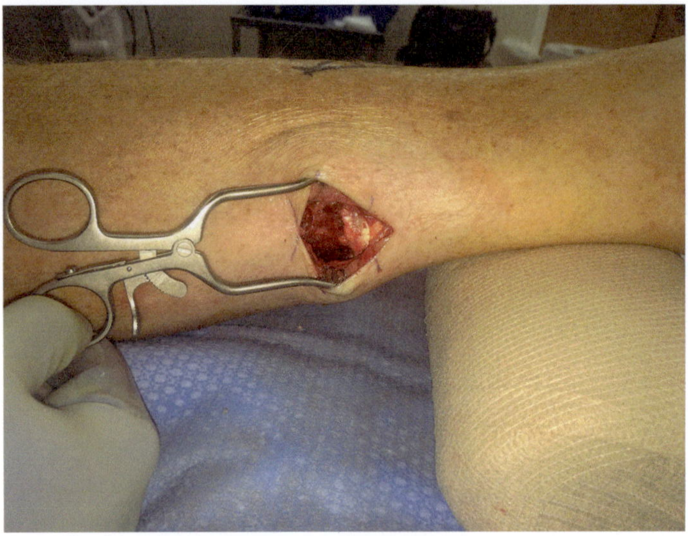

Fig. 4.7 With completion of the procedure, a gap is visible in the gastrocnemius tendon. The underlying soleus muscle fibers are also visualized

A careful layered closure is then performed (Fig. 4.8). The crural fascia may be closed with absorbable braided sutures. The subcutaneous layer is closed with 3–0 or 4–0 absorbable monofilament sutures and the skin closed with 3–0 nylon sutures. The extremity is immobilized with either a well-padded plaster splint or a pneumatic boot, depending on the anticipated weight-bearing status of the patient as well as the nature of other procedures performed.

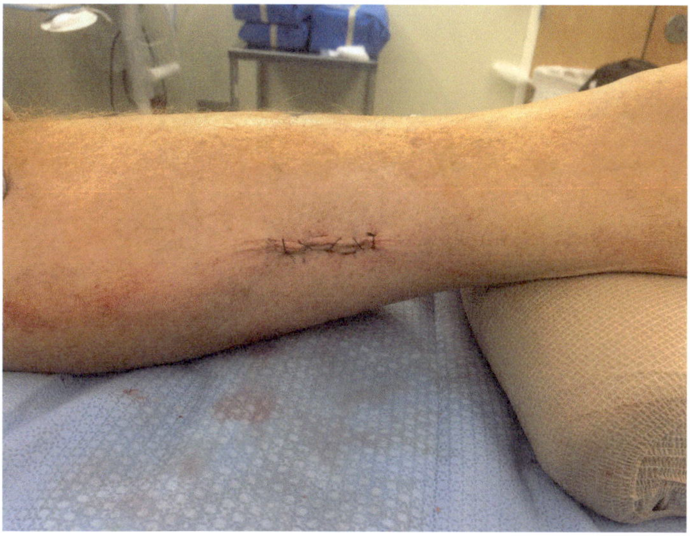

Fig. 4.8 Wound closure for the Strayer procedure

Triple Hemisection Achilles Lengthening

As with a Strayer procedure, the patient may be positioned supine or prone. Three percutaneous midline incisions are marked on the skin over the Achilles tendon (Fig. 4.9). These are separated by 2–3 cm and begin approximately 2 cm above the tendon insertion.

A #15 blade is inserted vertically through the distal incision and passed deep through the midline of the tendon. The scalpel is then rotated medially and turned perpendicular to the tendon. With the ankle gently dorsiflexed so that the tendon is under tension, the blade is brought back toward the skin, thus transecting the medial 50% of the tendon.

The middle incision is then percutaneously incised in a vertical fashion. The scalpel is again passed through the midline of the tendon, in line with the skin incision. This time, however, the blade is rotated *laterally* and brought back toward the skin to transect the lateral 50% of the tendon. The sural nerve is at risk with this step of the procedure, and care should be taken not to incise beyond the lateral tendon edge.

Finally, the most proximal incision is made. The scalpel is again inserted through the tendon and now again turned medial to release the medial tendon fibers. As with the prior tendon cuts, the ankle is continually dorsiflexed by an assistant.

With this, three alternating step cuts have been made in the tendon. Upon completion of the last cut the tendon typically elongates (Fig. 4.10). If it does not, pro-

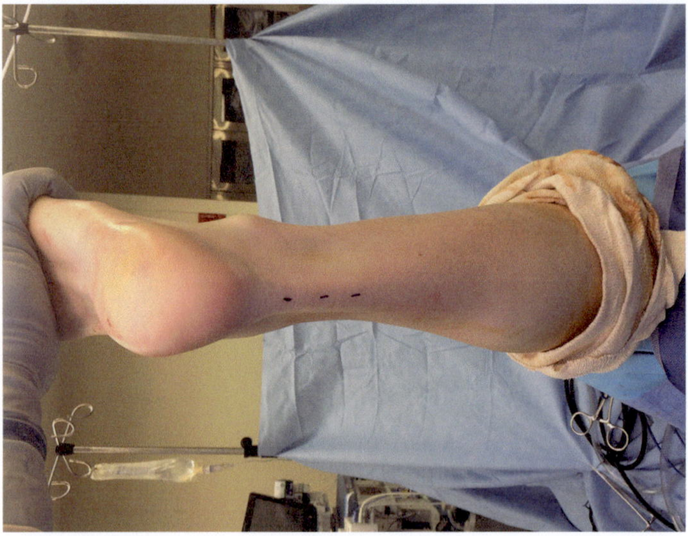

Fig. 4.9 Skin incisions for the Hoke procedure

Fig. 4.10 Illustration demonstrating elongation of the Achilles following a Hoke procedure

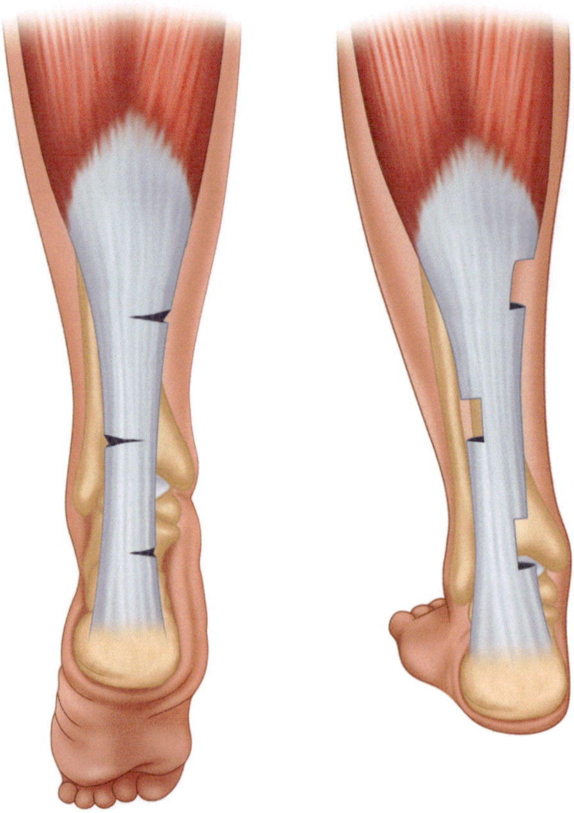

gressive dorsiflexion is applied. If the tendon does not release with this, the cuts are revisited to ensure that there are no intact peripheral fibers. If present, these should be released. If not, then the central portion of each cut can be slightly extended toward or beyond the midline to achieve lengthening.

The wounds are closed with nylon. As with the Strayer procedure, the extremity is immobilized with either a padded splint or a pneumatic boot.

Postoperative Protocol

Dressings and sutures are typically removed between 2 and 4 weeks postoperatively. As most patients with plantar wounds have diabetes, it is better to leave the sutures in for a longer period of time to minimize the risk of dehiscence. Following a Strayer procedure, heel weight-bearing is permitted as soon as possible, typically in a pneumatic boot or a postoperative shoe that offloads the plantar forefoot. With an Achilles lengthening, however, weight-bearing is typically restricted (either non-weight-bearing or partial weight-bearing) for 6 weeks in order to prevent tendon rupture. Nevertheless, active range-of-motion exercises are permitted at 2 weeks postoperatively.

Outcomes

There is fair clinical evidence to support the use of gastrocsoleus lengthening in neuropathic patients who have plantar forefoot ulcers that have not responded to nonoperative care [7, 8].

Mueller et al. reported the results of a prospective, randomized trial in which 64 patients with neuropathic plantar ulcers were treated with total contact casting alone or total contact casting combined with an Achilles lengthening [9]. All patients in the Achilles lengthening group healed, compared with only 88% of patients who were treated with casting alone. While this difference was not statistically significant, there was a significant difference in the ulcer recurrence rate (81% in the casting group compared with 38% of patients who underwent casting combined with Achilles lengthening).

Meanwhile, Laborde reported on 20 neuropathic plantar forefoot ulcers treated with a gastrocsoleus recession [10]. The procedure used was a Vulpius recession, in which the tendon release is v-shaped and slightly more distal than a Strayer. Patients with first metatarsal head ulcers also underwent Z-lengthening of the peroneus longus, while patients with ulcers under the fifth metatarsal head underwent fractional lengthening of the posterior tibial muscle. Ninety-five percent of ulcers healed at an average of 45 months. There were three recurrences, and these healed with repeat tendon lengthening.

Finally, Holstein and colleagues reviewed 68 patients with 75 neuropathic ulcers treated with an Achilles lengthening [4]. Ninety-one percent (68/75 feet) of patients healed at a median follow-up of 12 months. However, 10% of patients sustained an acute Achilles rupture. Further, transfer ulcers developed below the calcaneus in 47% of patients with complete anesthesia of the heel pad. Late heel ulceration occurred in another 14% of patients with ankle dorsiflexion >15°.

References

1. Firth GB, McMullan M, Chin T, Ma F, Selber P, Eizenberg N, Wolfe R, Graham HK. Lengthening of the gastrocnemius-soleus complex: an anatomical and biomechanical study in human cadavers. J Bone Joint Surg Am. 2013;95(16):1489–96.
2. Strayer LM Jr. Recession of the gastrocnemius; an operation to relieve spastic contracture of the calf muscles. J Bone Joint Surg Am. 1950;32-A(3):671–6.
3. Hoke M. An operation for the correction of extremely relaxed flat feet. J Bone Joint Surg Am. 1931;13:773–83.
4. Holstein P, Lohmann M, Bitsch M, Jørgensen B. Achilles tendon lengthening, the panacea for plantar forefoot ulceration? Diabetes Metab Res Rev. 2004;20(S1):S37–40.
5. Pinney SJ, Sangeorzan BJ, Hansen ST. Surgical anatomy of the gastrocnemius recession (Strayer procedure). Foot Ankle Int. 2004;25(4):247–50.
6. Salamon ML, Pinney SJ, Van Bergeyk A, Hazelwood S. Surgical anatomy and accuracy of percutaneous achilles tendon lengthening. Foot Ankle Int. 2006;27(6):411–3.
7. Lavery LA, Davis KE, Berriman SJ, Braun L, Nichols A, Kim PJ, Margolis D, Peters EJ, Attinger C. WHS guidelines update: diabetic foot ulcer treatment guidelines. Wound Repair Regen. 2016;24(1):112–26.
8. Tagoe MT, Reeves ND, Bowling FL. Is there still a place for Achilles tendon lengthening? Diabetes Metab Res Rev. 2016;32(Suppl 1):227–31.
9. Mueller MJ, Sinacore DR, Hastings MK, Strube MJ, Johnson JE. Effect of Achilles tendon lengthening on neuropathic plantar ulcers. A randomized clinical trial. J Bone Joint Surg Am. 2003;85-A(8):1436–45.
10. Laborde JM. Neuropathic plantar forefoot ulcers treated with tendon lengthenings. Foot Ankle Int. 2008;29(4):378–84.

Chapter 5
Operative Management of Pressure Injuries

Dennis P. Orgill

Background

Pressure injuries commonly occur in patients with neurologic impairment or in those who are frail and hospitalized for prolonged periods. Previously referred to as pressure ulcers or pressure sores, the term pressure injury is now used to refer to these conditions by the National Pressure Ulcer Advisory Panel [1]. Pressure injuries are theoretically preventable, although, practically, there are many pressure injuries in patients with comorbid diseases that may in fact not be preventable despite using the best available surfaces and nursing care [2]. In fact, many patients acquire pressure injuries near the end of life in which case comfort measures need to be considered in treatment algorithms. We recently reviewed pressure injury pathophysiology and treatment of pressure injuries [3].

The pathogenesis of pressure injuries relates to prolonged pressure and a skin injury that can be caused by direct pressure, shear forces, and/or moisture. Pressure injuries most commonly develop within the soft tissues that are between a support surface and a bone. Pressure within the tissues rises to a level greater than the pressure within capillaries, halting blood flow and making tissues ischemic. In patients that are neurologically intact, this causes pain and prompts movement to relieve pressure. This is well demonstrated in humans during sleep, naturally changing position several times throughout the night. We know from surgery that prolonged ischemia time can result in permanent necrosis. In the operating room, when performing surgery on an extremity, we let down tourniquets after about 2 h to allow for reperfusion of tissues. Ischemia can be prolonged with cooling which is used

Electronic Supplementary Material: The online version of this chapter (https://doi.org/10.1007/978-3-319-66990-8_5) contains supplementary material, which is available to authorized users.

D.P. Orgill, MD, PhD (✉)
Division of Plastic Surgery, Brigham and Women's Hospital Harvard Medical School, Boston, MA, USA
e-mail: dorgill@partners.org

D.P. Orgill (ed.), *Interventional Treatment of Wounds*,
https://doi.org/10.1007/978-3-319-66990-8_5

during cardiopulmonary bypass or in total circulatory arrest. Because of these observations, recommendations have been made to turn patients every 2 h; however, the evidence to support this recommendation, particularly when someone is on a well-designed support surface, is not direct.

Once a pressure injury occurs, it can be staged according to the NPUAP classification from Stage 1 (non-blanchable erythema in intact skin) to Stage 4, an ulceration down to the bone [4]. When a dry eschar is present and the depth cannot be easily recognized, these injuries are referred to as "unstageable pressure injury" (Fig. 5.1). The vast majority of pressure injuries that we see in our Wound Care Center are those that occur in patients with neurological injury such as spinal cord injuries, following stroke, or with debilitating neurological diseases such as multiple sclerosis. There is a smaller group of patients that have been critically ill and are neurologically intact that have the capacity to regain substantial movement. We find that many of these patients have a great capacity to heal these wounds once they have recovered from the initial medical conditions and are able to freely ambulate.

Initial Assessment

A large number of patients with Stage 3 and Stage 4 injuries will not completely heal without a surgical intervention(s). A comprehensive initial evaluation of patients with pressure sores is required to determine if patients are operative candidates. It is very important to understand why each patient develops a pressure injury in the first place. Unless these factors are resolved, recurrence rates are high. We have seen several patients that come in with multiple pressure injuries. These are a particularly challenging as they provide substantial evidence that the patient has been unable to effectively offload areas of pressure. Without correcting this preoperatively, patients will develop pressure sores after the operation, either in similar places or in other anatomic areas. Also, many patients are unable to tolerate being in the prone position, and we off-load the surgical site for 6 weeks following a closure operation. Operating on more than one pressure sore can make positioning very challenging. For patients that are unable to offload their ulcerations, closure with surgery can be a futile procedure as recurrences are almost guaranteed. In contrast, patients that are able to ambulate, walking is an ideal position for offloading.

Nutrition is a critical factor to allow healing. Many patients with pressure injuries are nutritionally depleted and will not heal wounds which can become larger and infected over time. Part of this is due to metabolic losses due to the large wounds. Operating on a patient with a poor nutritional status places them at a very high risk for complications. If there is no direct measurement of nutrition but a history of weight loss or loss of muscle mass, it should be concerning. When there is a question, we obtain serum levels of albumin and prealbumin. A high-protein diet can be helpful in correcting nutritional deficits (1.25–1.5 g/kg/day).

Other medical issues must be dealt with as well. Common conditions that we see in patients with pressure injuries include diabetes mellitus, peripheral vascular

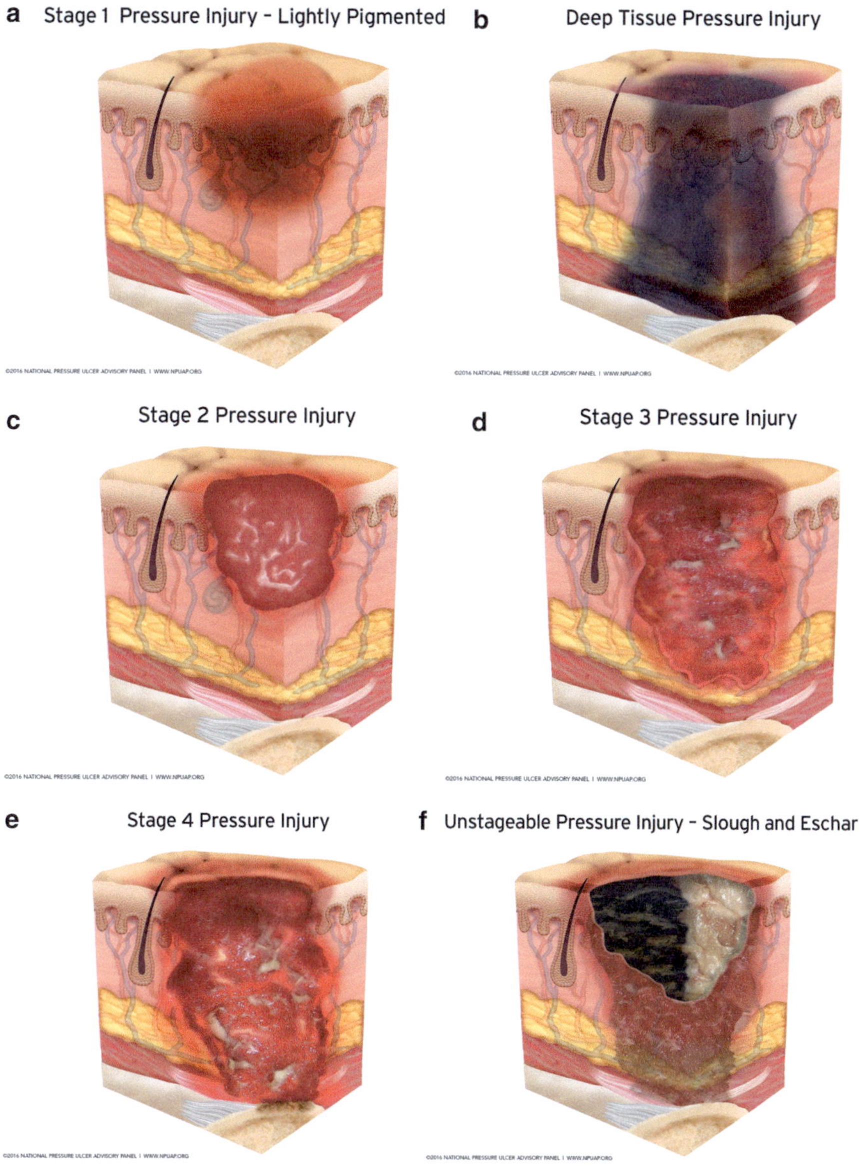

Fig. 5.1 (**a**–**d**) Stage 1–4 pressure injury. (**e**) Deep tissue pressure injury. (**f**) Unstageable pressure injury with slough and eschar (Adapted from the Pressure Injury Staging Illustrations in National Pressure Ulcer Advisory Panel [1]. National Pressure Ulcer Advisory Panel, European Pressure Ulcer Advisory Panel and Pan Pacific Pressure Injury Alliance [4]. Prevention and Treatment of Pressure Ulcers: Quick Reference Guide. Emily Haesler (Ed.). Cambridge Media: Osborne Park, Western Australia; 2014. Retrieved January 18, 2017, from http://www.npuap.org/resources/educational-and-clinical-resources/pressure-injury-staging-illustrations/)

disease, coronary artery disease, end-stage renal disease, and pulmonary dysfunction. Smoking has deleterious effects on wound healing, and we require patients having elective surgery to stop smoking and be off all nicotine products for 1 month prior to surgery. Optimization of these conditions is critical before pursuing surgery.

Urgent Debridement

Patients can develop abscesses and become septic from pressure injuries which often require emergent debridement in the operating room. In some cases, these can progress to necrotizing fasciitis or Fournier's gangrene. These latter conditions require an aggressive approach with often multiple trips to the operating room combined with broad spectrum antibiotics. The purpose of these procedures is to drain purulent fluid collections and remove devitalized tissue in order to stabilize patients. The vast majority of patients that we see present with chronic indolent pressure sores. Many of these patients can have serial debridement as outpatients while preparing the patient for definitive surgery.

Intraoperative Debridement

For pressure ulcerations that are grossly infected, they need to be drained and debrided until the infectious process is controlled. We often do this with the electrocautery to minimize bleeding. These patients are often hyperemic, and debridement needs to be taken with caution to avoid excessive bleeding.

Many patients benefit through the use of Negative-pressure wound therapy (NPWT) devices. These should be used with caution in an infected field and, if used, should be changed frequently. We will generally use traditional dressings until the wound is reasonably clean. In general, we like to shrink down the wound to a small sinus tract before attempting flap closure and to do these closures on an elective basis. This allows the patient to prepare for the surgery and make sure that the appropriate offloading and nutritional issues are resolved.

After applying a NPWT or other device for several weeks, the wound will often shrink down significantly (Fig. 5.2). This allows us to do a relatively small debridement and flap closure in these complex patients. For our closure procedures, we prefer to do a complete excision of the wound. This can be facilitated by painting the cavity with a dye such as methylene blue and taking about 5 mm of normal tissue around the entire cavity (Figs. 5.3 and 5.4). We then shave down any exposed bone with an osteotome removing all devitalized or grossly infected bone. We obtain deep bone cultures of visually normal bone using clean instruments and send these for microbiology to determine the type and length of antibiotic coverage necessary. We then copiously irrigate the wound using a gravity system often using a

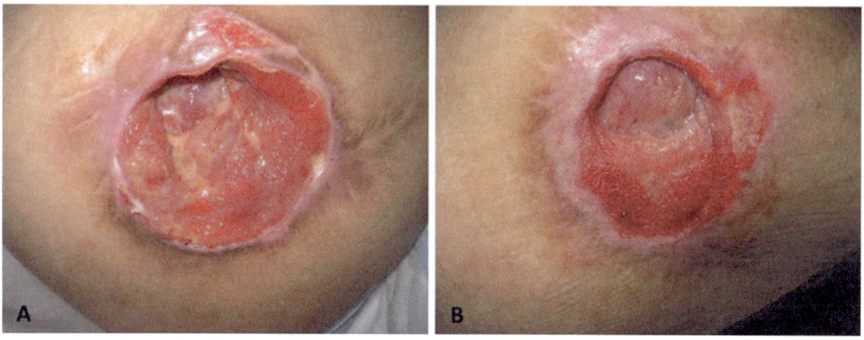

Fig. 5.2 Typical results of pressure injuries treated with NPWT. (**a**) Initial ischial pressure injury. (**b**) After 2 months of treatment, now ready for closure. Note the contraction of the wound, proliferation of granulation tissue, and removal of slough (Reproduced from Ricci et al. [3]. Copyright 2017 by Wolters Kluwer Health, Inc)

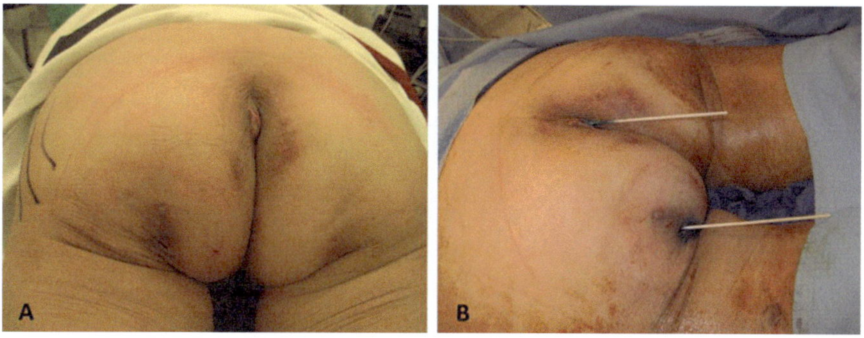

Fig. 5.3 (**a**) Pre-op photo of patient with sacral and ischial pressure injuries. (**b**) Wounds marked with *methylene blue* on cotton swaps to identify entire bursa (Reproduced from Ricci et al. [3]. Copyright 2017 by Wolters Kluwer Health, Inc)

combination of normal saline and antibiotic irrigation. Previously we have used a pulse irrigation system but now prefer to use the gravity system (Video 5.1).

Specific Anatomic Areas Flap Options

In this section, we will focus on Stage 3 and Stage 4 pressure injuries. We prefer to optimize the patient's medical condition and allow the wound to shrink down as much as possible prior to elective flap closure. By shrinking the wounds to small sinus tracts, it makes the flap design simpler. When considering various flap options, the surgeon always needs to think ahead and be prepared for another flap should a recurrence occur. In the literature, it suggests that recurrence rates around 50% are common. Therefore, the ability to re-rotate or readvance when possible should be

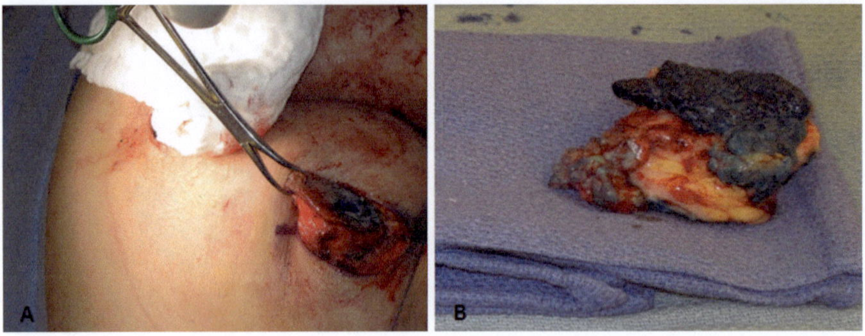

Fig. 5.4 (**a**) Intraoperative and (**b**) postoperative photos of complete en bloc resection of pressure injury bursa that is identified with *methylene blue* dye (Reproduced from Ricci et al. [3]. Copyright 2017 by Wolters Kluwer Health, Inc)

Table 5.1 Commonly used flaps for pressure injuries

Location of pressure injury	Flap
Sacrum	V to Y flap, rotation flap, gluteal perforator flap
Ischium	Posterior thigh flap, gluteal rotation flap
Trochanter	Tensor fascia Lata flap
Ankle	Local transposition flaps or perforator flaps
Heel	Local flaps, medial plantar flap
Scalp	Local flaps

considered. Flaps should take tissue from areas where there is excess tissue and transpose it to the wound avoiding tension. There are various flaps that are commonly used for specific anatomic locations which are listed in Table 5.1.

Sacral Wound Closure

Sacral pressure injuries are most common in elderly debilitated patients that spend most of their time in bed. Often they have some type of neurological impairment. During the closure operation, we first totally excise the wound, shave down the bone, and obtain deep bone biopsies for culture as described above. There are a wide range of flaps that have been successfully described for the closure of sacral wounds. For small to moderate sized wounds, we prefer V to Y flaps that are made fairly large to allow for readvancement should the wound recur. We excise through the skin and cut down and divide the fascia over the gluteus maximus muscle. This allows a very nice mobilization of the flap that can move medially. For additional mobilization, the flap can be dissected further to base this on a single large perforator through the gluteus maximus muscle that tracks to the superior gluteal system. The pedicle can be dissected through the gluteal muscles for additional length, but this generally is not necessary. We prefer to not connect the V incision to the wound

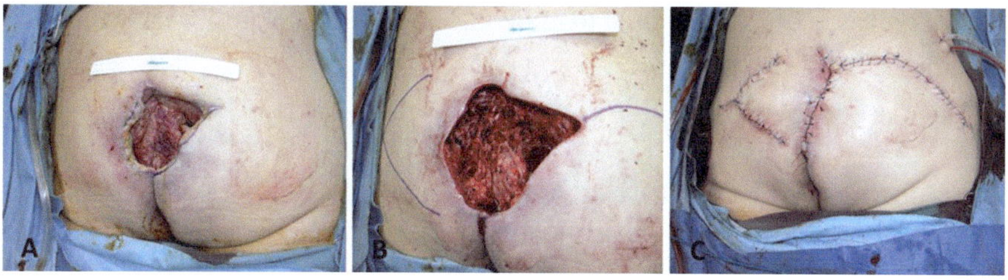

Fig. 5.5 (**a**) Initial sacral pressure injury, (**b**) after debridement, and (**c**) closure utilizing a fasciocutaneous gluteal V-Y advancement on the left side and a gluteal advancement rotation on the right side (Reproduced from Ricci et al. [3]. Copyright 2017 by Wolters Kluwer Health, Inc)

and have described a modified V to Y approach for these wounds [5]. This allows for closure without having any t-junctions to heal. Closure is accomplished by suturing the tissues in layers. We do the final layer with a permanent suture such as polypropylene which we leave in for about 6 weeks. When a closure is close to the anus, we will use a dissolvable suture. These flaps generally leave little dead space, and we often utilize one small suction drain that we usually remove 2 days following closure.

A transposition flap, based on a single gluteus maximus perforator, is also a nice option for closure and allows for transfer of tissue on the lateral aspect of the buttock to the central aspect of the buttock. These can be based on either the superior or inferior gluteal system. These flaps must be dissected with care, and postoperative positioning is critical to not avoid compression of the pedicle.

Another common option is the use of large rotation flaps. These generally utilize most of the buttock skin and can be either superiorly or inferiorly based. They have the advantage that they are easy to readvance should a recurrence occur. The disadvantage of these flaps is that they create a large dead space that require drains to be in place for several days following the operation and makes the complication of a seroma more apt to occur. Keeping patients off their back in the postoperative period for 6 weeks is important to reduce the risk of recurrences.

Ischial Wound Closure

We most commonly see these injuries in paraplegic's that are wheelchair bound. Because of the lack of sensation combined with the inability to move places them at high risk for these injuries. Making sure they have adequate padding and a proper wheelchair prior to doing an operation is essential. For many ischial pressures injuries, there is minimal skin deficit and with care, the wound can be debrided through a fairly small wound. In this case, we can cover the bone with the gluteus maximus muscle and simply close the skin. In cases where skin is required, we will often use posterior thigh flaps from below. These can be designed as V to Y advancement flaps, transposition flaps, or rotation flaps (Fig. 5.5). Large gluteal rotation flaps, superiorly based can also be used to close these deficits, similar to what is describe for sacral pressure injuries.

Trochanteric Wound Closure

These injuries are most common in bedridden patients and in spinal cord injury patients where excessive pressure is placed over the hip. Occasionally, we will see bilateral trochanteric injuries that make treatment challenging because of positioning. Similar to sacral and trochanteric injuries, these need initial wound care and debridement followed in conjunction with patient preparation. The most common flap for these is based on the tensor fascia lata although other flaps including the anterolateral thigh flap and a variety of perforator flaps can be designed.

Scalp Pressure Injuries

Scalp injuries most commonly occur on the posterior scalp in patients that have been lying in bed for a prolonged period, often in an ICU setting. Once they recover from their underlying injury, these ulcerations typically heal. When they don't heal, common reconstructive options include skin grafts, scalp rotation flaps, and trapezius myocutaneous flaps. Trapezius flaps can often reach the occiput.

Lower Extremity Pressure Injuries

We frequently see lower extremity pressure ulcerations over the knee, ankle, and heel. Very often these are associated with an underlying vascular disease. It is important to do a careful exam and additional diagnostic studies if palpable pulses are not present. There are many flaps that can be designed for each of these areas, often based on specific perforators (Fig. 5.6). Occasionally free tissue transfer can be used for limb salvage. In debilitated patients, amputation can often be the best option.

Postoperative Care

Patients particularly with spinal cord injuries tend to heal slowly. We try to design a protocol to completely offload the flap for 6 weeks following surgery. We use closed suction drains that are placed into the wound for several days and then removed.

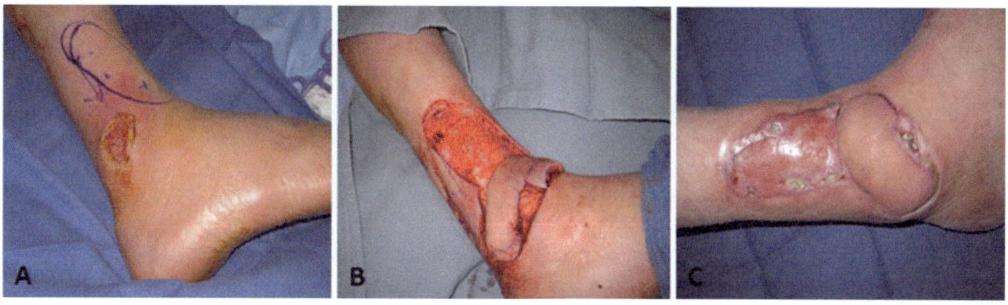

Fig. 5.6 (**a**) Pressure injury on the lateral malleolus with perforator-based propeller flap marked adjacent and (**b**) closure of wound by rotation of flap and skin grafting of the donor site to avoid undue tension on the closure. (**c**) Several weeks postoperatively (Reproduced from Ricci et al. [3]. Copyright 2017 by Wolters Kluwer Health, Inc)

Sutures stay in until the patient returns in 6 weeks for follow-up. We try not to see the patients, unless there is a problem, before 6 weeks to avoid transport to our clinic where they are at risk for wound disruption. We use digital photography as a communication tool for patients that live far away.

Recurrence

We believe that with proper selection and preoperative treatment and counseling, we can reduce the rates of recurrence substantially. However, particularly in the neurologically impaired patients, even with the best efforts, recurrence is sometimes unavoidable. We try not to do multiple operations in sequence. For recurrences early on, we have been able to get many of these to heal with dressing changes alone, often using a NPWT device and a renewed effort at offloading. For those that occur months or years after surgery, repeat surgery is often required.

Conclusions

Surgery to treat pressure injuries is one of the most challenging procedures that plastic surgeons can perform, due to the high rate of recurrence. An adequate preoperative assessment and counseling are critical to the long-term success of these operations. Nevertheless, with careful planning, these operations can be of tremendous benefit to these patients.

References

1. National Pressure Ulcer Advisory Panel. Available at http://www.npuap.org
2. Public Policy Committee and the Wound Subcommittee. Avoidable versus unavoidable pressure ulcers. Wound ostomy and continence nurses society. 2009. Available via http://c.ymcdn.com/sites/www.wocn.org/resource/resmgr/Publications/PS_Avoidable_vs_Unavoidable_.pdf. Accessed 1/7/2017.
3. Ricci JA, Bayer LR, Orgill DP. Evidence-based medicine: the evaluation and treatment of pressure injuries. Plast Reconstr Surg. 2017;139(1):275e–86e.
4. NPUAP Pressure Injury Stages. Available at http://www.npuap.org/resources/educational-and-clinical-resources/npuap-pressure-injury-stages/. Accessed 1/7/2017.
5. Hartzell TL, Orgill BD, Chan R, Mathy JA, Orgill DP. VY modification of a bipedicle perforator flap. Plast Reconstr Surg. 2009;124(1):167–70.

Chapter 6
Forefoot Operations

Paul J. Kim

Introduction

The foot is at particularly high risk for injury due to its remote anatomical location and functional requirements. Specifically, wounds can occur for a variety of reasons including acute or repetitive trauma (including burns) or as a direct consequence of a disease such as diabetes mellitus or autoimmune processes (e.g., rheumatoid arthritis) or as a consequence of a treatment for another condition (e.g., radiation, elective or nonelective surgery). Further, repetitive minor trauma can lead to the development and chronicity of a wound due to the forces encountered between the shoe and the foot or the foot and the ground. The forefoot is often the first location where wounds manifest in cases of systemic diseases. This is because of its remote location as well as the decreased soft tissue density covering the bony architecture in this area. The term "wound" and "ulcer" is often used interchangeably. However, more precisely a "wound" should be reserved to describe a soft tissue defect that is more acute, while an "ulcer" denotes a degree of chronicity.

Coverage or closure of a wound is not the only goal of surgical correction in the forefoot. Biomechanical abnormalities are often the underlying reason for development and chronicity of ulcers in the forefoot especially in the environment of underlying systemic diseases [1]. Wound prevention, targeted procedure selection, long-term durability at the wound site, and avoidance of transfer ulcers are all equally important. The surgical treatment of burns, radiation injury, and tumor

Electronic Supplementary Material: The online version of this chapter (https://doi.org/10.1007/978-3-319-66990-8_6) contains supplementary material, which is available to authorized users.

P.J. Kim, DPM, MS (✉)
Georgetown University School of Medicine, Washington, DC 20007, USA

Division of Wound Healing and Hyperbaric Medicine, Department of Plastic Surgery, MedStar Georgetown University Hospital, Bles 1st Floor, 3800 Reservoir Road NW, Washington, DC 20007, USA
e-mail: paul.j.kim@gunet.georgetown.edu

D.P. Orgill (ed.), *Interventional Treatment of Wounds*,
https://doi.org/10.1007/978-3-319-66990-8_6

resection will not be discussed in detail in this chapter. Each of these conditions has their own unique challenges and is out of the scope of this chapter. The focus of this chapter is on biomechanical forefoot surgery related to the chronic or nonhealing wound.

Successful outcome of biomechanical surgery cannot be determined in the operating room but can only be determined when the patient returns to weight bearing and ambulation. This is because the surgical correction addresses the *dynamic* processes during weight bearing and ambulation, while the immediate post-correction examination of the foot in the operating room is a *static* assessment. Maintaining or improving function is the primary goal of surgical correction [2]. This involves selecting the most appropriate procedure and identifying the most appropriate patient. Most wounds will heal with good conservative wound care including the use of dressings, topical ointments, and offloading/immobilization. However, for chronic wounds, surgical correction may be preferred or required to expedite healing and/or address the underlying biomechanical fault.

The fundamentals of patient care apply to forefoot operations including a thorough medical and wound history, a physical examine with a focus on the lower extremity, and an understanding of the patient's expectations for recovery (Table 6.1). The medical history will provide important information as to the healing capacity of the patient including any confounding conditions such as metabolic disorders, diabetes mellitus, renal disease, and cardiac disease. These preexisting conditions will influence procedure selection by limiting the kind of procedure selected based on the patient's capacity to heal and the course of their underlying diseases. A wound is often associated with these underlying conditions, and it should be thought of as one of the manifestations of the underlying disease. For example, a patient with diabetes mellitus may also have peripheral neuropathy and peripheral vascular disease. In this environment, an acute wound can progress to a chronic nonhealing ulcer. Underlying medical problems are important determinants in surgical selection which will be discussed in greater detail in the following paragraphs.

The patient's expectations should also be carefully considered. The patient is typically concerned about esthetic and functional outcomes of surgery. The surgeon should focus the discussion on achieving realistic functional goals. It is important to manage these expectations by having a frank discussion with the patient that biomechanical surgical correction of the forefoot is necessary to heal the ulcer or to prevent one from occurring. The patient may not understand the relationship between the ulcer and the planned biomechanical surgical procedure or understand the nuances of the deformity and the probability of ulcer occurrence. Thus, more time should be spent describing the pathological processes rather than the technical aspects of the surgical technique. Postoperative recovery time including the time needed for nonweight bearing and limited weight bearing should be clearly described. The likelihood of postoperative complications including infection and dehiscence, which occur at higher rates in the compromised population, should also be discussed [3]. Further, the fact that the long-term outcomes of biomechanical surgery are not always predictable and that additional surgeries may be required

Table 6.1 Critical preoperative planning

	Considerations	Comments
Medical history	Comorbidities and medications can contribute to the development and/or chronicity of a wound	Regardless of the treatment rendered, the wound may not heal if the underlying systemic disease is not addressed. An example of this is a patient with an autoimmune disease such as rheumatoid arthritis. In this case both the disease itself as well as medications used for its treatment may inhibit or delay postoperative healing. Communication with a rheumatologist to align good disease management with the surgical plan is critical
Wound history	Important questions need to be answered including why did the wound start, when did it start, what treatments have already been employed? Includes wound trajectory (through wound size and quality documentation) to determine whether healing can occur without surgical intervention	The lack of wound healing progress should trigger a deeper examination. Perhaps there is an infection or biofilm. Is there adequate perfusion to the wound site? Are biomechanics the key contributor? Is there a combination of factors that need to be addressed? Most often a combination of factors lead to wound chronicity
Physical examination	A thorough vascular, neurological, dermatological, and musculoskeletal exam with a focus on identifying biomechanical abnormalities is required The apex of the deformity must be identified and addressed	This examination should be performed with each visit and at the time of surgery. These aspects may change over time, especially with changes in underlying medical conditions and medications
Patient's goals and expectations	A quick surgical recovery and return to daily activities Maintain or improve the appearance of their foot. Maintain or improve their quality of life	A frank discussion is needed regarding what the surgery involves and the recovery time needed including periods of nonweight bearing and partial weight bearing The patient may have unrealistic expectations for the outcomes of surgery. Function should be the focus of the discussion with a clear description of the appearance of the foot after healing has occurred Despite good surgical planning and strict adherence to the treatment course, the outcome is not always predictable The patient should understand that there may be a need for accommodative devices including custom-molded inserts, braces, and shoes after healing has occurred

(continued)

Table 6.1 (continued)

	Considerations	Comments
Surgeon's goals and expectations	The goal of surgical intervention is to maintain or improve function	Surgical intervention may not a be a one-time event. A staged approach may be necessary and revision surgery may be required in the future Complications can occur, especially with patients with underlying comorbidities. These should be expected and addressed promptly

should be carefully explained to the patient. This is because surgical procedures are inexact in correcting the underlying biomechanical fault, and the physiology and the functional demands of the patient change over time. The patient may require life-long use of a modified shoe, custom-molded insert, ankle-foot orthoses, brace and the use of assistive devices (cane, crutches, walker, wheelchair). The management of the patient's expectations is as important as the surgical procedure itself.

Anatomy and Biomechanics

A critical piece of a focused lower extremity physical examination includes the assessment for perfusion. The ulcer may be the result of compromised perfusion due to an underlying disease process or loss of local vasculature. Hence, understanding the etiology is important. Further, the degree of perfusion may dictate the surgical procedure selected and the ultimate outcome. The foot is fed by three large arteries: anterior tibial (AT), posterior tibial (PT), and peroneal. All three arteries feed different angiosomes of the forefoot. An angiosome is a block of tissue fed by a named source artery [4]. The AT artery becomes the dorsalis pedis (DP) artery as it crosses the ankle and have multiple distal branches and feeds the dorsal aspect of the forefoot. The PT artery has two main branches, medial and lateral, which feeds the plantar forefoot. The DP and PT have arterial to arterial connections in the forefoot that is primarily located at the proximal interspaces of the metatarsals. This redundant blood supply in the forefoot is an important anatomical consideration if one of the main arteries are compromised. The peroneal artery feeds the lateral aspect of the forefoot.

The palpation of the main arteries is the critical first level of assessment for perfusion. These arteries should be further assessed utilizing an audible handheld Doppler. Peripheral arterial disease can progress from a triphasic to biphasic to monophasic and finally to no signal. More advanced noninvasive modalities including ankle-brachial index/toe-brachial index, transcutaneous oximetry, skin perfusion pressures, and noninvasive angiography should be considered if there is any suspicion of compromise [5]. Contrast angiography may be necessary to determine the degree of vascular compromise, for the purposes of intervention, or for surgical planning for open bypass. It is important when contrast angiography is utilized that the forefoot is also imaged in multiple planes. Ultimately, perfusion must be adequate enough to heal soft tissue and/or bone. Thus, identifying the level of perfusion as well as maximizing perfusion to the affected area is critically important in surgical planning of the forefoot.

The musculoskeletal anatomy of the foot is directly related to function (Table 6.2). The forefoot is defined as the anatomical structures distal to the metatarsal cuneiform joint (Lisfranc's joint). The toes consist of small long bones with articulations. The hallux has one interphalangeal joint, while toes 2–5 typically have 2 interphalangeal joints. The toes articulate with its corresponding metatarsals 1–5. Although sesamoids can occur anywhere in the foot, the tibial and fibular sesamoids under the first metatarsal head are consistently present and are responsible for changing the axis to enhance the mechanical advantage of flexor hallucis longus. The 1st metatarsal articulates with the medial cuneiform, the 2nd metatarsal with the middle cuneiform, the 3rd metatarsal with the lateral cuneiform, and the 4th and 5th metatarsal with the cuboid. Extrinsic (those that originate from the lower leg) and intrinsic (those that originate within the foot) muscles attach through tendons to the distal foot. The opposing muscles of flexors/extensors, invertors/evertors, and adductors/abductors work in concert to align the foot dynamically during ambulation for efficient shock absorption and propulsion. The skeletal architecture is bound by capsules and ligaments to provide structural rigidity while allowing a small degree of flexibility. Each joint has a unique articular configuration with an axis of rotation. Veins and lymphatics are also important in the foot with the importance of the arterial network discussed above.

The soft tissue envelope of the foot is specially designed to be durable. The skin on the dorsal aspect of the foot is different than the plantar aspect of the foot. The glabrous junction delineates the plantar and dorsal skin. The plantar skin consists of a thicker dermis with a more robust subcutaneous layer which envelops the foot in a moccasin distribution allowing for protection anteriorly/posteriorly and medially/laterally to a small degree. The epidermis and dermis of the plantar foot resist penetration, while the subcutaneous layer disperses shock [6].

The foot can be segmentally divided into sagittal plane columns which function as discrete collective units. The medial column includes the hallux, 1st metatarsal, and cuneiform, the central column consists of metatarsals 2 and 3 and their corresponding middle and lateral cuneiforms, and the lateral column includes the metatarsals 4 and 5 and the cuboid. This columnar division is both anatomical and functional. The medial and lateral columns are considered to have a greater degree of motion in the sagittal and frontal plane than the central column which has relatively less available excursion. This distinction becomes important for surgical procedure selection which will be further discussed in the following paragraphs. The anatomical relationship of the columns can be seen globally in the foot type. Pes planus refers (colloquially described as "flatfeet") to a foot type with a depressed or collapsed medial column, to a lesser degree the lateral column, which can be rigid or nonrigid and may have a valgus (everted) frontal plane rotation. The pes cavus foot type (colloquially described as "high-arched feet") refers to when the medial column, to a lesser degree the lateral column, is elevated which is generally rigid

Table 6.2 Musculoskeletal anatomy and function

	Anatomy	Function
Phalanges (digits)	Long bones with two interphalangeal joints with the exception of the hallux which has one interphalangeal joint Contains both intrinsic and extrinsic muscle tendon insertions	Primarily a sagittal plane range of motion The digits are important for balance and as well serving as a lever arm during propulsion The hallux is a critical digit for forefoot function
Metatarsals	Long bones that articulate with the digits distally and the cuneiforms or cuboid proximally The tibial and fibular sesamoid is located under the first metatarsal head. Other accessory bones can be present in other locations throughout the foot The intrinsic muscle tendon insertions are located about the metatarsal heads around the metatarsal phalangeal joint complexes. Direct extrinsic muscle tendon insertions to the 1st and 5th metatarsal bases	Primarily a sagittal plane range of motion with the 1st and 5th metatarsal with a smaller degree of frontal plane range of motion Significant forces are imparted through the metatarsals during the weight-bearing portion of the gait cycle This includes during the midstance phase of gait and especially during propulsion Pressure is isolated across the metatarsal heads (and to a lesser degree the digits) with heal lift The parabola of the metatarsals provides even pressure distribution
Cuneiforms	Three wedge-shaped bones that articulate with its corresponding metatarsals. Medial cuneiform with the 1st metatarsal, the middle cuneiform with the 2nd metatarsal, and the lateral cuneiform with the 3rd metatarsal Multiple ligamentous attachments exist across the Lisfranc's joint as well as direct tendon insertions from the anterior and posterior tibial muscles	The relative range of motion of the cuneiforms are limited Provides stability of the forefoot on the midfoot especially during propulsion Maintains the integrity of the medial column
Cuboid	A cube-shaped bone that articulates with the 4th and 5th metatarsals Has no direct tendon insertions; however, the peroneus longus traverses in a groove on the plantar aspect	Similar in function to the cuneiforms with less range of motion Maintains the integrity of the lateral column
Medial column	Includes the hallux, 1st metatarsal and medial cuneiform	Functional units that work collectively for maintenance of the medial arch during weight bearing, shock absorption during midstance, and stability during propulsion Has the greatest degree of axis of rotation as compared with the other columns

(continued)

Table 6.2 (continued)

	Anatomy	Function
Central column	Includes the 2nd and 3rd toes, 2nd and 3rd metatarsals, and middle and lateral cuneiforms	Functional units that work collectively for maintenance of stability with weight bearing Has the most limited degree of axis of rotation as compared with the other columns
Lateral ray column	Includes the 4th and 5th toes, 4th and 5th metatarsals, and the cuboid	Functional units that work collectively for maintenance of the lateral arch during weight bearing, shock absorption during midstance, and stability during propulsion Has the 2nd greatest degree of axis of rotation as compared with the other columns

and may have a varus (inverted) frontal plane rotation. Further segmentation of the columns is called rays which include the digit with its adjoining metatarsals. Beyond the sagittal plane columns, the foot can be further segmented into frontal plane segments: forefoot, midfoot, and hindfoot. For the purposes of this chapter, the forefoot has already been defined. However, it is important to recognize that the forefoot, midfoot, and hindfoot are functionally interdependent. Thus, the forefoot should not be viewed in insolation; the foot should be examined globally with the knowledge that the surgical correction will affect all segments of the foot.

The anatomy of the forefoot reflects the biomechanical requirements for efficient ambulation. This includes the ability to stand and balance in a stationary position and propel the body forward during ambulation. The foot is best described as both a flexible adaptor and a rigid lever which reflect the demands during the gait cycle. There are two phases of the gait cycle, swing and stance. The swing phase involves advancing one of the lower extremities forward through the air with each step, while the contralateral limb is in a fixed, stationary position. The extensor muscles below the knee contract to clear the forefoot from the ground by dorsiflexing the toes at the metatarsophalangeal joint and the foot at the ankle joint. The stance phase of the gait cycle begins with heel strike during which the heel impacts the ground. Midstance occurs when the entirety of the foot is in contact with the ground, and during this period the foot functions as shock absorber. Heel lift ends the stance phase of gait and begins the propulsive phase with active plantarflexion of the toes at the metatarsophalangeal joint and the contraction of the extrinsic and intrinsic plantarflexory muscles against the ground. The foot functions as a rigid lever for propulsion. During this period, the pressure is distributed focally across the balls of the foot (across the metatarsal heads) and to a lesser degree the toes with the heel off the surface of the ground. The body is propelled forward, and the gait cycle repeats itself. The physical examination should include evaluation of the lower extremity and any associated pathologies while standing and walking (Table 6.3).

Table 6.3 Deformity and examination

Deformity	Description	Examination	Wound location
Pes planus	Collapse of the medial arch	Can be either rigid or nonrigid with range of motion of the medial column Can affect the relative position and range of motion of the bones in the forefoot causing other structural conditions included in this table	In the rigid condition under the medial column and lateral columns Other wound locations related to the other pathologies list in this table
Pes cavus	Raised medial arch	Generally rigid with limited range of motion at the midfoot Can affect the relative position and range of motion of the bones in the forefoot causing other structural conditions included in this table	Can cause increase pressure across the plantar aspect of the metatarsal heads causing wound development and/or chronicity in these locations Wounds can occur on the dorsal aspect of the midfoot as well due to rubbing in shoes
Hammer toes	Flexion contracture of the digit at interphalangeal joint(s)	Manual range of motion should be conducted to assess the degree of reducibility at the interphalangeal joints Can cause retrograde buckling at the metatarsophalangeal joint	Digital ulcers at the distal tip is a common location Dorsal interphalangeal joint ulcers can occur from rubbing in shoes Sub-metatarsal head ulcers can occur due to the retrograde buckling
Hallux abducto valgus (bunion)	Abduction of the hallux and medial deviation of the 1st metatarsal	1st metatarsal phalangeal joint deviation or subluxation causes limitation of range of motion at this joint Limited to no reducibility of the medial deviation and dorsal excursion of the 1st metatarsal	Medial aspect of the 1st metatarsal head Plantar medial aspect of the hallux interphalangeal joint Sub-2nd metatarsal head due to pressure transference
Tailor's bunion	Lateral deviation of the 5th metatarsal typically associated with a abductovarus rotated 5th digit	The dorsolateral eminence is obvious and is easily palpable due to the relatively thin soft tissue coverage in this area	Lateral aspect of the 5th metatarsal head Lateral aspect of the 5th toe if the digit is rotated Sub-4th metatarsal head due to pressure transference

(continued)

Table 6.3 (continued)

Deformity	Description	Examination	Wound location
Hallux rigidus	Degenerative process of the 1st metatarsal phalangeal joint	Limitation or absence of dorsiflexion with crepitus with range of motion Palpable dorsal or dorsomedial bone spurs	Sub-1st metatarsal head Plantar aspect of the hallux interphalangeal joint
Parabola asymmetry	Irregular length of digits, metatarsals or rays/columns	The physical examination may not reveal this condition. Plain film radiographs are typically needed to evaluate for relative bone or segment length differences	Distal toes Sub-metatarsal heads A short segment can cause adjacent segment wounds A long segment typically causes wounds directly along this segment

Forces are experienced by the foot with weight bearing and ambulation. In the case of wound caused by an acute trauma in an otherwise healthy patient, it may not be as important to consider the forces experienced in the foot. In the compromised patient, repetitive minor trauma may lead to the development and chronicity of ulcers. Thus, deleterious forces must be analyzed and addressed. These forces are experienced between the foot and the shoe or the foot and the ground. This is classically seen in the diabetic patient with peripheral neuropathy. In the insensate foot, the normal mechanism of protecting or offloading the traumatized area in response to noxious stimuli is limited or absent. Therefore, repetitive trauma to the skin goes unrecognized by the patient. This is especially dangerous in the environment of ischemia in the compromised host [7].

Prolonged, excessive, or repetitive forces can cause skin breakdown. There are two important types of forces encountered in the foot. The sagittal plane and shear force. The sagittal plane force is a downward force of the foot to the surface of the shoe or ground. These sagittal plane forces in the foot are referred to as peak plantar pressures which can be measured with an off-the-shelf device [8]. A focal callous is often the precursor to ulceration [9]. The callous is part of the reparative process of the skin and is formed in response to repetitive sagittal plan forces. Shear forces are experienced in the transverse and/or frontal plane between the underlying bone and the skin envelop and/or the skin and the surface of the shoe or ground. This is a force experienced in a side-to-side, front-to-back, or rotational direction [10]. Their forces are more difficult to measure, and there is no commercially available platform for its detection. The classic physical sign of a shear force is the formation of a blister where the epidermis is separated from the dermis. A broad callous can also signify abnormal shear forces. Sagittal and shear forces manifest in a characteristic ulcer shape. The sagittal plane-induced ulcer is typically symmetrical and circular in shape (e.g., 2 × 2cm). Shear force ulcers are typically asymmetrical and oval in shape (e.g., 2 × 3cm). The forefoot experiences these forces when weight bearing and during ambulation. Once the predominant deforming force is identified, the most appropriate surgical procedure can be selected to address it.

Operative Preparation

The success or failure of an operation is less dependent on the technical aspects of the procedure itself but more on the perioperative preparation. The perioperative preparation has several aspects including appropriate patient selection, the physical examination of the deformity, relevant laboratory and imaging, and intraoperative considerations. All of these variables should be carefully considered prior to performing the procedure.

The patient's expectations are important, but it is also the responsibility of the surgeon to identify potential challenges to a successful outcome. In other words, procedure selection should be based on what is the best fit for the patient. This includes the rehabilitation capacity of the patient and adherence to the postoperative plan. Rehabilitation potential is based on factors including age, body mass index (BMI), muscle strength, comorbidities, home environment, and socioeconomic factors. Some patients have a decreased capacity to heal or on medications that delay healing (e.g., long-term steroid use, or other disease modifying medications). The patient may also have a high BMI which may cause difficulties in offloading.

Medical optimization includes nutrition optimization, blood glucose control, short-term reversal of anticoagulation, and stabilization of chronic disease processes (e.g., cardiac function). Thus, coordination with the patient's primary care provider is important beyond that of obtaining a medical clearance for surgery. All operations have inherent risk due to anesthesia even though most forefoot surgeries are not lengthy and can be conducted with monitored anesthesia care with local anesthetic blocks. Further, if the underlying etiology of the wound is a consequence of an underlying medical condition, and this condition is not addressed, the surgical procedure will fail. For example, if a rheumatoid patient has a digital ulcer and is not medically managed, the incision will not heal, or the procedure may succeed in the short term but may not be a durable correction. Friend and family support dynamics and their willingness to assist the patient in recovery are also important. A less appreciated but perhaps a significant factor includes the patient's socioeconomic status. For example, the patient's insurance coverage and access/transport for the follow-up clinic visits and to physical therapy may impact the surgical outcome.

Beyond the vascular assessment discussed in the previous section, the reducibility of the deformity will dictate procedure selection [11]. The reducibility of the deformity is related to the anatomical and biomechanical aspects discussed above. The concept of reducibility (flexibility) is dependent on whether the deformity can be realigned (reduced) into a biomechanical neutral (rectus) position that decreases the deforming force(s). A nonreducible deformity is one that is rigid and cannot be manually manipulated into a rectus position. There is a spectrum of reducibility so

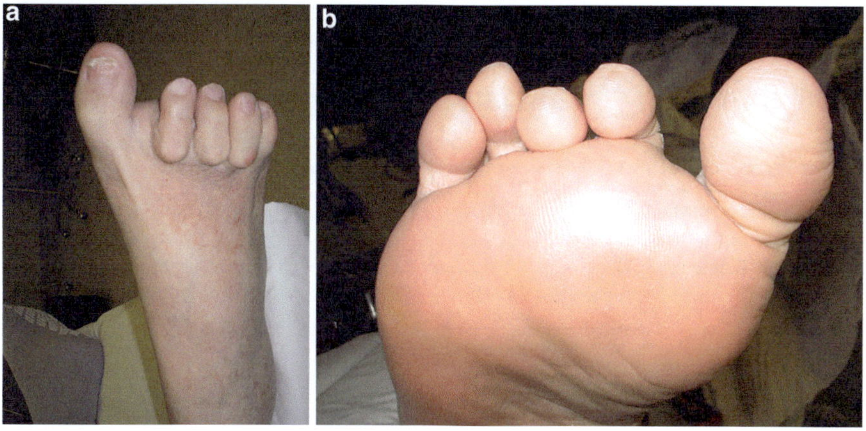

Fig. 6.1 (**a**) A dorsal view of the forefoot. There is deviation of the hallux and contractures of the toes. Note the erythema over the dorsal aspect of the proximal interphalangeal joint of the 4th toe due to rubbing in the shoe. (**b**) A plantar view of the same patient. Note the retrograde buckling at the metatarsophalangeal joint caused by the digital contractures causing an increased pressure across the balls of the foot

it is not absolutely in one state or another. The physical examination includes the assessment of the range of motion of the joints of the foot which will assist in determining the reducibility of the deformity (Fig. 6.1). For example, if a patient has a medial deviation of the first metatarsal (e.g., hallux abducto valgus deformity) and it cannot be laterally displaced with manual manipulation, then this deformity is considered fixed or rigid.

The general approach for procedure selection based on the concept of reducibility is the that a reducible deformity can be addressed using soft tissue correction, whereas a nonreducible deformity requires osseous correction (Fig. 6.2). The exception is when there is gross joint instability wherein an osseous correction is indicated. A deformity may require a combination of soft tissue and osseous correction because the deformity may contain both reducible and nonreducible components. However, a nonreducible deformity can rarely be surgically corrected with a soft tissue correction alone. Further, the apex of the reducibility or nonreducibility should be identified and should be the target of the correction. There may be multiple apices of the deformity which requires a sequential reduction of the deformity at each of these locations. The physical examination should include viewing the unshod patient while standing and walking which may accentuate the deformity. In other words, the deformity may be uncovered under these conditions. For example, on the examination table, the medial arch may be high, but with weight bearing, the medial arch may collapse which would indicate a reducible deformity. This is important to procedure selection.

Imaging is also helpful for surgical planning to determine the degree of reducibility, anatomical relationships around the deformity, and detect the presence of infection or other pathological processes. Plain film radiographs should be taken as

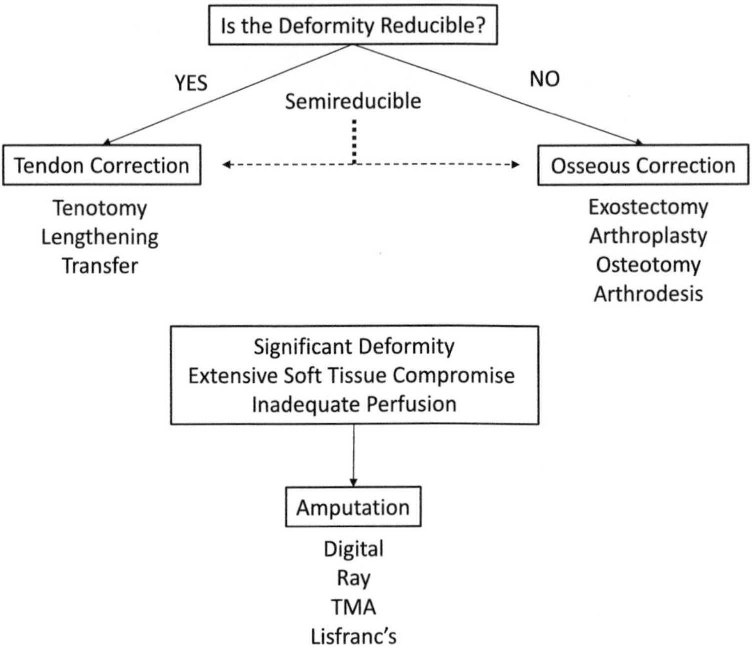

Fig. 6.2 A simple algorithm for procedure selection in the forefoot based on a biomechanical exam focused on the reducibility of a deformity

the initial imaging modality with advanced imaging as necessary. The plain films should be preferably weight bearing, three views (anterior-posterior, oblique, lateral), which includes the entirety of the foot. Other plain films include three views of the ankle and coned-down forefoot views as necessary. Anatomical variations can be readily identified including differences in metatarsal length and joint morphology. Pathological processes identified by the plain films including joint degeneration and infection which will also guide the surgical plan. Of note, joint degeneration is often related to a nonreducible deformity which again will assist in understanding the deformity and in the most appropriate procedure selection.

There are unique intraoperative considerations due to the anatomical location of the forefoot. Local anesthetic blocks are very effective in the foot for intraoperative and postoperative pain control and will speed postoperative recovery [12]. An ankle block involves anesthetizing the posterior tibial, anterior tibial, and peroneal nerves as they cross the ankle. In the case of the forefoot, a more distal block may be all that is required. For example, an isolated digital block may be all that is needed thereby limiting the region of anesthesia. It is important to coordinate the sedation that is provided by the anesthesiologist with the administration of the local anesthetic. The choice of local anesthetics includes Lidocaine and Marcaine. The author recommends the use of 0.5% Marcaine plain due to its tolerability and longer duration of activity although there is delay in onset of activity for 10–15 min. The use of epinephrine is not needed for hemostasis in forefoot surgeries and can be a complicating factor for the vascularly compromised patient. Preoperative and postoperative antibiotics in the compromised host should be conducted routinely; the presence of wound in the non-compromised host is in itself an indication for antibiotics especially if internal fixation is used. An ankle tourniquet set at 250 mmHg for no greater than 1.5–2 contiguous hours is safe and useful for efficiency but is not absolutely necessary [13]. For the vascularly compromised patient, the use of a tourniquet can compromise the ability to visualize the degree of local perfusion. Further, depending on the kind of anesthesia used, the patient may not be able to tolerate inflation of an ankle tourniquet. In the case where an ankle tourniquet is used, it may be necessary to communicate with the anesthesiologist that a deeper level of sedation is needed. It is recommended that the tourniquet be deflated prior to incision closure to obtain hemostasis to prevent hematoma formation. Other specialized equipment for forefoot surgery includes mini or small bone fragment fixation trays and sagittal saw with smaller blades (101 or smaller). Pulsatile or nonpulsatile irrigation prior to closure utilizing antibiotic or surfactant impregnated or unimpregnated solution prior to closing the soft tissue is recommended. Closed suction drains may be helpful to be prevent hematomas and seromas particularly after partial foot amputations. Drains are not typically necessary for any other types of forefoot procedures. Deep venous thrombosis prophylaxis should also be considered due to potentially prolonged immobilization after forefoot surgery.

Surgical Procedures

General surgical principles apply to forefoot surgery. This includes gentle tissue handling and meticulous dissection. Wound bed preparation is especially important in the presence of a chronic ulcer. This includes infection/biofilm eradication, maximization of perfusion, and local edema control. Excisional debridement of the wound should be conducted to remove nonviable and senescent tissue [14]. In the presence of active infection, a staged surgical approach through initial decompression, serial debridements, followed by the definitive procedure is recommended. This is especially important if the surgical plan includes the use of internal fixation because any remaining infection can proliferate in the presence of internal hardware. It is reasonable to make an incision through the wound in order to perform surgical procedures in the forefoot. If it is not clear whether or not the wound is free of infection/biofilm, a separate incision should be made at a different location. Ideally the wound is excised in its entirety allowing for removal of nonviable tissue, infection/biofilm, and for direct access to the surgical site.

Fixation of bone can include internal and external constructs. The general principles of bone fixation apply including maintaining as much of the periosteum as possible, adequate preparation of opposing bone surfaces, and stabilization. The use of internal fixation utilizing wires, screws, and plates are used in the forefoot. External fixation utilizing a mini-rail that spans the bone segments with pins that percutaneously penetrate the skin is sometimes necessary if internal fixation is not desired.

The goal of biomechanical surgery is to reduce the deformity to a neutral position where forces are more evenly distributed. In this way, the wound heals, remains healed in the long term, and prevents the development of new wounds in other locations. Often a combination of procedures that include soft tissue, tendon, osseous, and amputations are performed in concert to address the wound and the underlying deformity. A detailed technical description of each of the procedures is out of the scope of this chapter. The focus of the remaining sections will be on the important principles and rationale for the more commonly performed procedures.

Soft Tissue Plastic reconstructive principles apply to the forefoot including primary closure and the use of grafts. Healing through secondary intention after operative excisional debridement is possible with or without the use of an adjunctive negative pressure wound therapy device. Primary closure or coverage of the wound is often the preferred method. Primary closure should be conducted under little to no tension across the incision line. Local tissue advancement flaps including bilobed, V to Y, and transpositional techniques can be used to close wounds by utilizing the surrounding tissue.

Grafts can be autologous, allografts, or animal-derived tissue which can be used to terminal epithelialization. Autologous grafts should be the considered as the first option in most cases. The split-thickness skin graft (STSG) can be harvested from the thigh, calf, or medial arch. STSG should be pie crusted to allow for evacuation of fluid to prevent a hematoma or seroma. Fenestration utilizing a mesher is usually not necessary for the forefoot because the wounds are generally smaller so there is not a need for STSG expansion to increase its surface area. STSG can be applied to the plantar surface of the forefoot, but dressings and offloading devices should be used to attempt to eliminate shearing of the graft from the surface of the recipient site. A STSG can be applied to deeper wounds with exposed muscle and tendon. However, with contraction of the muscle, the STSG may shear off. Typically, a dermis is necessary to cover deeper exposed tissue prior to the application of a STSG. A choice of human cadaver allograft or animal-derived tissue containing a collagen matrix can be used to build a neodermis. If either are utilized, the application of the STSG should be conducted after the production of a vascularized neodermis which typically takes between 3 and 4 weeks. Other bioengineered alternative tissues are available for surgical use [15]. This includes a variety of processed tissues (e.g., intestinal submucosa, pericardium, tendon, cartilage) harvested from mammals and fish. Further, human fetal foreskin, amniotic tissue, amniotic/placental tissue, and cultured cells containing growth factors and mesenchymal stem cells have been described [16]. Their clinical effectiveness has not been fully elucidated and have been used almost exclusively in the clinic setting. Free tissue transfers are also a viable option in the forefoot for larger defect coverage and will be discussed in another chapter.

Tendon Procedures Tendon surgery is broadly categorized into tenotomies, lengthenings, and transfers (Table 6.4). Certainly, soft tissue deformity includes ligament

Table 6.4 Tendon procedures

Indication example	Procedure	Comment
Digital contractures	Tenotomies	Complete transection of the tendon through percutaneous or open technique
Digital contracture with retrograde buckling at the metatarsophalangeal joint contracture	Tendon lengthening	Typically, the tendon is lengthened by hemisectioning at two locations, one distal and one proximal, along the tendon substance in opposite directions with a midline incision connecting the medial and lateral incision. This creates the Z configuration
Hallux contracture with associated retrograde buckling and plantarflexion of the 1st metatarsal head	Tendon transfer (e.g., Jones tenosuspension)	The extensor hallucis longus is detached at its insertion and rerouted through the neck of the 1st metatarsal and anastomosed onto itself. This tendon essentially functions as a sling by elevating the distal aspect of the 1st metatarsal

and capsular contractures caused by its adaptation to its deformed position. These can be addressed through incisions through the capsule and/or ligaments thereby releasing the contractures during the surgical procedure. As discussed in the previous section, the effectiveness of tendon procedures is predicated on a reducible deformity. A contracted joint can be caused by a biomechanical imbalance of the opposing muscle groups. Thus, diminishing the deforming force through tendon surgery can reduce this imbalance [17]. The physical exam of the forefoot can reveal a taut or bowstrung tendon which is more obvious for the extensor tendons versus the flexor tendons due to the relative thin soft tissue coverage dorsally. The outcome of these procedures cannot be readily predicted on the operating room table. There is a misconception that an increase in the range of motion on the operating room table signifies success. However, since these procedures address the dynamic imbalance, the ultimate outcome is observed during weight bearing during ambulation. A healed wound without recurrence or relocation is the definitive indicator that the procedure was correctly chosen.

A tenotomy is a procedure that completely transects the tendon. This technique is used frequently and effectively for reducible flexion contraction deformities of the toes (e.g., claw toes, hammer toes) [18]. These deformities result in digital tip ulcers and/or ulcers on the dorsal aspect of the interphalangeal joints. Traditionally, a small blade is introduced into the plantar IPJ crease percutaneously or through a small open incision, and the flexor digitorum longus and brevis are transected.

Tendon lengthening typically involves hemisectioning the tendon in a more controlled fashion. This procedure can be performed percutaneously or open. The typical incision into the tendon is conducted in a frontal or sagittal plane Z orientation (Fig. 6.3, Video 6.1). The tendon can be anastomosed side-to-side or end-to-end in the new elongated position. A commonly conducted example of this type of

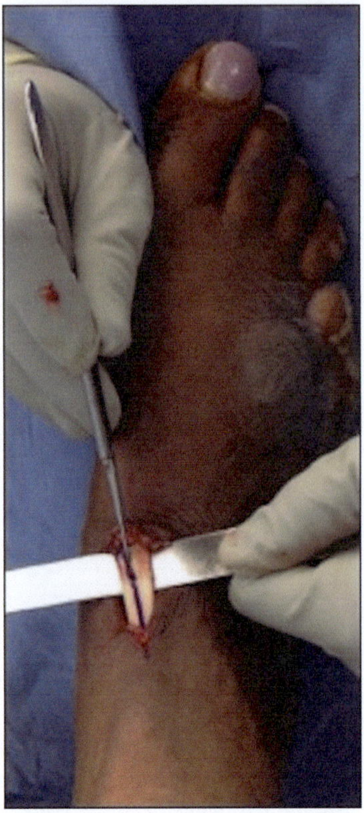

Fig. 6.3 An intraoperative photograph of a tibialis anterior tendon lengthening open sagittal plane Z lengthening. The proximal and distal incisions have already been conducted. The photograph depicts the midline central incision being conducted. This procedure was performed for a patient with plantar 5th metatarsal head ulcer caused by a reducible varus loading on the lateral column

procedure is the Achilles tendon lengthening (TAL). The TAL can be conducted percutaneously or in an open fashion along the distal 1/3 of the Achilles tendon. This procedure is performed to heal plantar forefoot ulcers by decreasing the plantarflexory force of the posterior leg muscle group [19]. This technique utilizes a triple hemisectioning approach commonly performed percutaneously through three incisions into the tendon alternating from midline lateral-medial-lateral.

The tendon transfer involves rerouting a tendon from one location to another. This procedure involves detaching part or all of a tendon from its insertion and relocating and reattaching via anchor or screw (with or without a washer) to the surface of another bone. Alternatively, if the tendon is long enough, the tendon can be rerouted through the bone and anastomosed onto itself. The concept is to decrease the deforming force in one location and augment the opposing force. An example of this kind of procedure is the Jones tenosuspension [20]. This procedure is used when retrograde buckling of the hallux occurs, and there is an increase in the pressure under the 1st metatarsal head causing ulcer formation or chronicity. In this case, the extensor hallucis longus tendon is one of the major causes of this buckling. This tendon is transected near its insertion and rerouted through the 1st metatarsal neck and anastomosed to itself. This tendon now functions as a sling and elevates the first ray as well as eliminating the retrograde buckling of the hallux. The interphalangeal joint is fused at the same time to prevent hallux claw toe contracture.

Osseous Procedures Osseous procedures involve the removal or realignment of bone or fusion of joints (arthrodesis) (Table 6.5). Any one of these procedures or the combination of these procedures can be conducted for the same surgical case. Thus, the selection of the most appropriate procedure depends on other factors as discussed in the previous paragraphs. Osseous procedures are typically performed for nonreducible (rigid) deformities or for joint instability in the case of fusion of joints. The use of plain film radiographs and/or advanced imaging is helpful for these procedures to determine osseous relationships for surgical planning. A radiopaque marker placed at the wound site allows for visualization of the wound in relation to the underlying bony structures. Abnormal angular relationships between osseous structures in the forefoot can be identified and templated for correction utilizing plain film radiographs or computerized tomography (CT). The degree of technical complexity advances from exostectomies, arthroplasties, and osteotomies to arthrodesis.

Bone resection procedures include exostectomies and arthroplasties. An exostectomy is utilized to remove a bony prominence which can be located plantarly, dorsally, medially, or laterally. A plantarly located bony prominence is particularly problematic causing the development of a wound or contribute to the chronicity of the wound. Although this procedure is simple in concept and execution, if there is continued underlying instability of the bone segment or joint, the ulcer will recur with weight bearing. An example is a collapse of the medial column at the 1st metatarsal cuneiform joint causing a plantar ulcer. An exostectomy can be performed to remove the prominence. However, if the joint is unstable there will be further collapse with weight bearing causing the area to become prominent again thereby leading to ulcer recurrence [21]. An arthroplasty refers to procedures that remove segment of bone around joints most often including the cartilaginous surface. An example in the forefoot is resecting the head of the proximal phalanx of a digit for the correction of a nonreducible hammertoe deformity with an overlying ulcer at the proximal interphalangeal joint or distal tip of the toe. Percutaneous fixation with a Kirschner wire can be used to maintain correction until the surrounding soft tissue adapts to its new position. An isolated metatarsal head resections or multiple metatarsal head resections can be conducted for ulcers on the balls of the feet.

Osteotomies are procedures that involve cutting through and realigning bone. The bone segment is then fixated in its new position using internal and/or external hardware. Osteotomies can correct for angular deformities or shorten or lengthen bone segments. For example, a long 2nd metatarsal creates an abnormal parabola which can cause a focal area of pressure on the plantar aspect of the foot [22]. The altered pressure distribution may result in a nonhealing ulcer. Shortening of the metatarsal by cutting through the metatarsal obliquely and shifting the segment proximally will reduce the area of increased pressure. Typically, fixation is required using a wire, screw, or plate.

Table 6.5 Osseous procedures

Indication	Procedure	Comment
Pes planus		The selected procedure will depend on the degree of deformity. Midfoot and rearfoot surgery is often needed for more complex deformities
	Exostectomy	Exostectomies are most effective for less complex, stable (without progressive collapse) deformities of the medial column
	Arthrodesis	Arthrodesis of the 1st metatarsal cuneiform joint can be performed with angular cuts to reduce the deformity or through the use of wedge-shaped bone grafts
Pes cavus	Osteotomy	Dorsally based osteotomies of the metatarsals can elevate the metatarsals. The apex of the deformity has to be identified which may be in the midfoot and/or rearfoot. In this case, metatarsal osteotomies would be ineffective
	Arthrodesis	Arthrodesis can be performed for more severe deformities utilizing a dorsally based wedge resection across the Lisfranc's joint
Hammer toes	Exostectomy	Exostectomy can be effective for removal of prominent condyles or bone spurs that may underlie the ulcer
	Arthroplasty	Removal of the head of the proximal or middle phalanx of the toe will allow for reduction of a nonreducible digital contracture deformity
	Arthrodesis	This may include resection of the base of the corresponding more distal phalanx to perform an arthrodesis
Hallux abducto valgus (bunion)	Exostectomy	An exostectomy of the dorsomedial eminence does not directly address the biomechanical problem. However, the resection of the bony prominence may be all that is required to heal the overlying wound
	Osteotomy	An osteotomy at the head, shaft, or base of the 1st metatarsal can be performed to reduce the medial deviation
	Arthrodesis	An arthrodesis with angular osteotomies at the 1st metatarsal cuneiform can be conducted to reduce the deformity
	Arthroplasty	Arthroplasty (removal) of the head of the 1st metatarsal (arthroplasty) should be reserved for severe deformities, the bone infection, complex hosts, or limited functional demand due to the significant impact this has to the function of the foot

(continued)

Table 6.5 (continued)

Indication	Procedure	Comment
Tailor's bunion	Exostectomy	An exostectomy of the dorsolateral eminence does not directly address the biomechanical problem. However, the resection of the bony prominence may be all that is required to heal the overlying wound
	Osteotomy	Similar to the hallux abducto valgus, an osteotomy can be performed, and distal portion of the osteotomy can be reduced in the medial corrected position
	Arthroplasty	Arthroplasty (removal) of the 5th metatarsal head is less biomechanically impactful than at the 1st metatarsal but again should be reserved for more complex deformity, bone infection, complex hosts, or limited functional demand
Hallux rigidus	Exostectomy	An exostectomy of the dorsal spur does not directly address the biomechanical problem. However, the resection of the bony prominence may be all that is required to heal the overlying wound
	Arthroplasty	Arthroplasty is typically performed at the base of the hallux to decompress the joint to reduce retrograde buckling on the 1st metatarsal or to allow for some range of motion in this nonfunctional joint
	Arthrodesis	Arthrodesis creates absolute stability across the metatarsophalangeal joint. However, without any motion of this joint, the corrected position may cause ulcer recurrence or transfer ulcers if not placed in the ideal position
Parabola asymmetry	Exostectomy	Exostectomy can be performed to remove the plantar bony prominence for the digits or metatarsals
	Arthroplasty	An arthroplasty (removal) of the head of a long metatarsal can be effective; however, pressure will be redistributed to adjacent metatarsal resulting in transfer ulcers
	Osteotomy	An osteotomy is the preferred method to shorten a long metatarsal by creating an oblique osteotomy at the head/neck and sliding the capital fragment proximally. This can be done in a controlled manner to the desired position with or without fixation

Arthrodesis (fusion) is performed across joint surfaces in cases of joint instability or rigid deformities. An underlying wound can occur in both cases. The joint cartilage is typically resected and prepared for healing across the joint to occur. Angular corrections can be conducted at the same time by making angular bone cuts to realign the bone segments in a more neutral position (Fig. 6.4). Internal and/or external fixation is utilized and provides stability until the joint fuses. Again, the prior paragraphs example of an ulcer under the first metatarsal cuneiform joint due to a collapse of the medial column is an illustration where arthrodesis may need to be performed. A complex case is one that involves Charcot neuroarthropathy (CN) in the diabetic foot. CN typically involves significant bone fractures and dislocations

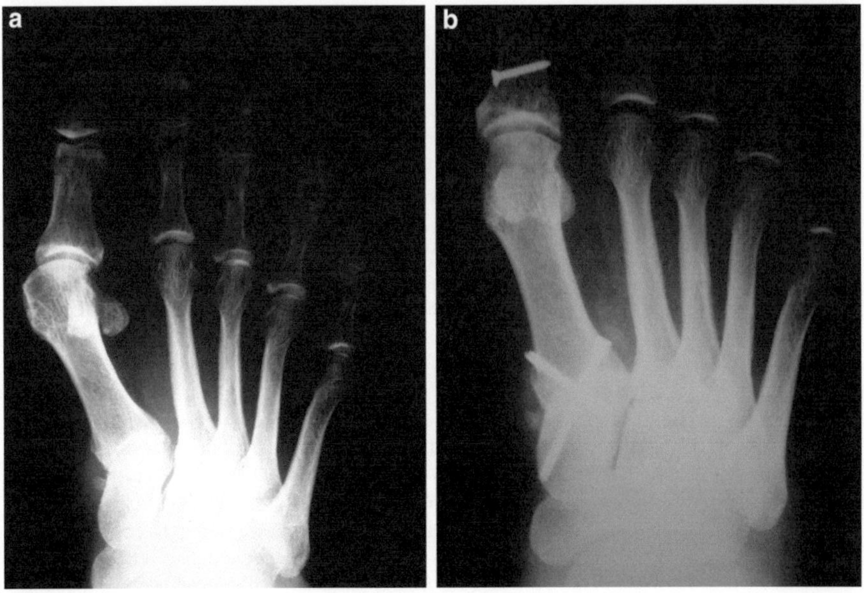

Fig. 6.4 (**a**) A preoperative weight-bearing anterior-posterior projection plain film radiograph of a patient with a severe hallux abducto valgus deformity with medial deviation of the 1st metatarsal causing an ulcer on the medial aspect. (**b**) A postoperative weight-bearing anterior-posterior projection plain film radiograph of the same patient. Note the apex of the deformity was at the 1st metatarsal cuneiform joint. Hence, an arthrodesis was performed with an angular osteotomy to reduce the deformity

with a potentially high rate of surgical complications [23]. The surgical reconstruction typically includes realignment and arthrodesis across multiple joint segments. The medial column is reduced to a neutral position, and an arthrodesis is performed to maintain the correction. For osseous procedures, the internal fixation is typically not removed after bone healing unless it becomes an issue such as backing out of a screw causing skin irritation or causing a wound.

Amputation Procedures Amputation can be functional and is a viable option in some patients (Table 6.6). Partial digital, digital, partial ray, ray, transmetatarsal (TMA), and Lisfranc's amputations are the procedures performed in the forefoot. Typically, forefoot amputations are performed due to extensive soft tissue loss from infection and/or ischemia. Amputations reduce functional ability of the foot by decreasing the efficiency due to a shortened lever arm. Further, a transfer of plantar pressure occurs which can result in ulcers in other locations. Partial and complete digital amputations do not significantly impact overall foot function. However, a shortened or absent toe alters the parabola and transfers more pressure to adjacent toes and also effects balance. In the diabetic population, a cascade of serial toe amputations may result [24]. If more than two toes are amputated including the hallux, the remaining toes will deviate and be a nidus of chronic ulcers (Fig. 6.5). Thus,

Table 6.6 Amputation procedures

Procedure	Description	Functional impact
Partial digital	At least the base of the proximal phalanx remains	Minimal with possible transverse deviations of adjacent digits due to the loss of a buttress from the partially amputated toe. Minimal impact on function
Digital	Disarticulation at the level of the metatarsophalangeal joint	Transverse deviations of adjacent digits to be expected. Balance and propulsion is compromised
Pan digital	Disarticulation of all digits at the level of the metatarsophalangeal joint	Can be functional as long as the metatarsal parabola is normal
Partial ray	Includes the digit and part of the associated metatarsal	Loss of intrinsic stability since the metatarsophalangeal joint complex is compromised. Transfer lesions can occur due to the resultant uneven pressure distribution
Ray	Includes the digit and the entirety of the metatarsal	Likelihood of transfer ulcers high if not appropriately accommodated. Medial and ray resections can be the most problematic with the loss of insertion from extrinsic muscle insertions
Transmetatarsal	Includes the digits and distal metatarsal	Can be highly functional with the use of accommodative inserts and rigid shank with a rocker-bottom shoe
Lisfranc's	Disarticulation at the Lisfranc's joint	Significant impact due to shortened lever arm and irregular parabola

a pan digital amputation may be the preferred option rather than leaving isolated remaining toes.

Partial or complete ray resections are most often conducted in the presence of osteomyelitis when there is compromise to the structure of the bone. These procedures also create more mobility of the surrounding soft tissue in order to close a defect primarily. Ray resections significantly alter the pressure distribution on the plantar aspect of the foot. The forces that are normally dispersed across the five metatarsal heads, and to a lesser degree, the corresponding digits are altered with ray resections. The effect is less impactful if one ray, or a central ray, is resected. Complete ray resections of the 1st and 5th metatarsals are particularly biomechanically impactful due to the insertion of portions of the anterior tibial and posterior tibial tendons on the 1st metatarsal and the insertion of the peroneus brevis at the base of the 5th metatarsal. The loss of these insertions results in the overpowering of the opposing muscle groups. This biomechanical compromise causing significant alterations in sagittal and shear forces experienced in the foot leading to high reamputation rates [25]. If two or more rays are resected, a TMA should be considered as a more biomechanically stable construct.

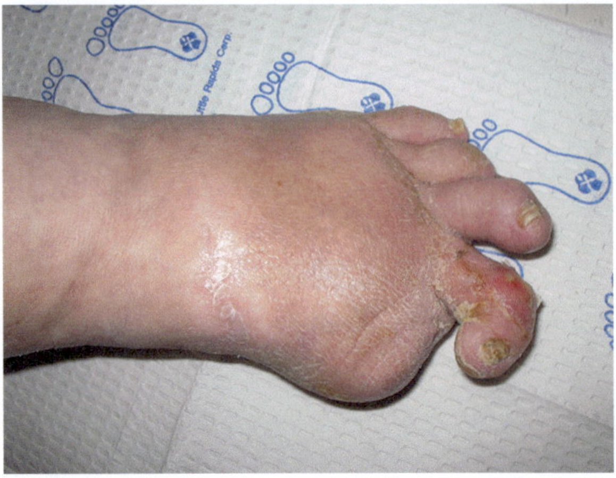

Fig. 6.5 A photograph of a foot with a prior healed hallux amputation. Note the deviation of the 2nd toe with an ulceration due to altered biomechanics

Symmetry at the amputation site is important. Specifically, the maintenance of parabolas is a central concept to successful forefoot amputations. For TMAs, osteotomies performed on the 2nd or 3rd metatarsals should be the longest as compared with the other metatarsals. Further, the osteotomies of the metatarsal should be conducted in an oblique fashion (30°–45°) to the weight-bearing surface to create a rocker-bottom effect at the distal aspects of the metatarsals. An equinovarus deformity due to the overpowering of the posterior muscle group can occur after a TMA is performed due to the loss of the opposing long extensor insertions on the toes. Thus, a TAL or gastrocnemius recession should be conducted as an adjunctive procedure with the TMA to prevent distal plantar ulcer development. The TMA has been demonstrated to be a durable amputation with acceptable long-term results [26]. The plantar skin and underlying adipose tissue should be preserved if possible and dorsally rotated for durability of the amputation when weight bearing. However, the rotation of tissue for closure should be based on which artery provides the best blood supply to the incisional area. A Lisfranc's amputation is not a preferred procedure due to the lack of symmetry and loss of anatomical parabola. Further, the lever arm necessary for propulsion is very short; thus, the Lisfranc's amputation has limited functional capacity. This procedure should be reserved for situations in which a TMA is not an option due to the lack of soft tissue coverage. If a Lisfranc's amputation procedure is chosen, an Achilles tenectomy (complete transection) should be performed to prevent the development of the equinovarus deformity.

Postoperative Care

As with preoperative planning, the immediate and long-term postoperative care is critical to achieving good outcomes. Immediate postoperative care after forefoot surgery includes edema control, adequate immobilization, and modification of weight bearing. Edema control decreases tension along the incision and reduces the likelihood of hematoma/seroma formation. The patient should be instructed to elevate the lower extremity above the level of the heart for the first 2–3 weeks postoperatively for the majority of the time. Compression dressings will assist in edema control when the lower extremity is in a dependent position which is applied in the operating room and can be reapplied at every dressing change. Immobilization of the extremity after forefoot surgery includes the use of a surgical shoe, surgical boot, splint, or cast. Specially designed surgical shoes and boots are available with multidensity inserts and a rocker bottom for ischemic or neuropathic patients. The degree of immobilization needed will dictate which type of immobilization device is selected. The purpose of immobilization is to protect the surgical site from trauma and to limit the range of motion surrounding the surgical site. If the surgery is limited to the digits, then a surgical shoe may be adequate. If an osteotomy is performed, or a more proximal amputation is performed in a compromised host, then a greater degree of immobilization is needed utilizing a surgical boot or cast. A posterior splint is an option that immobilizes and allows for easy access to the surgical site if necessary. However, a posterior splint is a less rigid construct as compared with a surgical boot or cast and should not be used for weight bearing.

Immediate postoperative weight-bearing status is very important. Full, unlimited weight bearing should be discouraged in all cases. Limited weight bearing is permissible for (1) digital surgery; (2) small soft tissue defect coverage or closure; (3) distal tenotomies, lengthenings, and transfers; (4) metatarsal osteotomies with limited need for fixation; and (5) digital amputations. Nonweight bearing on the surgical extremity is preferred for the following conditions:(1) plantar incisions, (2) large soft tissue defect coverage or closure, (3) more proximal tenotomies, lengthenings, and transfers, (4) tenuous fixation, and (5) partial ray, ray, TMA, or Lisfranc's amputations. Nonweight bearing is difficult even with the use of assistive devices such as crutches or a walker. The patient's upper body strength and balance will dictate whether a wheelchair is a preferred method. For forefoot surgery, heel weight bearing for transfers is acceptable. However, during ambulation, heel weight bearing is not realistic because the weight will shift forward on the foot during propulsion regardless of how compliant the patient. The author is not in favor of the use of forefoot offloading wedge surgical shoes because it is difficult for the patient to maintain balance on only the heel and tend to slap the forefoot onto the ground with each step. The duration of limited to nonweight bearing is dictated by the surgery performed and patient factors including age and comorbidities. As a general rule, soft tissue will heal faster than bone. Typically, 4–6 weeks of immobilization and modified weight bearing is necessary after forefoot surgery. A progression to less rigid immobilization and advancing to greater degree of weight bearing should be conducted over time. Prolonged immobilization causes muscle atrophy and joint rigidity; thus, physical therapy may be necessary for full rehabilitation. For procedures involving bone, serial plain film radiographs should be taken during the postoperative course to ensure progressive healing.

It is important to recognize that the foot has been structurally changed after surgery. The structural change will alter the biomechanics of not only the foot but the

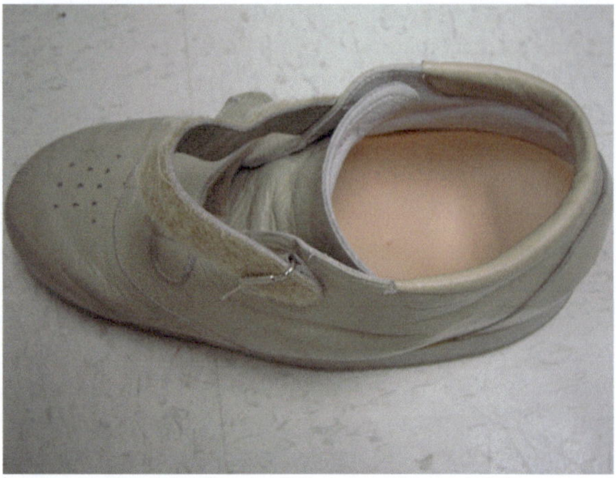

Fig. 6.6 A custom shoe for a diabetic patient after forefoot surgery. The shoe is constructed to provide stability and assist in ambulation. Note the custom accommodative insert to distribute pressure on the plantar aspect of the foot

entire body. Long-term accommodation may be necessary after forefoot procedures. This includes the use of custom-molded inserts, braces, or ankle-foot orthoses. Custom-molded inserts may include toe or forefoot fillers (after amputation) to reduce or prevent movement in a shoe (Fig. 6.6). The diabetic patient with peripheral neuropathy requires special attention with the use of trilaminate multidensity materials to better distribute the forces experienced on the plantar foot. A specially modified shoe with a seamless interior and a rigid shank and a rocker bottom may also be necessary to assist in more efficient ambulation. Further, knee- or thigh-high compression hose may also be indicated for long-term edema control.

Discussion

The forefoot deserves special attention because of its terminal anatomical location and its propensity for injury leading to wounds. The demands of ambulation require an understanding of the biomechanics of the foot especially when considering surgical intervention. The majority of noncomplex wounds will heal without the need for surgical intervention. However, surgery may be necessary for larger, deeper wounds with possible bone involvement. Surgical intervention for the acute complex wound in a non-compromised host still requires attention to biomechanics because the selected procedure may affect the biomechanics of the foot especially when bone is resected or altered which changes the architecture of the foot. Further, in the cases of chronic ulcers, there is almost always an underlying biomechanical fault leading to its development and chronicity.

The maintenance or improvement of function should be the central goal in procedure selection. Forefoot surgery may address the underlying biomechanical component of the wound and/or decreases the likelihood of future development, recurrence, or transfer. This is conducted through an array soft tissue, tendon, and/or bone procedures. The determinants of success or failure of forefoot surgery are no different than any other surgery. Appropriate patient selection, accurate deformity identification, proper procedure selection, and diligent perioperative care will dictate the outcome.

References

1. Cavanagh PR, Ulbrecht JS, Caputo GM. New developments in the biomechanics of the diabetic foot. Diabetes Metab Res Rev. 2000;16(Suppl 1):S6–S10.
2. Attinger CE, Brown BJ. Amputation and ambulation in diabetic patients: function is the goal. Diabetes Metab Res Rev. 2012;28(Suppl 1):93–6.
3. Wukich DK, McMillen RL, Lowery NJ, Frykberg RG. Surgical site infections after foot and ankle surgery: a comparison of patients with and without diabetes. Diabetes Care. 2011;34(10):2211–3.
4. Attinger CE, Evans KK, Bulan E, Blume P, Cooper P. Angiosomes of the foot and ankle and clinical implications for limb salvage: reconstruction, incisions, and revascularization. Plast Reconstr Surg. 2006;117(7 Suppl):261S–93S.
5. Forsythe RO, Hinchliffe RJ. Assessment of foot perfusion in patients with a diabetic foot ulcer. Diabetes Metab Res Rev. 2016;32(Suppl 1):232–8.
6. Dalal S, Widgerow AD, Evans GR. The plantar fat pad and the diabetic foot – a review. Int Wound J. 2015;12(6):636–40.
7. Peters EJ, Armstrong DG, Lavery LA. Risk factors for recurrent diabetic foot ulcers: site matters. Diabetes Care. 2007;30(8):2077–9.
8. Yavuz M, Erdemir A, Botek G, Hirschman GB, Bardsley L, Davis BL. Peak plantar pressure and shear locations: relevance to diabetic patients. Diabetes Care. 2007;30(10):2643–5.
9. Arosi I, Hiner G, Rajbhandari S. Pathogenesis and treatment of callus in the diabetic foot. Curr Diabetes Rev. 2016;12(3):179–83.
10. Davis B, Crow M, Berki V, Ciltea D. Shear and pressure under the first ray in neuropathic diabetic patients: implications for support of the longitudinal arch. J Biomech. 2017;52:176–8.
11. Frykberg RG, Bevilacqua NJ, Habershaw G. Surgical off-loading of the diabetic foot. J Vasc Surg. 2010;52(3 Suppl):44S–58S.
12. Urfalioglu A, Gokdemir O, Hanbeyoglu O, Bilal B, Oksuz G, Toker M, et al. A comparison of ankle block and spinal anesthesia for foot surgery. Int J Clin Exp Med. 2015;8(10):19388–93.
13. Lichtenfeld NS. The pneumatic ankle tourniquet with ankle block anesthesia for foot surgery. Foot Ankle. 1992;13(6):344–9.
14. Cardinal M, Eisenbud DE, Armstrong DG, Zelen C, Driver V, Attinger C, et al. Serial surgical debridement: a retrospective study on clinical outcomes in chronic lower extremity wounds. Wound Repair Rregen. 2009;17(3):306–11.
15. Cook EA, Cook JJ, Badri H, Mostafa J. Bioengineered alternative tissues. Clin Podiatr Med Surg. 2014;31(1):89–101.
16. Lavery LA, Fulmer J, Shebetka KA, Regulski M, Vayser D, Fried D, et al. The efficacy and safety of Grafix((R)) for the treatment of chronic diabetic foot ulcers: results of a multi-centre, controlled, randomised, blinded, clinical trial. Int Wound J. 2014;11(5):554–60.
17. Garwood CS, Steinberg JS. Soft tissue balancing after partial foot amputations. Clin Podiatr Med Surg. 2016;33(1):99–111.
18. Scott JE, Hendry GJ, Locke J. Effectiveness of percutaneous flexor tenotomies for the management and prevention of recurrence of diabetic toe ulcers: a systematic review. J Foot Ankle Res. 2016;9:25.

19. Mueller MJ, Sinacore DR, Hastings MK, Strube MJ, Johnson JE. Effect of Achilles tendon lengthening on neuropathic plantar ulcers. A randomized clinical trial. J Bone Joint Surg Am. 2003;85-A(8):1436–45.
20. Dayer R, Assal M. Chronic diabetic ulcers under the first metatarsal head treated by staged tendon balancing: a prospective cohort study. J Bone Joint Surg Br. 2009;91(4):487–93.
21. Laurinaviciene R, Kirketerp-Moeller K, Holstein PE. Exostectomy for chronic midfoot plantar ulcer in Charcot deformity. J Wound Care. 2008;17(2):53–5, 7–8.
22. Molines-Barroso RJ, Lazaro-Martinez JL, Aragon-Sanchez J, Garcia-Morales E, Carabantes-Alarcon D, Alvaro-Afonso FJ. The influence of the length of the first metatarsal on the risk of reulceration in the feet of patients with diabetes. Int J Low Extrem Wounds. 2014;13(1):27–32.
23. Eschler A, Gradl G, Wussow A, Mittlmeier T. Prediction of complications in a high-risk cohort of patients undergoing corrective arthrodesis of late stage Charcot deformity based on the PEDIS score. BMC Musculoskelet Disord. 2015;16:349.
24. Chu YJ, Li XW, Wang PH, Xu J, Sun HJ, Ding M, et al. Clinical outcomes of toe amputation in patients with type 2 diabetes in Tianjin. China Int Wound J. 2016;13(2):175–81.
25. Izumi Y, Satterfield K, Lee S, Harkless LB. Risk of reamputation in diabetic patients stratified by limb and level of amputation: a 10-year observation. Diabetes Care. 2006;29(3):566–70.
26. Thorud JC, Jupiter DC, Lorenzana J, Nguyen TT, Shibuya N. Reoperation and reamputation after transmetatarsal amputation: a systematic review and meta-analysis. J Foot Ankle Surg. 2016;55(5):1007–12.

Chapter 7
Hindfoot Operations

Alec A. Macaulay and Jeremy T. Smith

Background

Etiology of Hindfoot Wounds

Wounds about the hindfoot can be caused by a number of problems and are often multifactorial in nature. Heel ulcers represent, by far, the most common category of hindfoot wounds. These ulcers develop for a number of reasons, often due to excess pressure on the heel, a poor healing environment, and decreased protective sensation. Cited risk factors for the development of heel pressure ulcers include diabetes mellitus, old age, living in a nursing home, immobility, spinal cord injury, malnutrition, renal impairment, cigarette smoking, peripheral neuropathy, and peripheral vascular disease [1–3]. The heel is second only to the sacrum as the most common site of pressure ulcer formation, with about one-third of all pressure ulcers being at the heel [1, 4]. Heel pressure ulcers represent a very serious problem; the 6-month mortality rate in patients with advanced heel pressure ulcers has been shown to be as high as 70% [1, 2].

Post-traumatic and postsurgical wounds represent two other categories of hindfoot wounds. Open fractures of the talus or calcaneus, as well as degloving injuries, can lead to significant hindfoot soft tissue loss as well as damage to the remaining soft tissue envelope. Surgical incisions about the hindfoot, most notably for calcaneus fractures and Achilles tendon procedures, also can lead to hindfoot wounds. The anatomy of the hindfoot, particularly the posterior aspect of the heel where

---

Electronic Supplementary Material: The online version of this chapter (https://doi.org/10.1007/978-3-319-66990-8_7) contains supplementary material, which is available to authorized users.

A.A. Macaulay, MD • J.T. Smith, MD (✉)
Department of Orthopedic Surgery, Brigham and Women's Hospital, Harvard Medical School, Boston, MA, USA
e-mail: jsmith42@partners.org

D.P. Orgill (ed.), *Interventional Treatment of Wounds*,
https://doi.org/10.1007/978-3-319-66990-8_7

there is very little tissue between the Achilles-calcaneus complex and the overlying dermis, makes this region particularly susceptible to wound problems [1]. By contrast, the inferior aspect of the heel has far greater soft tissue protection and is therefore far less susceptible to wound problems.

Assessment of Hindfoot Wounds

An important first step when evaluating any hindfoot wound is to determine the underlying cause(s) and any perpetuating factors. Listed below are important parts of the assessment of a hindfoot wound:

- *Overall health and status of the patient* – Overall health and physiologic reserve, living situation, and cognitive status are important factors for assessing and treating hindfoot wounds. Many patients who present with hindfoot wounds have medical comorbidities that have contributed to the development of the wound, ranging from systemic disease such as diabetes to biomechanical factors leading to pressure ulcers.
- *Nutrition* – The nutritional state of the patient is important to assess, as optimal nutrition is critical for wound healing. In addition to the general appearance of the patient, serum albumin and prealbumin can be used to screen for malnourishment. The services of a nutritionist should be sought in the setting of poor nutrition.
- *Wound location* – Is the wound inferior, posterior or on either side of the hindfoot? Location is important due to the anatomic implications, blood flow and treatment options of various hindfoot wounds. The location of the wound may give clues as to its etiology, with pressure ulcers typically located at the posterior heel, for example. Foreign-body-related wounds, in contrast, are often at the plantar surface of the foot.
- *Blood flow* – Assessment of the vascular supply to the wound is a key part of any wound assessment. There is a high correlation between peripheral vascular disease and heel ulcers [2]. Vascular supply to the hindfoot consists of two angiosomes arising from branches of the posterior tibial and peroneal arteries [1]. There is a watershed area between these two vascular supplies at the lateral hindfoot that is prone to postsurgical wound-healing problems. Similarly, the lateral hindfoot is a common site of pressure ulcers. To adequately heal a hindfoot wound, ample vascular supply from either these arteries or from collateral circulation is necessary. The initial assessment of blood flow starts with the appearance, color and warmth of the skin, presence of hair, and assessment of pulses. If there is any concern for inadequate blood flow, more advanced assessment with vascular studies and the involvement of vascular surgery should be initiated. Vascular studies may include ankle-brachial indices, toe-brachial indices, segmental leg pressures, pulse volume recordings, transcutaneous oxygen pressures, or advanced imaging with angiography.

- *Sensation* – The presence of sensory neuropathy and the loss of protective sensation are important to assess with 5.07 Semmes-Weinstein monofilament testing. If a patient has peripheral neuropathy of unclear etiology, involvement of a neurologist should be requested.
- *Infection* – The presence of infection is important when assessing a wound about the hindfoot. Systemic signs of infection, such as fever, chills, or generalized malaise can suggest an infection associated with a hindfoot wound. Abnormalities in laboratory work such as elevated erythrocyte sedimentation rate (ESR), C-reactive protein (CRP), and white blood cell (WBC) count all may be suggestive of infection. The general appearance of the wound, presence of purulence or erythema, and any odor from the wound are important additional initial assessments. Plain x-rays, either of the foot, ankle, or calcaneus, may reveal bony destruction which would be highly concerning for infection. At times, the use of advanced imaging, such as magnetic resonance imaging (MRI) or tagged white blood cell scan, can assist in determining the presence and extent of infection.
- *Wound extent (size, depth)* – Is the wound limited to the dermis and superficial tissues or does it extend to the muscles, tendons, and bone? It is important to sterily probe the wound to evaluate its depth as just visualizing the wound very commonly leads to an underestimation of wound depth [5]. Furthermore, wounds that probe to bone in the diabetic foot ulcer population have been shown to have a high incidence of underlying osteomyelitis [5]. Exposed tendon, often the Achilles, or bone is very problematic and typically requires treatment with debridement of the exposed tissue and attempts at wound coverage.
- *Pressure on the wound* – Pressure is often a contributing cause of hindfoot wounds and can also be a perpetuating factor for recurrent wounds. It is important to assess for any external source of pressure on the skin and wound, such as might be caused by ill-fitting shoe wear, as well as any internal source of pressure on the skin and wound, such as from underlying bony deformity. At times, there is no definable external or internal source of pressure other than immobilization. This is frequently the cause of hindfoot wounds in patients with limited ability to mobilize, as seen in some elderly patients or those with certain neurologic deficits.
- *Imaging* – Imaging is a very important adjunct to the assessment of hindfoot wounds. Imaging can provide insight into the extent of the wound, other pathology in the area, and the presence and extent of infection. Radiographs can show bony injuries (such as an underlying calcaneus fracture) and can also show bony changes suggestive of underlying osteomyelitis. Computed tomography (CT) better shows bony detail and can show some soft tissue pathology as well. MRI is usually the imaging modality of choice to assess the extent of soft tissue involvement and the presence of infection in either the soft tissues or bone. Tagged white blood cell scans can also be useful to determine the presence of infection, especially when MRI is contraindicated.
- *Wound etiology* – It is critical to determine the cause of the wound, as treatment options may vary depending upon the cause. For example, wounds due to

abnormal bony morphology with normal vascular supply are typically managed differently than those with normal bony anatomy yet with vascular insufficiency.

Treatment of Hindfoot Wounds

Non-operative Treatment of Hindfoot Wounds

Many hindfoot wounds can be effectively treated with non-operative measures. The first step in non-operative treatment is to promote a favorable healing environment by off-loading pressure on the wound, optimizing nutrition, ensuring adequate vascular supply, treating infection if present, and achieving tight glucose control in the case of diabetes. This often requires a multidisciplinary team approach that includes representatives from orthopedic surgery or podiatry, nutrition, vascular surgery, infectious diseases, wound care, endocrinology, primary care, nursing, and orthotics/prosthetics.

There are a variety of ways to offload pressure on a hindfoot wound, including heel elevation and pneumatic boots when in bed and heel off-loading shoes, braces, and orthotics when out of bed and ambulatory. If these measures are inadequate, then the patient may require restricted weight bearing on the affected limb. This can be done with the help of external supportive devices including crutches, a walker, or a wheelchair.

Proper wound care is essential to promote healing. The principles of this include the debridement of any nonviable or infected tissue and keeping the wound clean and protected. There are many dressing supplies available to help with this endeavor, and subatmospheric pressure dressings can be particularly useful.

If the hindfoot wound is infected, antibiotic use is very important. Deep tissue cultures are useful to guide antimicrobial therapy, whereas superficial wound cultures are often polymicrobial and misleading [6].

Operative Treatment of Hindfoot Wounds

Hindfoot wounds are more difficult to treat surgically than many wounds in the midfoot or forefoot. One reason for this is that procedures that reduce pressure on the midfoot and forefoot, namely, Achilles tendon lengthening procedures, do not have the same effect on the hindfoot. Additionally, it is feasible to heel weight bear while treating a midfoot or forefoot wound, but it is much more difficult to forefoot weight bear only while treating a hindfoot wound. And furthermore, the forefoot and midfoot are naturally off-loaded when the lower extremity is elevated or when lying supine in bed, while the hindfoot may continue to receive pressure in these positions. Therefore it is not surprising that healing times, results, and limb salvage rates are inferior for hindfoot wounds and ulcers when compared to midfoot and forefoot wounds and ulcers [1, 7].

The initial surgical treatment of many hindfoot wounds is a thorough debridement of devitalized or infected tissue. It is important to debride the wound to healthy margins of tissue. This allows characterization of the wound, and in the setting of infection, allows for deep tissue biopsies for microbiology culture. Unfortunately, at times this involves removal of tendon or bone. This may compromise function later but is often a necessary step in effective treatment. Reconstructive efforts, such as tendon transfer to supplement for a compromised Achilles tendon, may be undertaken at a later time when and if the wound has been effectively treated.

Given the high association of hindfoot wounds and peripheral vascular disease, revascularization procedures may be necessary. Revascularization procedures are ideally performed prior to more advanced local surgical treatments beyond a debridement. Revascularization procedures may also be necessary in the setting of traumatic injuries with vascular disruption.

In certain circumstances, bony procedures can be helpful to promote healing of hindfoot wounds. If there is pressure on the skin or wound by underlying bone, then removal of the offending bone can help with the healing process. Additionally, bone removal may be an important part of the treatment if osteomyelitis is present. Bone resection procedures of the hindfoot take three main forms: plantar exostectomy, partial calcanectomy, and total calcanectomy. These three options are presented below.

Plantar Exostectomy

Plantar exostectomy may be performed when there is bony pressure from the calcaneus at the plantar foot, contributing to an ulceration or wound. This excess pressure can occur when there is loss or attenuation of the plantar fat pad and associated soft tissues. Excess pressure can also occur following events that cause abnormal architecture of the calcaneus bone itself, as can be seen with Charcot neuroarthropathy or malunion of calcaneus fractures. A plantar exostectomy removes a prominent part of the calcaneus, typically at the weight-bearing surface, to relieve pressure on the overlying wound or skin.

Case Example
A 63-year-old woman with neuropathy and recurrent foot ulcers presented with a wound at the plantar hindfoot that had been present for more than a year. The plantar hindfoot ulcer persisted despite extensive nonsurgical treatment, including local wound care, prolonged heel off-loading, and the use of custom orthotics with a cut out under the ulceration. She had palpable pulses and no evidence of vascular insufficiency. Plain x-rays and an MRI did not reveal deep infection or osteomyelitis (Fig. 7.1a, b). She underwent a plantar exostectomy of the calcaneus to take pressure off of the hindfoot ulcer. This procedure involved a medial hindfoot incision at

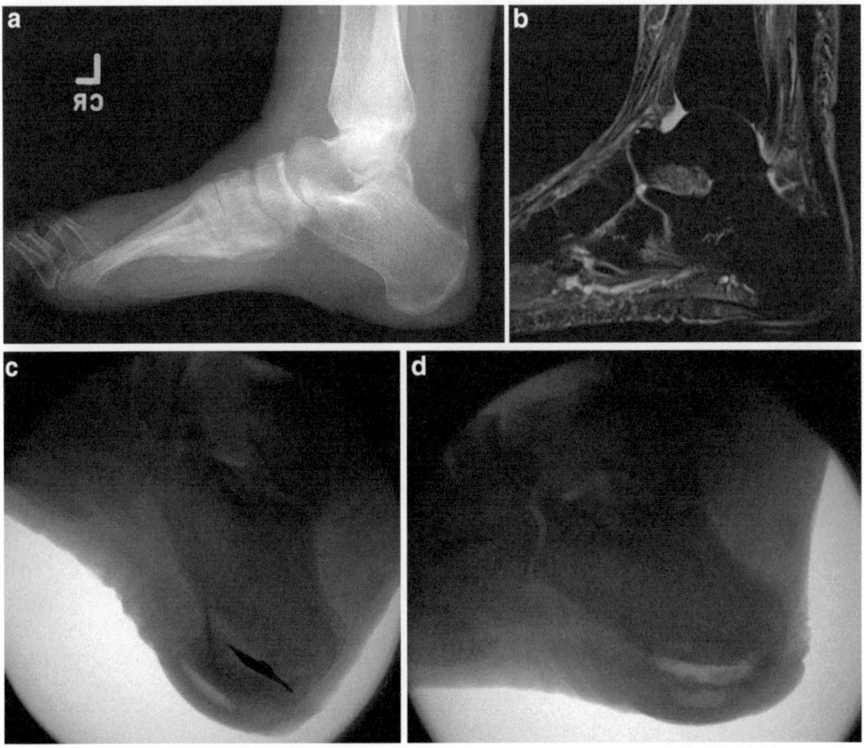

Fig. 7.1 Plantar exostectomy. (**a**, **b**) Preoperative x-ray and MRI without osteomyelitis of the calcaneus. (**c**) Intraoperative fluoroscopic image showing planned level of exostectomy using a small saw. (**d**) Fluoroscopic image after plantar exostectomy

the glabrous/non-glabrous skin junction and the use of a small saw to remove the plantar portion of the calcaneus deep to the ulceration (Fig. 7.1c, d).

Partial Calcanectomy

There are scenarios when a simple plantar exostectomy is insufficient and a larger bony procedure is necessary. At times, to allow for a tension-free closure of a large hindfoot wound, a substantial amount of bone must be resected. Soft tissue coverage options, such as flaps or skin grafts, are often limited at the hindfoot. This is due to a number of factors, including the relatively poor vascular supply to this area and the reality that many of these wounds occur in patients with multiple comorbidities that make flap or skin graft coverage unlikely to be successful. In this setting, a partial calcanectomy may be considered to achieve a tension-free closure. Similarly, if osteomyelitis is present, then a partial calcanectomy may be required to remove infected bone.

Partial calcanectomy involves detachment or excision of the terminal Achilles tendon and excision of a substantial, yet subtotal, amount of the calcaneus. When performed in conjunction with an ulcer excision and skin closure, this procedure is eponymously known as a Gaenslen procedure [8]. Case series have shown this procedure to lead to successful wound healing 75–100% of the time, although subsequent procedures are often needed [9–12]. A longer time to wound healing and higher failure rates have been noted in patients with diabetes [12, 13]. Rates of subsequent below-knee amputation have been reported to be 0–29% [9–12, 14]. Although the Achilles is detached and a substantial amount of the calcaneus is excised, overall functional mobility, with the use of a specialized ankle-foot orthosis, has been found to be similar to preoperative function [9, 11, 12]. Postoperative function does not seem to differ much based on whether more or less than half of the calcaneus is excised [14].

Case Example
A 92-year-old woman was admitted to the hospital with a non-healing posterior hindfoot pressure ulcer. She was largely non-ambulatory due to a prior cerebrovascular accident. On examination, the posterior aspect of the calcaneus was exposed with bone easily palpable. Plain radiographs and an MRI revealed extensive osteomyelitis of the calcaneus (Fig 7.2a, b). She underwent an excision of the ulcer and partial calcanectomy (Gaenslen procedure). The wound was approached from straight posterior, excising the margins of the ulceration and using a saw to remove the infected bone (Fig. 7.2c). The proximal part of the incision was closed primarily and the distal part received a subatmospheric pressure dressing. She was treated with postoperative culture-specific intravenous antibiotics.

Total Calcanectomy

Excision of the calcaneus in its entirety is necessary when the extent of osteomyelitis does not allow for the salvage of any of the bone or when a hindfoot wound is so large that the entire calcaneus must be removed to facilitate subsequent closure. There are far fewer cases of total calcanectomy reported in the literature than partial calcanectomy. What can be gleaned from the available cases, however, is that patients are left with a less stable and likely a less functional foot [15]. Midtarsal instability can occur after a total calcanectomy and may require subsequent stabilization [13, 15].

Case Example
A 47-year-old man with diabetic peripheral neuropathy developed a large non-healing hindfoot ulcer. He presented to the hospital with areas of skin necrosis at the hindfoot and exposed calcaneus (Fig. 7.3a). Plain radiographs and an MRI revealed osteomyelitis of the entire calcaneus and part of the talus (Fig. 7.3b, c). Vascular studies were performed, and he was deemed to have adequate vascular supply to heal a hindfoot surgical procedure. A total calcanectomy was performed by using a

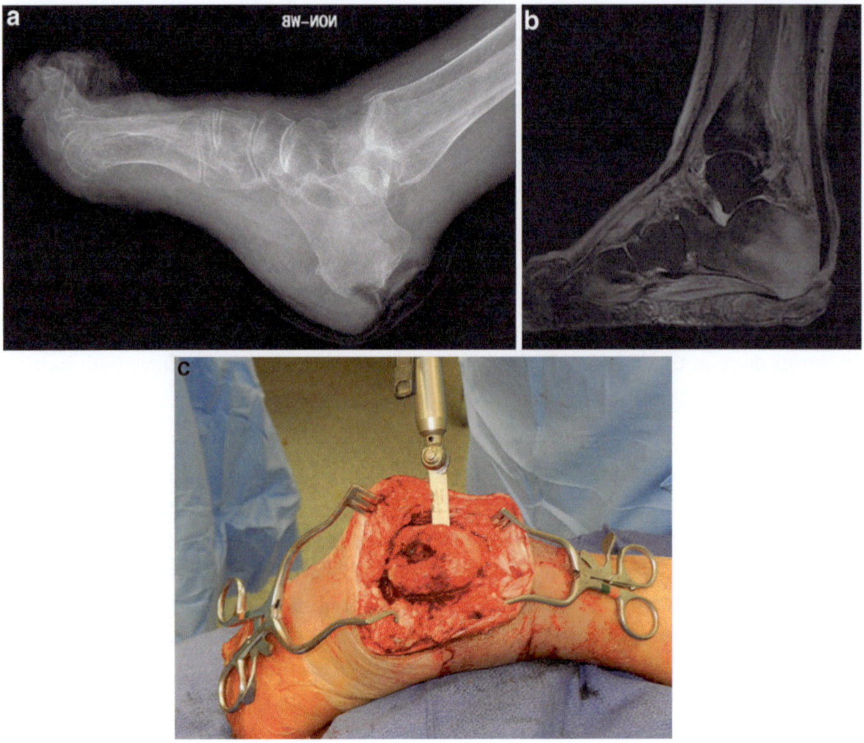

Fig. 7.2 Partial calcanectomy. (**a**, **b**) Preoperative x-ray and MRI showing soft tissue loss of the posterior hindfoot and extensive changes to the calcaneus consistent with osteomyelitis. (**c**) Intraoperative picture showing resection of part of the calcaneus

posterior incision with removal of all devitalized soft tissue, removal of the entirety of the calcaneus, and primary closure (Fig. 7.3d, e). A surgical drain was left in place for several days, and he received culture-specific intravenous antibiotics for 6 weeks. The wound healed well, and he is now ambulating in a specialized prosthetic to accommodate the atypical shape of his hindfoot (Fig. 7.3f).

Amputations

Length-sparing amputations are rarely indicated for the treatment of hindfoot wounds. In fact, most length-sparing amputations rely on either a healthy hindfoot or at least maintenance of the heel fat pad. Yet, several length-sparing amputations involve the hindfoot, and therefore we have chosen to include them in this discussion of hindfoot operations. Importantly, these procedures are typically used for treatment of unsalvageable midfoot or forefoot wounds, not hindfoot wounds.

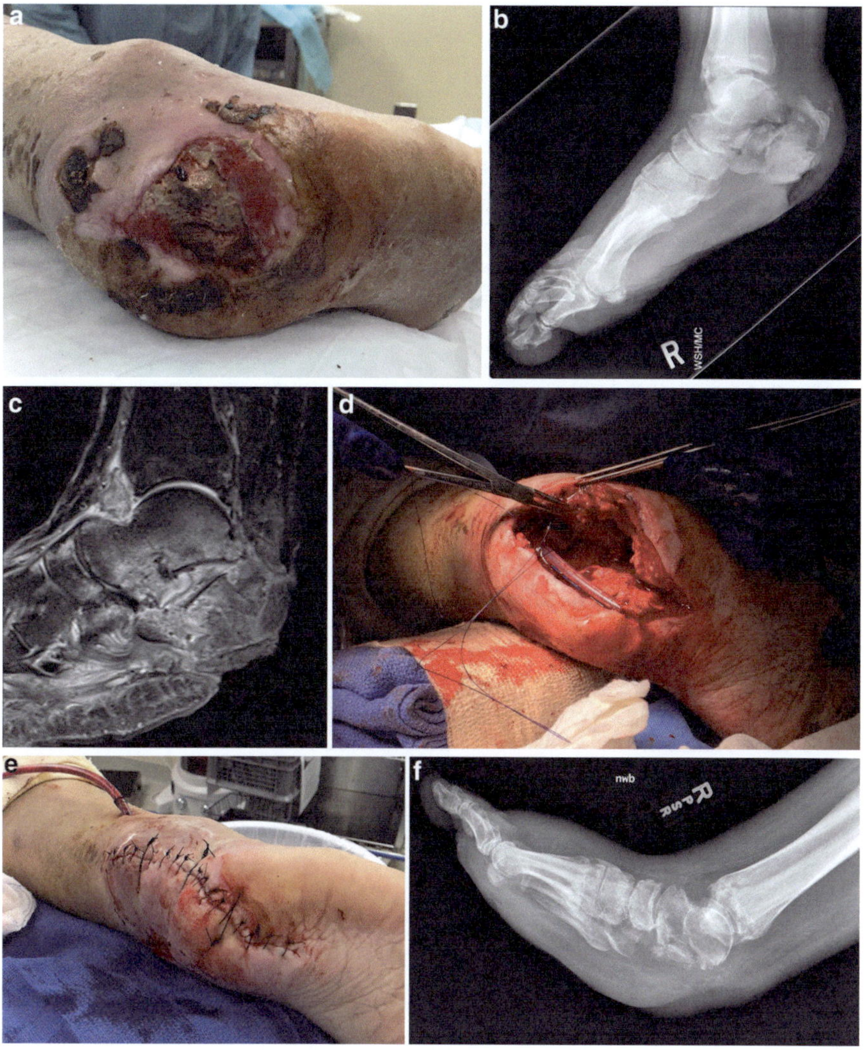

Fig. 7.3 Total calcanectomy. (**a**) Clinical picture showing the hindfoot wound with areas of necrotic soft tissue and bone. (**b**, **c**) Preoperative x-ray and MRI showing extensive underlying calcaneal destruction from osteomyelitis. (**d**, **e**) Intraoperative pictures showing resection of the necrotic soft tissue and entire calcaneus. The wound was closed primarily over a drain. (**f**) Postoperative x-ray showing resection of the entire calcaneus

The Pirogoff amputation involves an arthrodesis (fusion) of the calcaneus to the tibia with removal of the entire midfoot, forefoot, and talus. This procedure has the advantage of preserving most of the length of the lower extremity.

Case Example

A 67-year-old woman with diabetic peripheral neuropathy developed midfoot Charcot arthropathy with collapse of the midfoot (Fig. 7.4a). She developed a chronic plantar ulceration at the midfoot with extensive osteomyelitis of her

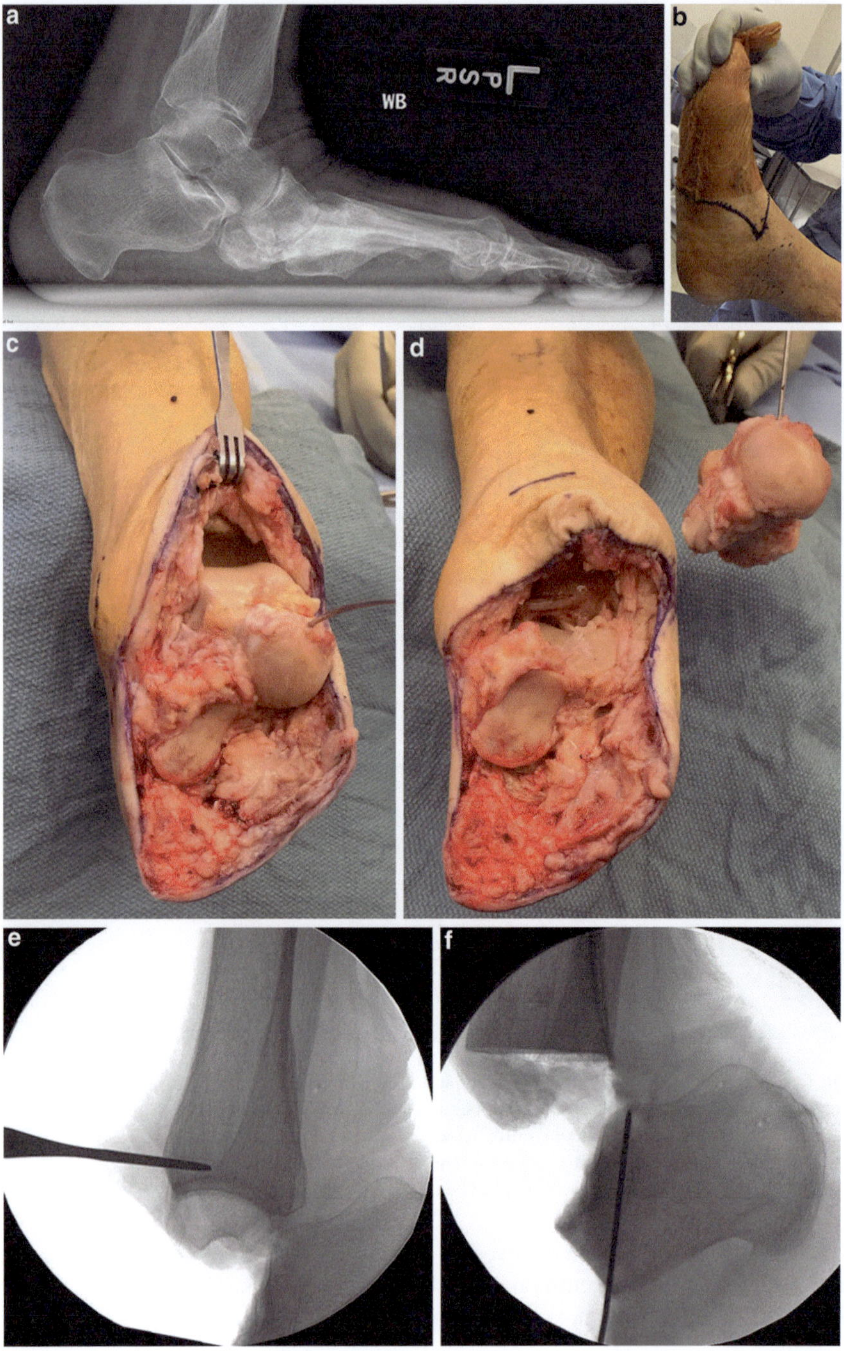

Fig. 7.4 Pirogoff amputation. (**a**) Preoperative x-ray showing midfoot collapse and deformity. (**b–d**) Intraoperative pictures showing the incision, disarticulation through the transverse tarsal joint, and resection of the talus. (**e, f**) Intraoperative fluoroscopic images showing the osteotomies

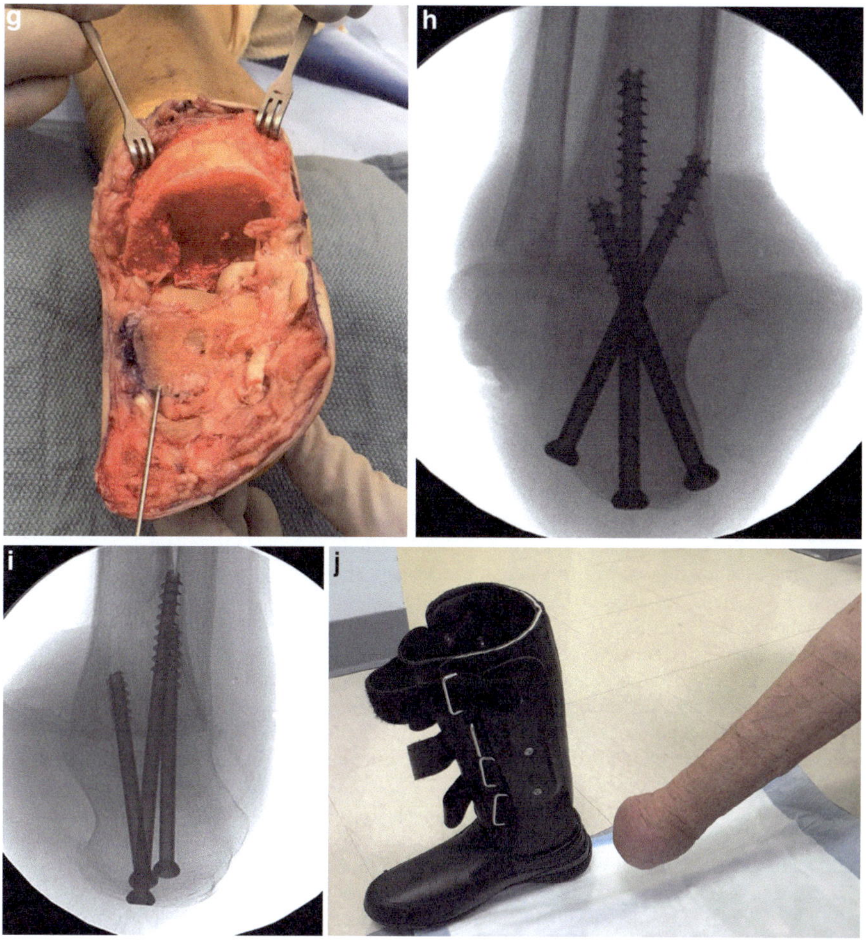

Fig. 7.4 (continued) of the tibial plafond and calcaneus in preparation for arthrodesis. (**g**) Intraoperative picture showing the tibia and calcaneus prepared for arthrodesis. (**h**, **i**) Intraoperative fluoroscopic images showing the tibiocalcaneal arthrodesis. (**j**) Postoperative clinical picture showing the healed amputation with custom made brace

midfoot. She underwent a Pirogoff amputation, which involved a fish-mouth-shaped incision and subsequent disarticulation of the foot through the transverse tarsal joint (Fig. 7.4b, c). The talus was subsequently removed (Fig. 7.4d) and the tibia and calcaneus cut to facilitate the tibiocalcaneal arthrodesis (Fig. 7.4e–g). Large diameter screws were used to fix the arthrodesis site (Fig. 7.4h, i). She healed well and at 5 months postoperatively was ambulating with the use of a custom brace (Figure 7.4j).

Another length-preserving amputation is a Syme amputation, which is an amputation at the level of the ankle joint. With this procedure, the foot is removed, and the distal tibia is beveled to become a weight-bearing stump. The calcaneal fat pad and plantar hindfoot are then secured to the distal tibia, becoming the weight-bearing portion of the extremity. Thus, as with a Pirogoff amputation, a Syme amputation requires an intact heel pad.

The most common and useful amputation for the treatment of hindfoot wounds is a below-knee amputation. This can be considered as the initial procedure in the case of an extensive hindfoot wound deemed unsalvageable or a hindfoot wound associated with significant infection, neurovascular injury, or extensive bony injury. Below-knee amputation is also useful when limb salvage surgery has failed to give the patient a satisfactory result. Below-knee amputation can lead to a better and more functional result than extensive limb salvage and thus should not necessarily be viewed as a failure.

References

1. Bosanquet DC, Wright AM, White RD, Williams IM. A review of the surgical management of heel pressure ulcers in the 21st century. Int Wound J. 2016;13(1):9–16.
2. Malik R, Pinto P, Bogaisky M, Ehrlich AR. Older adults with heel ulcers in the acute care setting: frequency of noninvasive vascular assessment, surgical intervention, and 1-year mortality. J Am Med Dir Assoc. 2013;14(12):916–9.
3. Cichowitz A, Pan WR, Ashton M. The heel: anatomy, blood supply, and the pathophysiology of pressure ulcers. Ann Plast Surg. 2009;62(4):423–9.
4. Vangilder C, Macfarlane GD, Meyer S. Results of nine international pressure ulcer prevalence surveys: 1989 to 2005. Ostomy Wound Manage. 2008;54(2):40–54.
5. Grayson ML, Gibbons GW, Balogh K, Levin E, Karchmer AW. Probing to bone in infected pedal ulcers. A clinical sign of underlying osteomyelitis in diabetic patients. *JAMA*. 1995;273(9):721–3.
6. Mutluoglu M, Uzun G, Turhan V, Gorenek L, Ay H, Lipsky BA. How reliable are cultures of specimens from superficial swabs compared with those of deep tissue in patients with diabetic foot ulcers? J Diabetes Complicat. 2012;26(3):225–9.
7. Pickwell KM, Siersma VD, Kars M, Holstein PE, Schaper NC. Diabetic foot disease: impact of ulcer location on ulcer healing. Diabetes Metab Res Rev. 2013;29(5):377–83.
8. Gaenslen FJ. Split-heel approach in osteomyelitis of Os Calcis. J Bone Joint Surg Am. 1931;13(4):759–72.
9. Smith DG, Stuck RM, Ketner L, Sage RM, Pinzur MS. Partial calcanectomy for the treatment of large ulcerations of the heel and calcaneal osteomyelitis. An amputation of the back of the foot. J Bone Joint Surg Am. 1992;74(4):571–6.
10. Lin CT, Chen SG, Chen TM, Chang SC. Partial calcanectomy facilitates wound closure of heel defects in high-risk patients. Ann Plast Surg. 2016;76(6):688–92.
11. Isenberg JS, Costigan WM, Thordarson DB. Subtotal calcanectomy for osteomyelitis of the os calcis: a reasonable alternative to free tissue transfer. Ann Plast Surg. 1995;35(6):660–3.
12. Bollinger M, Thordarson DB. Partial calcanectomy: an alternative to below knee amputation. Foot Ankle Int. 2002;23(10):927–32.
13. Crandall RC, Wagner FW Jr. Partial and total calcanectomy: a review of thirty-one consecutive cases over a ten-year period. J Bone Joint Surg Am. 1981;63(1):152–5.
14. Oliver NG, Steinberg JS, Powers K, Evans KK, Kim PJ, Attinger CE. Lower extremity function following partial calcanectomy in high-risk limb salvage patients. J Diabetes Res. 2015;2015(4):1–7.
15. Baumhauer JF, Fraga CJ, Gould JS, Johnson JE. Total calcanectomy for the treatment of chronic calcaneal osteomyelitis. Foot Ankle Int. 1998;19(12):849–55.

Chapter 8
Skin Grafting

Jillian L. Fortier, Charles L. Castiglione, and Lifei Guo

History of Skin Grafting

Skin grafting has been a tool in the reconstructive surgeon's armamentarium since the mid-nineteenth century. The first biologic transfer of skin was reported in 1869 by Swiss surgeon Jacques Louis Reverdin, who while working in Paris harvested thin slices of full-thickness dermis using a lancet in an attempt to cover a forearm wound with skin islands, from which he postulated an outgrowth of epidermis would be stimulated [1]. This technique was attempted by several surgeons of the time, and the first case series describing skin grafting was published in 1870 by G.D. Pollack in London, in which he reported success in 8 of 16 cases using the Reverdin technique [2]. George Lawson presented three cases of full-thickness skin grafts (FTSGs) before the Clinical Society of London in 1870 [3]. The first description of intermediate-thickness skin grafts and FTSGs in the literature was published by L. X. E. L. Ollier of Lyon in 1872 [4]. In the aftermath of the Franco-Prussian War of 1870–1871, accomplished microscopist Carl Thiersch of Leipzig reported on experimental work on skin grafting and concluded that very thin split-thickness grafts had the highest survival rate [5]. Additional reports of FTSGs were published by J. R. Wolfe of Glasgow, in 1875 [6], and Fedor Krause of Germany, in 1893 [7].

The first description of large split-thickness skin grafts was published by Vilray P. Blair and James Barrett Brown of St. Louis in 1929 [8]. The invention of the

Electronic Supplementary Material: The online version of this chapter (https://doi.org/10.1007/978-3-319-66990-8_8) contains supplementary material, which is available to authorized users.

J.L. Fortier, MD • L. Guo, MD, PhD, FACS (✉)
Department of Plastic Surgery, Lahey Hospital & Medical Center,
41 Mall Road, 6 West, Burlington, MA 01805, USA
e-mail: Lifei.guo@lahey.org

C.L. Castiglione, MD, FACS
Department of Surgery, Hartford Hospital, Connecticut Children's Medical Center,
Hartford, CT, USA

D.P. Orgill (ed.), *Interventional Treatment of Wounds*,
https://doi.org/10.1007/978-3-319-66990-8_8

dermatome by Earl Padgett and George Hood in 1939 further popularized this technique. In the beginning of World War II, reconstruction in Europe was largely dependent on tubularized flaps. Sir Archibald McIndoe, a plastic surgeon from New Zealand, used skin grafts in addition to tubed flaps for the treatment of pilots from the Royal Air Force who were horrifically burnt in the Battle of Britain [9]. With the advent of harvesting large STSGs with a dermatome and with improvements on the Blair knife, which was largely used in burn wound debridement, skin grafting became a more common technique throughout Europe for reconstruction of wounds that previously had been managed with tubed flaps [2]. Modern advances in the harvesting and preparation of skin grafts with techniques such as meshing and negative pressure wound therapy have helped establish skin grafting as a permanent rung of the reconstructive ladder.

Wound Suitability for Skin Grafting

Wounds with significant skin loss should prompt consideration for skin grafting for coverage. Small wounds with skin loss will often close spontaneously via secondary intention if kept clean and moist with regular dressing changes. The treating surgeon should evaluate all wounds and consider the mechanism of injury, chronology, location, and presence of underlying structures or necrotic tissue prior to attempting skin grafting. Excessive bleeding, infection, presence of necrotic or fibrinous tissue, and exposure of underlying bone without periosteum or tendon without paratenon all preclude skin grafting since skin graft take is unlikely under these circumstances. Furthermore, systemic conditions such as uncontrolled diabetes and peripheral vascular disease would significantly decrease blood supply to the wound bed and inhibit adequate skin graft take. These conditions should be addressed prior to skin grafting with control of bleeding, debridement of necrotic, infected or fibrinous tissue, and optimization of systemic disease with control of diabetes, peripheral arterial revascularization, or compression therapy for chronic extremity edema. Skin grafts require a vascularized, clean wound bed with granulation tissue that will provide a surface for early skin graft imbibition and eventual revascularization (see Fig. 8.1). Premature skin grafting without optimization of the wound bed and control of underlying systemic disease may lead to skin graft failure and creation of an additional donor site wound without achieving closure of the primary wound.

More complicated wounds or wounds with exposed structures such as bone without periosteum, tendon without paratenon, cartilage without perichondrium, or exposed vasculature will require more complicated surgical closure techniques such as local or distant flaps, often in combination with skin grafting. The size and location of the donor site should be considered in operative planning of large wounds. Radiated wound beds typically require flap closure since irradiation causes tissue fibrosis and endothelial damage within the microvasculature, inciting hypoperfusion, thus impeding skin graft take [10]. The incorporation of vacuum-assisted closure devices in the preparation of wounds has made skin grafting a viable option for

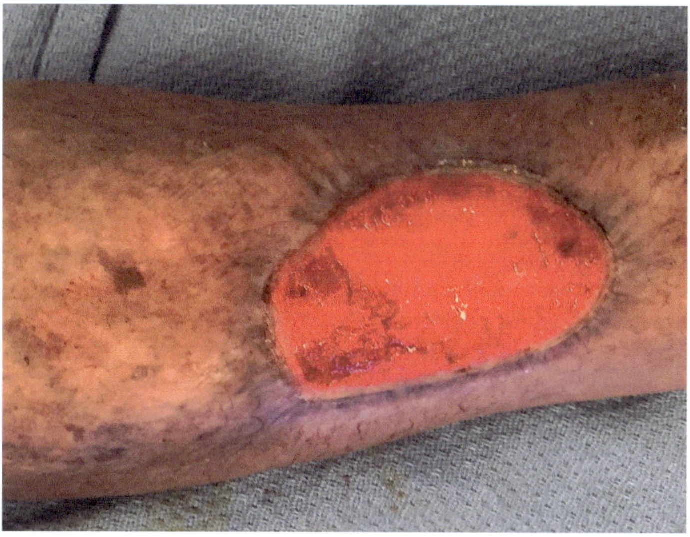

Fig. 8.1 Wound on right forearm with healthy bed of granulation tissue

wounds that previously would have required local or free tissue transfer for coverage. Parrett et al. reported in 2006 that once they began to utilize vacuum-assisted closure for open tibia-fibula fractures, there was a trend down the reconstructive ladder, using fewer free flaps and more delayed closures and skin grafts for definitive closure. The resultant decreased tissue edema, decreased wound circumference, and increased granulation tissue provided a favorable recipient bed for skin grafting without change in the infection, amputation, or malunion/nonunion rates and a decrease in reoperation rate with at least a 1-year follow-up [11].

Classification of Skin Grafts

Classically, a graft is tissue that is completely removed from the body, separated from its blood supply, and placed in another location without an axial blood supply. Skin grafts are classified based on the level at which they are harvested from the underlying tissue. Split-thickness skin grafts (STSGs) include epidermis and varying thickness of the underlying dermis, whereas full-thickness skin grafts (FTSGs) consist of the epidermis and the entirety of the dermis, including accessory structures such as capillaries, sebaceous and sweat glands, and hair follicles. Operative planning for the type of skin graft typically depends on the size of the defect to be covered and the thickness and nature of coverage that is desired for a particular area [12].

Split-Thickness Skin Grafts (STSGs)

Split-thickness skin grafts are typically used to cover defects in locations where the final cosmetic appearance is not a primary concern and when the size of the defect is too expansive to be covered by a full-thickness skin graft. STSGs are classified as thin (0.008–0.012 inch in depth), medium (0.012–0.018 inch in depth), and thick (0.018–0.030 inch in depth). The thickness of the graft is dependent upon the extent of the dermal component that is included. The dermal thickness of a graft is inversely proportional to the amount of contraction of the graft, with thicker STSGs having the least amount of wound contraction. Accordingly, thicker grafts including more of the dermal layer will heal with a more normal contour, whereas thin skin grafts appear attenuated or stretched after healing due to the decreased thickness of the dermal layer in addition to the absence of subcutaneous fat. Thin STSGs may be harvested from any area in the body, though the most common donor site is the anterior thigh given its broad, flat surface in a proximal location on the extremity with reliable blood supply, which is typically free from dependent edema and has minimal pressure points (see Fig. 8.2). STSGs take more rapidly and reliably in comparison to FTSGs due to the decreased time to revascularization of the thinner dermal component [8].

Meshing a skin graft increases the surface area of the graft by providing expansion of the graft, minimizes the collection of fluid under the graft which would preclude graft apposition, and increases the epidermal migration front, thereby accelerating healing. After meshing, healing of the epithelium proceeds from the islands of dermis across the graft filling in the vacant spaces of the mesh. By expanding the useful size of a given graft, meshing concomitantly decreases the size of the

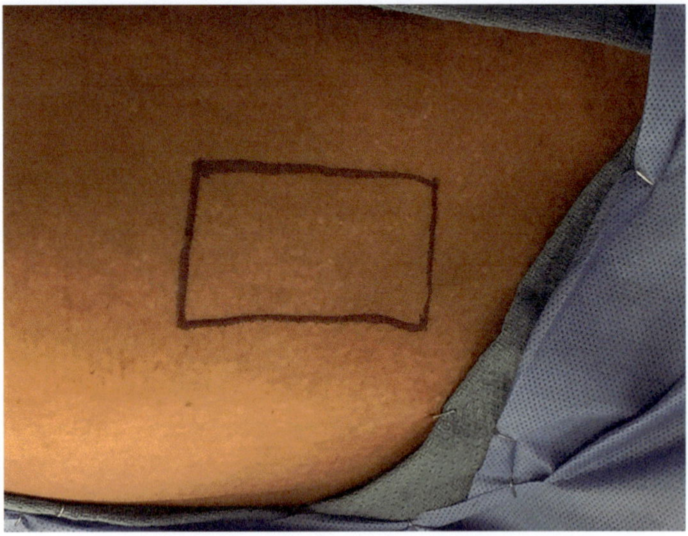

Fig. 8.2 Donor site on right lateral thigh marked with defect size

donor site that is necessary to close a particular defect. A disadvantage of meshing includes the fishnet appearance of the healed skin. The utilization of vacuum-assisted wound closure (VAC) aids in contraction of the wound bed, thereby minimizing the defect and necessary donor site. In patients with few available donor sites and extensive wounds, such as burn patients, the utilization of thin STSGs will enable re-harvest of the same donor site. After healing, the remaining dermis of the donor site can provide several thin STSGs until the supply of the dermis is exhausted [12].

Full-Thickness Skin Grafts (FTSGs)

Full-thickness skin grafts (FTSGs) include both the epidermis and the entire dermis and are usually used to cover smaller wounds in situations where there is a greater concern for aesthetic appearance. FTSGs are commonly used to cover defects of the face, the hand, joint extensor surfaces, or other openly visible areas since they have less contraction than STSGs and have a superior cosmetic result. Closure of the donor site is required and should be a consideration in donor site selection, with incisions placed along natural skin tension lines in locations where they will not distort the surrounding structures.

The most common donor sites for FTSGs are the posterior auricular region, upper eyelids, neck, hypothenar eminence, and groin. In older patients, where skin laxity is abundant, donor site choices become more ample. Because FTSGs include the dermal appendages, they maintain the hair pattern of their original location even after transplantation to the recipient site. Both the pigmentation of the donor site as well as the hair pattern should be considered in operative planning to achieve satisfactory cosmetic appearance after healing.

The thinner the FTSG, the easier it is for the graft to have adequate take. When harvesting thin FTSGs, care must be taken to exclude the underlying adipose tissue that is typically adherent to the deep surface of the dermis. FTSGs are not usually meshed, but can be pie-crusted with sequential stab incisions to prevent accumulation of fluid underneath the graft and to promote increased epidermal migration.

Furthermore, the quality and characteristics of the recipient site are of utmost importance in deciding which type of skin graft to utilize. While a graft has the potential to take on any site that is free of infection and necrotic tissue and has adequate vascularization, a thicker graft may be preferred in locations that are subject to pressure or overlying vital or mobile structures. Viable recipient tissues include granulation tissue, adipose tissue, muscle, and well-vascularized fascia, periosteum, perichondrium, and paratenon [13]. For recipient wounds that are lacking a well-vascularized surface, temporary wound coverage and preparation with a dermal substitute or VAC device may be utilized for optimization prior to skin graft coverage.

Dermal Substitutes

Dermal substitutes may be used in situations where the wound is so expansive that there is insufficient donor site for grafting or as a temporizing measure to develop a wound bed that is suitable for placement of a STSG. They are frequently placed over clean, debrided tissue that lacks its own microcirculation, such as bone without periosteum or tendon lacking paratenon.

Skin allografts are derived from cadaveric or neonatal donors, whereas xenografts are derived from bovine or porcine donors. These grafts may include only dermal elements or may include two layers to simulate the dermal and epidermal layers of native skin. Grafts may be characterized as acellular or cellular, depending on whether living cells are retained during graft processing. Cellular grafts can only be obtained from a human source and are often cultured from neonatal foreskin. They may stimulate elements of immunogenic host response in certain individuals. Acellular grafts, however, are immunologically inert and usually harvested from a decellularized cadaveric source. Xenografts must be acellular to prevent a strong immunogenic host response.

Acellular dermal matrix (ADM) is a common dermal substrate used by reconstructive surgeons to reinforce soft tissues and facilitate wound healing. It is created of nonliving dermal components, including collagen, elastin, laminin, and glycosaminoglycans and may be harvested from either an allogenic or xenogenic donor. It generally incorporates well into host tissue, and revascularization is often noted as early as 1–2 weeks after implantation [14]. It is commonly used in breast reconstruction to provide additional support and coverage of the inferior pole of a breast implant and to provide additional strength in hernia repairs and to bridge large abdominal wall defects. It has been used in chest wall reconstruction by providing a bridge to definitive STSG coverage of exposed vital structures, or may serve as a regenerative tissue matrix for chronic wounds [15].

Xenogenic ADMs, such as Strattice (LifeCell) and XenMatrix (CR Bard), are harvested from a porcine or bovine source and require processing to inhibit collagen degradation and to reduce immunogenicity. Acellular bilayered matrices, such as Integra (Integra LifeSciences, Plainsboro, NH), are composed of collagen framework cross-linked with shark glycosaminoglycans, which is covered by a silicone top layer that helps to prevent desiccation of the product during neovascularization of the dermal component. Neovascularization takes approximately 3 weeks, and once this is complete, the silicone layer is removed, and a thin autologous STSG can be placed over the vascularized dermal layer. This product is useful in creating a vascularized wound bed over exposed structures such as the bone, tendon, or joint and has the benefit of "off the shelf" availability. It also enables the surgeon to harvest a much thinner skin graft than would otherwise be needed, which permits the use of the same donor site for the harvesting of thin STSGs multiple times if adequate donor tissue is scarce. An additional layer of dermal collagen matrix may be used to add thickness to a depressed defect. Disadvantages of using acellular bilayered matrices include the considerable expense of the product, in addition to the classically described two-stage reconstruction of a defect [16].

Another variation of this concept includes engineered cellular matrices. For example, Dermagraft (Advanced Tissue Sciences, La Jolla, CA) is composed of fibroblasts from neonatal foreskins prepared on a polyglactin mesh and is indicated for non-infected full-thickness diabetic foot ulcers. Cellular bilayered matrices, such as Apligraf (Organogenesis, Canton, MA) and TransCyte (Advanced BioHealing, La Jolla, CA), are composed of both the dermal and epidermal layers and are indicated for use in diabetic ulcers and burn wounds, respectively. Regardless of which type of engineered cellular matrices is used, these products all act as a scaffold for ingrowth of neodermal tissue and prevent wound desiccation in the early stages of healing. However, for the products containing the engineered epidermal component, they all lack the typical stratification of squamous cells present in the epidermis of native skin and thus are largely friable, susceptible to shear forces, and at times unstable [16].

Cultured epidermal autografts (CEAs) are often used in burn patients to expand an individual's skin when there is not sufficient dermis available for split-thickness skin grafting. CEAs require biopsy of an individual's skin, which is then processed in the lab to isolate, expand, and culture the autologous keratinocytes, along with co-cultured murine keratinocytes, in sheets of tissue for grafting. Smaller surface areas can be cultured in as few as 16 days, though larger sheets of autologous keratinocytes can take up to 4 weeks to culture. Disadvantages of this technique include the considerable cost of the individualized bioengineered product in combination with the time required to produce the product, its lack of off the shelf availability, and the fragility of the final product with an exceedingly thin epidermal layer [16].

Operative Technique: STSG

After selection of an appropriate donor site, the skin graft is harvested with a power-driven or free-hand dermatome or alternatively with a Humby knife. Some surgeons opt to infiltrate local anesthetic or insert a local anesthetic pump for prolonged analgesia of the donor site. Others opt to infiltrate the subcutaneous tissue with normal saline to make the dermis more prominent for ease of harvest. If using a dermatome, the surgeon must select the appropriately sized guard based on the defect size, and the blade and guard should be inserted into the machine and adjusted to the desired thickness of the graft (see Fig. 8.3). Mineral oil, Vaseline-based lubrication, or Surgilube is applied to the donor site, and tension should be provided to the donor site with manual traction by an assistant or with a tongue depressor. This creates a friction-free surface between the dermatome and skin surface during harvesting [8].

The operation of the dermatome is often likened to the analogy of flying an airplane; the dermatome is turned on while hovering over donor site and slowly lowered down to the skin surface at a 45-degree angle for a smooth, gradual landing. Constant downward and forward pressure is applied to the dermatome as it is

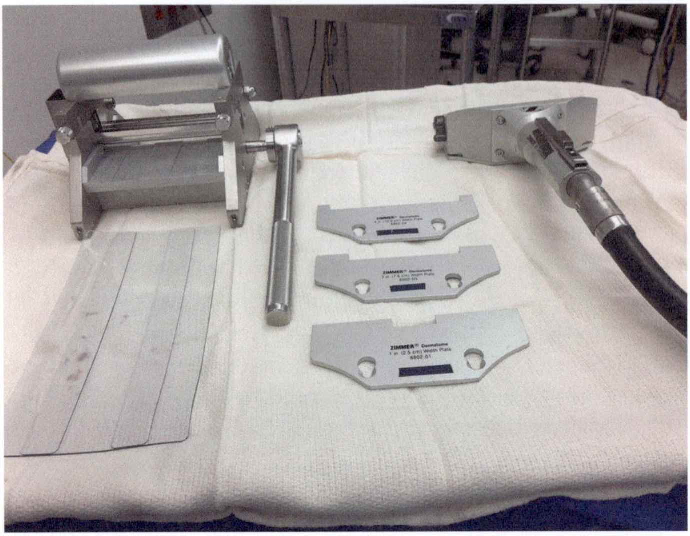

Fig. 8.3 Mesher on *left*, electric dermatome on *right* with different sized guards

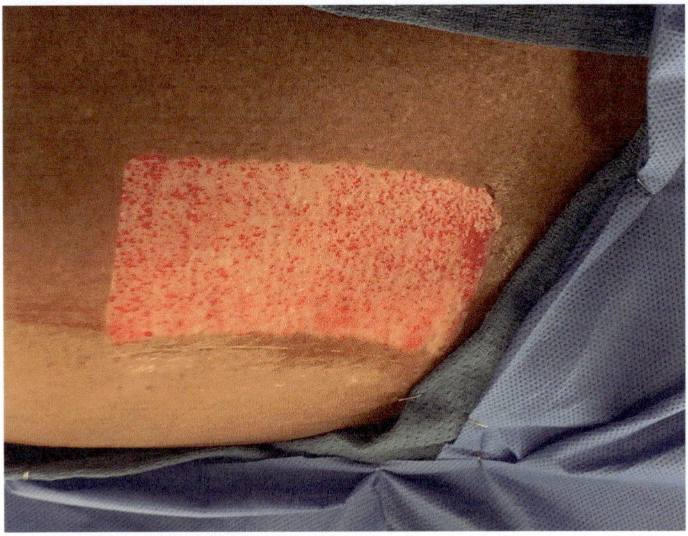

Fig. 8.4 Donor site after STSG harvested with dermatome

steadily advanced down the length of the donor site, with an assistant providing pressure on either side of the runway in order to keep the dermal surface taut. When the desired graft has been harvested, the dermatome is gradually lifted off the donor site with the machine still engaged, much like an airplane taking flight off a runway. This will truncate the harvested graft from the donor site (see Fig. 8.4). Alternatively,

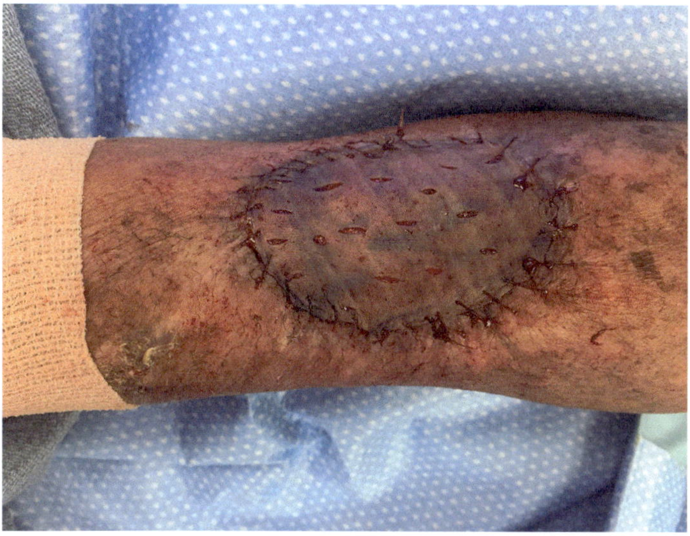

Fig. 8.5 Pie-crusted STSG secured to recipient site with chromic sutures

the surgeon can opt to disengage the dermatome without lifting off the donor site and can truncate the skin graft manually with sharp scissors (see Video 8.1).

If the surgeon opts to harvest a graft with a Humby knife, it should be held with the blade at a 45-degree angle to the skin and maneuvered back and forth in long, even strokes over the taut donor site to separate the graft from the underlying dermis. When the desired length of graft is harvested, the wrist is supinated in a back and forth motion to elevate off the donor site and separate the graft from the dermis [17].

Many surgeons choose to mesh the harvested STSG, which expands the surface area of the graft while also allowing drainage of any fluid that pools under the graft once secured to the donor site. Any collection of serum or blood underneath the graft can prevent imbibition of the dermal cells to the underlying microvasculature of the wound bed, preventing graft take. Grafts with meshing also have multiple points of contact with the underlying wound bed, thereby increasing the adhesion to the wound bed and preventing disruption of the graft by shear forces. Meshed skin grafts are therefore recommended for wound beds with irregular contour, since they are more likely to drape in close opposition to the peaks and valleys of the surface. In wounds with particularly irregular surfaces, vacuum-assisted wound closure can optimize the close apposition of the STSG to the underlying surface while also providing conforming qualities to the underlying wound bed. The disadvantages of meshing grafts include the "stocking net" appearance of healed skin after reepithelialization and the higher rate of wound contraction with higher ratios of meshing. Some surgeons will forego graft meshing and instead "pie-crust" the graft with multiple stab incisions in the graft to allow drainage of underlying effluent and necessary draping over the wound bed (see Fig. 8.5). Pie-crusting, while effective at allowing drainage of fluid, is not nearly as useful for expansion of the surface area of the skin graft in comparison to meshing [17].

Most STSGs are meshed with an expansion ration of 1.5 or 2:1, though this can be altered to as high as 6:1 based on the size of the defect and available graft donor site. The higher the ratio of meshing, the higher the rate of reepithelialization which is necessary for wound coverage, and the more expandability is achieved to cover the defect. To mesh the defect, the graft is placed on a rigid plastic sheet and passed through the meshing device, where it rolls through metal cutters to create the uniform meshed pattern across the skin graft [18]. Singh et al. described a technique in which they minced a STSG to dimensions of 0.3 × 0.3 mm (pixel sized), which are then suspended within a moist wound bed without consideration of the dermal side being up or down. They noted fast rates of epithelialization, decreased wound contraction, and increased mechanical stability compared with non-grafted wounds. While this technique has not become widely practiced, pixel grafting may be useful in treatment of the patient with extensive skin loss and limited donor sites [19].

The wound bed must be prepared prior to grafting with thorough debridement of any necrotic, infected, or fibrinous material. A thin coat of methylene blue can be painted on the defect surface, so that adequate debridement can be determined when all of the methylene blue has been eradicated. Debridement is often performed sharply with the edge of a scalpel, thereby disrupting the capillaries of the underlying granulation tissue [20]. Alternatively, hydrosurgical dissection with the use of a VersaJet (Smith & Nephew, Largo, FL) or similar device is an effective tool for gentle but adequate debridement of devitalized material while simultaneously minimizing the debridement of healthy, vital tissue [21]. A healthy bed of tissue that easily bleeds with gentle manipulation is optimal, as this will support the graft in the first days by permitting the necessary imbibition of the graft and diffusion of nutrients required for early graft take. Any excessive bleeding should be controlled to prevent collection of hematoma underneath the STSG, which would preclude apposition of the graft and may enable it to shear off the wound bed with any horizontal force.

The STSG is then placed on the wound bed with the shinier, dermal side facing downwards onto the wound. The STSG should drape gently over any contour irregularities of the wound bed and may be secured with quilting sutures to prevent tenting of the graft over wound depressions. The edges of the graft are then secured to the wound with absorbable sutures, staples, or with a thin layer of fibrin glue which may be sprayed on the surface of the wound just before placing the graft on the wound bed. Although the use of fibrin glue is beneficial in securing the graft in a timely fashion without need for sutures, it adds expense to the operation and precludes the ability to stretch a graft across a defect, thereby making a larger donor site necessary. The graft should be secured by suturing in a "ship to shore" fashion without ripping or strangulating the edges of the meshed graft. Excess STSG that overlies the edges of the wound should be trimmed to ensure minimal overlap [18].

There are a variety of dressings suitable to secure a STSG. Commonly, a layer of antibiotic ointment and a nonstick iodine-impregnated gauze is placed over the graft, followed by a layer of antibiotic ointment. This is secured with a light pressure

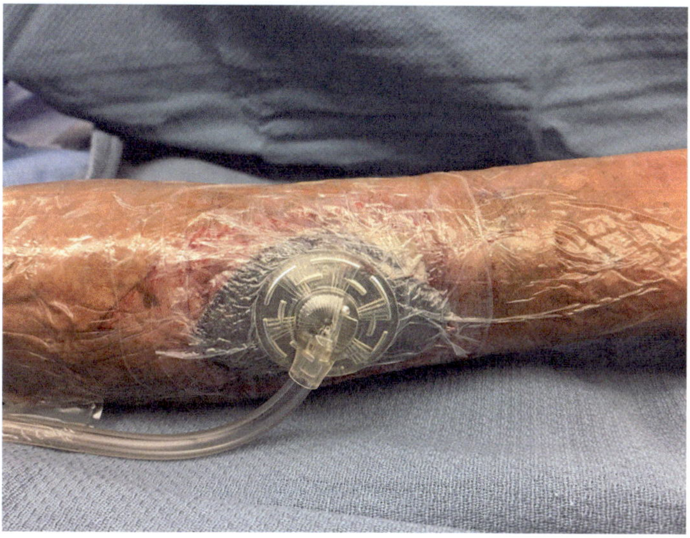

Fig. 8.6 STSG kept in close apposition to wound bed with vacuum-assisted closure device

dressing or nonstick gauze-wrapped cotton bolster providing 10–20 mmHg pressure to enhance graft adherence without causing pressure necrosis. Vacuum-assisted wound closure (VAC) has been shown to be effective at promoting adherence of the graft, providing surface conformity, and reducing the shearing forces while also draining any exudate, thereby reducing the rate of seroma formation (see Fig. 8.6). Patients treated with VAC have also been shown to ambulate earlier and have overall decreased length of inpatient hospitalization in comparison to patients managed without VAC [22].

The operative dressing is usually taken down on postoperative day 5–7 unless there is suspicion for early wound infection which would require earlier evaluation of the wound. When the operative dressing is first taken down, the surgeon must take care to prevent shearing the graft away from the recipient bed while lifting the VAC or bolster off, a process made easier by the initial layer of antibiotic ointment at the time of surgery. After the first dressing change, daily dressing changes with application of antibiotic ointment and nonstick iodine-impregnated gauze, and dry sterile dressing keeps the graft clean and moist in the initial phases of healing. The graft may be exposed to open air with daily application of a moisturizing cream or antibiotic ointment once it appears adherent to the wound bed. The patient should take care to keep the wound out of direct exposure to the sun and apply sunscreen once it is fully epithelialized, usually starting 3 weeks postoperatively (see Fig. 8.7a–e) [20].

After harvesting the STSG, the donor site may be dressed with an occlusive dressing which allows the accumulation of sterile serous fluid underneath the dressing, thereby stimulating the underlying dermis to reepithelize (see Fig. 8.8). Usually, a moist occlusive dressing such as large Tegaderm or Tegasorb (3 M Medical,

Maplewood, MN) preserves a sterile environment while minimizing patient discomfort in comparison to a dry dressing. Alternatively, some surgeons opt to dress the donor site with nonstick iodine-impregnated gauze, a layer of antibiotic ointment and dry sterile dressing. The operative dressing is typically left in place

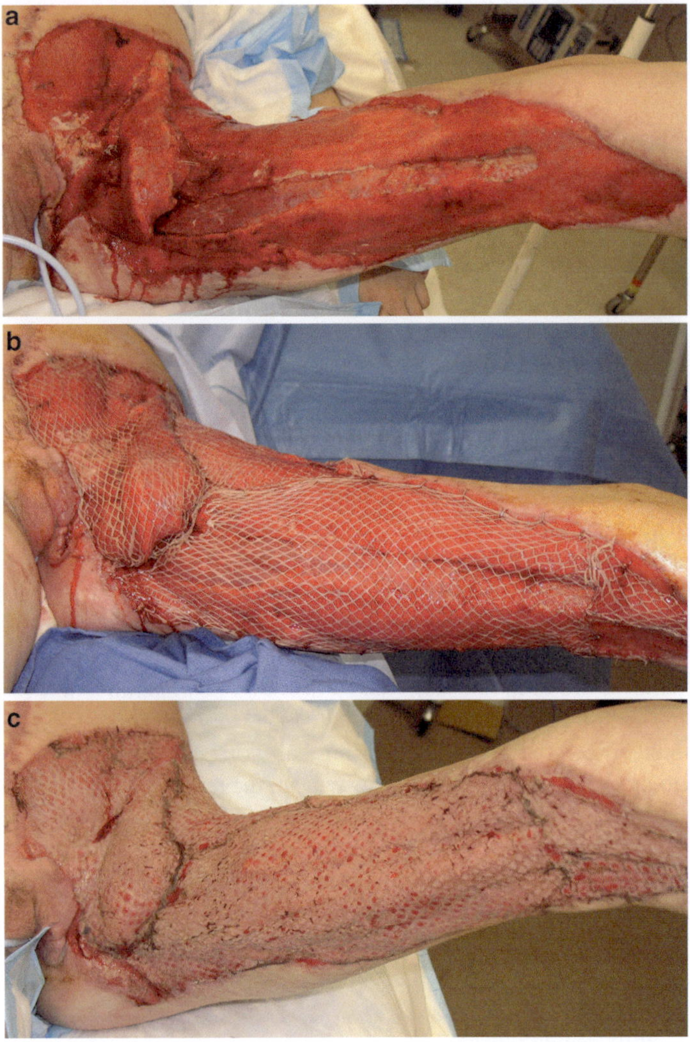

Fig. 8.7 (**a**) Left thigh and groin wound status post serial debridement of necrotizing soft tissue infection demonstrating clean, viable wound bed with granulation tissue. (**b**) Wound covered with STSG with 4:1 meshing ratio. (**c**) Healing STSG with good take after vacuum-assisted closure device removed on postoperative day 7. (**d**, **e**) Healed STSG 3 months postoperatively. Reconstruction with STSG provided durable coverage and definitive closure

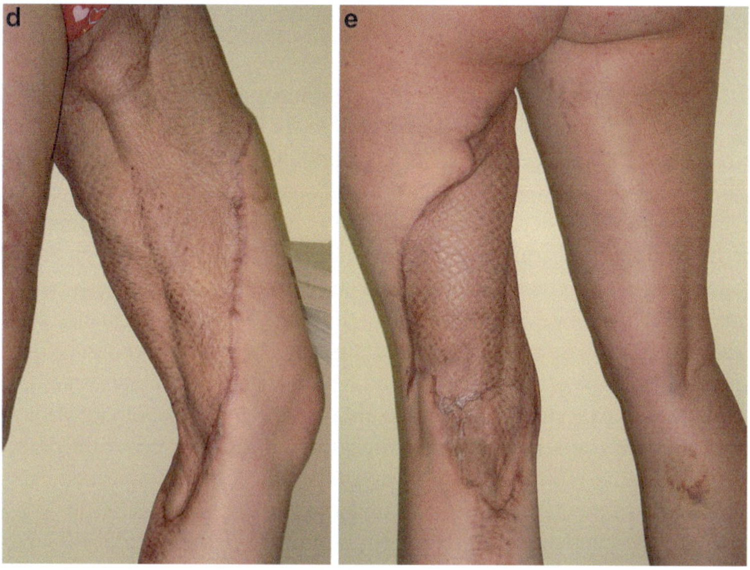

Fig. 8.7 (continued)

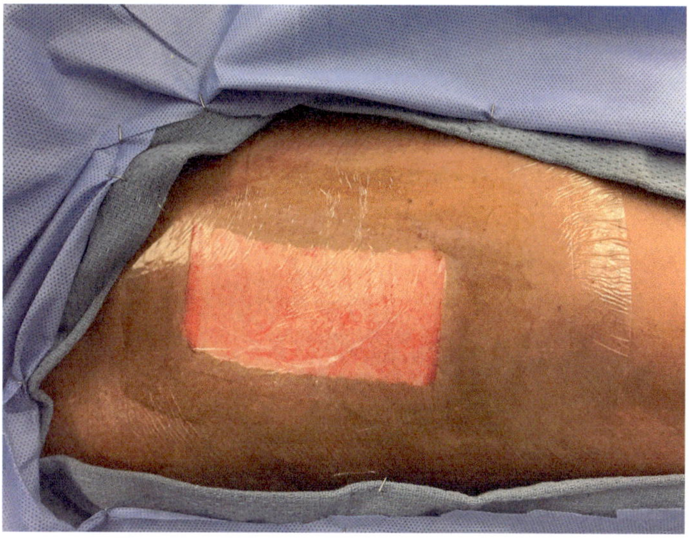

Fig. 8.8 Donor site dressed with occlusive Tegaderm dressing

until reepithelialization is complete, or the surgeon may opt to remove it earlier if the occlusive dressing leaks or appears concerning for infection. If the donor site is dressed with nonstick gauze, it is usually left in place with the overlying gauze changed as needed, until the edges of the nonstick gauze start to lift off the underlying, healing epidermis. At this time, the edges of the gauze can be serially trimmed until it is completely removed at the time of complete reepithelialization [20].

Operative Technique: FTSG

FTSG donor site selection is paramount in ensuring appropriate match of pigmentation, dermal thickness, texture, and hair growth for the recipient wound. Common donor sites for FTSGs used for coverage of facial wounds include the posterior auricular skin extending toward the mastoid process, skin of the upper eyelid, supraclavicular region, or posterior triangle of the neck. For larger, non-facial wounds, skin of the thigh, medial arm, groin, or abdomen may be suitable, though the existing hair pattern should be considered. Skin of the hypothenar eminence or antecubital fossa may be used to cover small defects on the hand. Donor site skin laxity and ease of closure should also be considered at the time of donor site selection [23].

The size and shape of the defect should be evaluated, and many surgeons find it helpful to create a pattern of the defect to aid in marking the donor site prior to graft harvest. An ellipse is marked incorporating sufficient tissue to cover the defect. The subcutaneous tissue is infiltrated with normal saline or local anesthetic to aid in hydrodissection of the dermis off of the underlying subcutaneous tissue. The FTSG is then incised and undercut, taking the entirety of the dermis while leaving behind the subcutaneous tissue. Any stippling of adipose tissue that remains attached to the dermis is sharply excised with scissors prior to FTSG inset. Pie-crusting of the FTSG is often performed to increase graft conformity and allow efflux of any fluid that gathers underneath the graft, thereby precluding its close apposition with the wound bed. The FTSG is then secured to the edges of the prepared recipient wound bed with absorbable sutures, fibrin glue, or staples. A light pressure bolster dressing or VAC is then applied to the wound in a similar fashion as described for STSGs. The donor site is closed primarily in layers, or if there is too much tension, a local tissue advancement or STSG may be necessary for definitive closure of the donor site [20].

Graft Healing

Skin graft healing requires adequate adherence of the graft to a recipient site with intact microvasculature and subsequent immobilization of the graft to support early graft neovascularization. In the first stage of graft healing, a fibrin network permits adherence of the graft to the recipient site, thereby providing close apposition to allow the cells of the graft to receive nourishment from the underlying tissues through the capillary action of plasmatic imbibition. This stage dominates wound healing for the first 24–48 h after graft apposition. If evaluated during the initial stage of healing, the graft appears white and edematous. Survival rates of thin STSGs are higher than survival of thick STSGs because of the difference of diffusion of metabolites and oxygen required during this initial process of cell imbibition [23].

By 48–72 h following graft apposition, a fibrin network is secreted between the graft and recipient bed. This allows for the ingrowth of vascular buds from the microvasculature of the recipient site into the fibrin network. The evolving vascular bed at the interface of the graft and recipient site develops anastomoses with pre-existing and newly forming blood vessels in the graft-recipient interface. This represents the inosculation phase of graft healing, which continues for up to 7 days after graft apposition. During the inosculation phase, the graft may appear mottled or have an erythematous to cyanotic hue. The success of wound healing during this phase is directly related to the microvasculature of the recipient bed, from which the vascular buds emerge. Additionally, the absolute immobilization of the graft by the postoperative dressing is essential to prevent shearing forces, which may otherwise disrupt the emerging vascular connections. Neovascularization is thought to initiate from both the base and the periphery of the recipient bed and in a healthy recipient bed will be established in the graft by postoperative day 7 [23].

Lymphatic vessels within the graft grow parallel to the microvasculature. Lymphatic flow develops within the wound bed by postoperative day 5 or 6, at which time the inflammatory effluent is drained from the wound and thereby decreases edema within the recipient site from postoperative days 7–9.

Reinnervation of the graft occurs later in the healing process but usually begins within the first 28 days postoperatively. Sensation returns to the periphery of the graft initially and gradually proceeds medially to the interior of the graft. Because there is a greater number of donor site nerve endings present in FTSGs, full return of sensation is more likely in FTSGs compared to STSGs [23].

Healing of the donor site of STSGs is characterized by reepithelialization, in which the epithelial cells from dermal appendages migrate across the islands of exposed dermis to establish a new epidermis. The more dermis that remains within the donor site after graft harvest, the faster the donor site heals since the process of epithelialization begins from multiple foci of present dermis and its appendages. Thus, donor sites of thin STSGs heal quicker than donor sites of thick STSGs. The donor site is completely reepithelized, and the epithelial cells are fully differentiated within 3–4 weeks of STSG harvest (Fig. 8.9) [23].

Factors Affecting Graft Take

There are three conditions necessary to support skin graft take: close apposition of the skin graft to the recipient site in order for the graft to receive nutrients via imbibition, the formation of nascent vasculature ingrowth from the recipient bed to the graft, and absolute sterility to reduce risk of infection. Any conditions that disrupt these processes from which the graft receives nutrients will reduce the chance of graft take. Pooling of seroma or hematoma lifts the graft away from the recipient bed, thereby decreasing the rate of diffusion of nutrients and avulsing the nascent vascular connections that are forming at the graft/recipient bed interface. Meticulous hemostasis, meshing of the graft, and bolstering or VAC placement over the graft

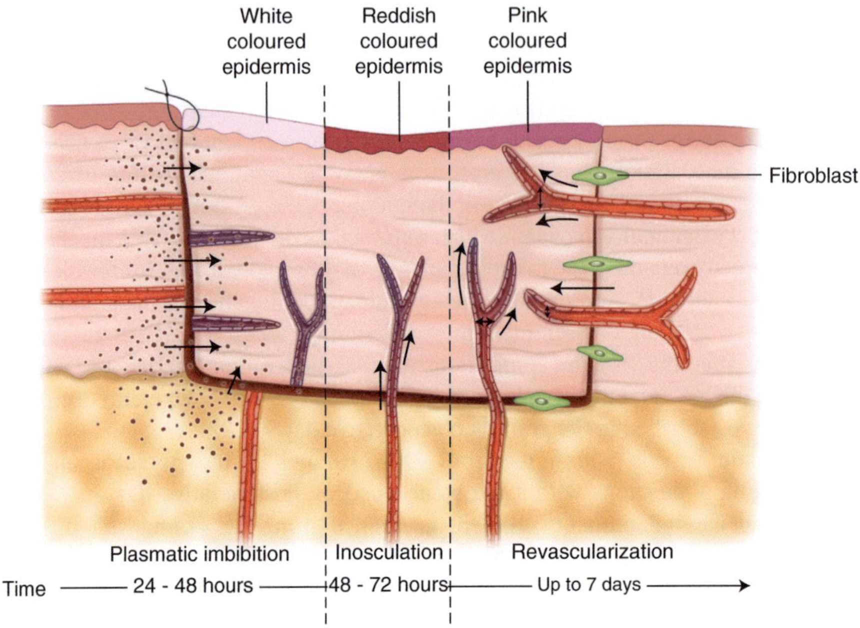

Fig. 8.9 Diagram illustrating the three stages of graft healing. For the first 48 h after grafting, the graft survives by plasmatic imbibition from the underlying wound bed, during which a gradient supports diffusion of molecules into the graft. From 48 to 72 h, the graft is nourished via inosculation, where there is ingrowth of vascular buds from the microvasculature of the recipient site into the fibrin network, forming anastomoses between the existing vascular network and nascent blood vessels. By 7 days after grafting, neovascularization occurs as there is ingrowth of new vasculature from the base and periphery of the skin graft (Adapted from Chang J, Neligan P. Plastic Surgery, 3rd ed. Elsevier, 2012)

site all serve to prevent the accumulation of fluid under the graft and preserve the early means of graft nourishment. Wounds situated on chronically edematous extremities of patients with lymphedema or chronic venous stasis disease provide a difficult environment for wound grafting since their level of baseline edema may prevent sufficient diffusion of nutrients from the wound bed to the graft in the early stages of wound healing. In patients with peripheral vascular disease and decreased perfusion of the affected limb, revascularization should be performed prior to elective skin graft or wound reconstruction to ensure adequate wound healing postoperatively [23].

Shear forces, which shift the skin graft horizontally in relation to the wound bed, may disrupt the delicate vascular ingrowth of the skin graft from the underlying recipient bed. Graft immobilization with bolstering or VAC in addition to minimization of movement of an adjacent joint is essential to prevent disruption of the nascent blood vessels. Many surgeons choose to immobilize skin grafts overlying a joint by splinting the joint for the early postoperatively period to protect the ingrowth of neovasculature [12]. In small defects (1 cm or less) overlying exposed surface without intrinsic vasculature, the graft may still take as a result of radial growth of the epithelium from the healthy edges of the wound bed surrounding the defect, as long as the epithelial cells do not completely outstrip their blood supply from the periphery.

Premature skin grafting in the presence of a contaminated or infected wound bed will significantly reduce the likelihood of skin graft take. During infection, high levels of inflammatory mediators including nitric oxide, interleukins, and cytokines lead to destruction of the fibrin bonds between skin graft and recipient bed. In particular, B-hemolytic streptococcal and pseudomonal infections produce high levels of plasmin and other proteolytic enzymes that disrupt the fibrin bonds characteristic of early wound healing. In wounds that have previously been infected, it is recommended that preoperative wound cultures be obtained to evaluate for colonization of the wound bed. In wounds with culture proven $>10^5$ organisms per gram of tissue, skin grafting is not recommended without further debridement and treatment of the bacterial colonization [24].

After initial removal of the operative dressing, the graft should be evaluated for percentage of graft adherence or "graft take." In wounds with partial graft loss, any nonadherent, nonviable tissue should be gently debrided and the resultant defect left to close by secondary intention. If the ensuing defect is large, additional skin grafting may be attempted after thorough evaluation of the likely causes of graft failure and after corrective steps have been taken to increase the likelihood of graft take. With partial graft loss, there is a higher rate of scarring, contracture, and contour deformities within the healed wound bed [17]. In certain situations, one may even attempt to regraft the area of untaken recipient site graft and achieve some viability and graft take the second time around when conditions are optimized.

Factors Effecting Wound Healing

As a general principle, wound healing requires effective delivery of oxygen and nutrients to the tissue while removing toxic metabolites and excess exudative fluid. Any condition, whether innate or acquired, which inhibits this process may lead to delayed wound healing. Oxygen delivery can be negatively impacted by systemic factors such as poor cardiac output, peripheral vascular disease, or anemia. In addition, factors that affect the local vasculature of the wound bed can have equally deleterious effects. One of the most common offenders is patient smoking or tobacco use. Smoking stimulates vasoconstriction of the microvasculature causing impaired oxygen delivery to the wound bed, in addition to releasing free oxygen radicals and toxic metabolites into circulation. Smokers are commonly found to have elevated carboxyhemoglobin levels compared to nonsmokers, which reduces the oxygen-carrying capacity of erythrocytes, stimulates endothelial changes, and increases platelet adhesiveness. Counseling on the risks of smoking especially related to wound healing complications, infection, and graft loss should be an essential component of the preoperative discussion [13].

Radiation therapy to tissue stimulates an initial inflammatory response, often causing desquamation of the targeted cells in a dose-dependent manner. As part of the inflammatory response, normal cells on the periphery of the radiated field migrate into the damaged tissue to initiate healing. Irradiated fibroblasts contribute to the synthesis of excess collagen in a wound bed with decreased density of microvasculature, thinned epidermis, and damaged and dysfunctional sweat and sebaceous glands. Irradiated tissues become stiff and fibrotic, with an increased infection risk and high likelihood of delayed healing. For this reason, irradiated tissue is not a suitable recipient wound bed for skin grafting, and flap reconstruction should be considered for all radiated wound beds. Furthermore, patients with skin graft reconstruction of oncologic defects should be allowed to heal for at least 6 weeks before undergoing radiation therapy to a grafted field [10].

Since malnutrition and chronic wounds go hand in hand, the patient's general nutritional state should be evaluated and optimized prior to wound reconstruction with skin grafting. Patients with hypoalbuminemia have a limited supply of essential amino acids necessary to stimulate collagen synthesis in a healing wound. Vitamin C is the essential cofactor for lysine and proline hydroxylation during collagen creation and cross-linking, and vitamin A is required for the process of epithelialization and normal bone metabolism and function. Zinc is an obligate cofactor for DNA polymerase and reverse transcriptase and therefore essential for the cellular proliferation that characterizes wound healing. Patients with marked malnutrition or suspected gross vitamin or mineral deficiencies should be optimized prior to considering elective wound reconstruction with skin grafting [13].

Certain medications can also have an adverse effect on the wound healing process. Chemotherapeutic agents may impair wound healing by inhibiting cellular proliferation, and frequently a chemotherapy-free period is requested prior to undertaking skin grafting. Cancer patients on Avastin may present with less than ideal vascular beds and may have difficulties in supporting adequate skin graft take. Similarly, long-term use of adrenocortical steroids delays wound epithelialization and collagen cross-linking, ultimately inhibiting wound contraction. Patients who take chronic steroids have been found to have decreased levels of cytokines prompting decreased macrophage migration, fibroblast proliferation, collagen synthesis, and angiogenesis, leading to a weakened incision. Studies have shown that the pre- and postoperative administration of vitamin A 25,000 IU/day minimizes and can reverse the deleterious effects of steroids on wounds [18].

Potential Complications of Skin Grafting

Infection is the single most destructive postoperative complication for nascent skin grafts. The inflammatory milieu that characterizes infection devitalizes the wound bed and commonly leads to skin graft failure. For this reason, it is essential that only a fully debrided wound bed free of infection be considered for skin grafting. Impeccable intraoperative sterility is essential to limit the risk of perioperative infection.

Skin graft contracture can impart functional limitations and an unsatisfactory aesthetic result in the grafted wound. Primary contraction is caused by the immediate recoil of the existing elastin fibers within the dermis of a harvested skin graft. The degree of primary contraction in a skin graft is directly proportional to the amount of dermis in a graft. The action of myofibroblasts within the newly harvested graft induces secondary contraction of a skin graft, which is inversely proportional to the dermal content of the skin graft. Therefore, STSGs have lower rates of primary contraction, but higher rates of secondary contraction in comparison to FTSGs [18].

Specialized functions such as the secretion of sweat, sebum, and the provision of hair growth within a skin graft are directly related to the thickness of dermis and the number of epithelial appendages present in the graft. Sweat glands require reinnervation by the sympathetic nervous system, whereas sebaceous gland secretion is directly related to the number of glands transferred within the graft. For this reason, thin STSGs are often noted to be drier and require regular moisturization compared to thick STSGs. FTSGs also boast improved return of sensory innervation compared to STSGs because its thicker dermal layer contains greater numbers of neurilemmal sheaths and hair follicles necessary for end organ sensory reception [18].

Pigmentation and texture difference between skin graft and recipient site is a well-known complication of skin grafting, though every effort should be made to select a donor site with similar skin tone and thickness to the healthy tissue surrounding the wound. In aesthetically sensitive locations where insufficient amount of similarly pigmented and textured skin is available for grafting, local tissue rearrangement or locoregional flap reconstruction should be considered [20].

References

1. Reverdin JL. Skin grafts – experience derived from the service of Dr Guyon at hospital Necker. Bull Imp Soc Chir Paris. 1869;10:511–5.
2. McDowell F. The source book of plastic surgery. Baltimore: Lippincott Williams & Wilkins; 1977.
3. Lawson G. On the transplantation of portions of skin for the closure of large granulating surfaces. Trans Clin Soc Lond. 1871;4:49–53.
4. Ollier LXEL. Autogenous skin grafts. Bull Acad Med Paris. 1872;1:243–6.
5. Thiersch C. About the fine anatomical changes in the healing of skin over granulations. Ver Dets Ges Chir Berlin. 1874;3:69–76.
6. Wolfe JR. A new method of performing plastic operations. BMJ. 1875;2:360–6.
7. Krause F. The transplantation of large unpedicled skin flaps. Ver Dtsch Ges Chir Berlin. 1893;22:46–52.
8. Blair VP, Brown JB. The use and uses of large split skin grafts of intermediate thickness. Surg Gynecol Obstet. 1929;49:82–97.
9. Andrew DR. The Guinea pig club. Aviat Space Environ Med. 1994;65(5):428.
10. Haubner F, Ohhman E, Pohl F, Strutz J, Gassner HG. Wound healing after radiation therapy: review of the literature. Radiat Oncol. 2012;7(1):162.
11. Parrett B, Matros E, Pribaz J, Orgill D. Lower extremity trauma: trends in the management of soft-tissue reconstruction of open tibia-fibula fractures. Plast Reconstr Surg. 2006;117(4):1315–22.

12. Shimizu R, Kishi K. Review article: skin graft. Plast Surg Int. 2012:1–5.
13. Thorne C. Grabb and Smith's plastic surgery. 1st ed. Philadelphia: Wolters Kluwer; 2015.
14. Nahabedian M. Acellular dermal matrices in primary breast reconstruction: principles, concepts, and indications. Plast Reconstr Surg. 2012;130:44S–53S.
15. Janie JE, O'Neill AC, Ahmad J, et al. Acellular dermal matrices in abdominal wall reconstruction: a systematic review of the current evidence. Plast Reconstr Surg. 2012;130(5 Suppl 2):S183–93.
16. Shores J, Gabriel A, Gupta S. Skin substitutes and alternatives: A review. Adv Skin Wound Care. 2007;20(9):493–508.
17. Buchanan P, Kung T, Cederna P. Evidence based medicine: wound closure. Plast Reconstr Surg. 2016;138:257S–70S.
18. Semer N. Practical plastic surgery for nonsurgeons. 1st ed. Philadelphia: Hanley & Belfus; 2001.
19. Singh M, Nuutila K, Kruse C, Dermietzel A, Caterson E, Eriksson E. Pixel grafting: an evolution of mincing for transplantation of full-thickness wounds. Plast Reconstr Surg. 2015;137(1):92e–9e.
20. Hazani R, Whitney R, Wilhelmi B. Optimizing aesthetic results in skin grafting. Am Surg. 2012;78:151–4.
21. Bibbo C. VERSAJET hydrosurgery technique for the preparation of full thickness skin grafts and the creation of retrograde split thickness skin grafts. J Foot Ankle Surg. 2010;49(4):404–7.
22. Gupta S. Optimal use of negative pressure wound therapy for skin grafts. Int Wound J. 2012;9:40–7.
23. Disa J, Halvorsen E, Hidalgo D. Chapter 303: open wound requiring reconstruction. In: Soube WW, editor. ACS surgery: principles and practice. New York: Decker Publishing; 2005.
24. Brown DL, Buchman SR, Cederna PS. Greenfield's surgery: scientific principles and practice. 5th ed. New York: Lippincott, Williams & Wilkins; 2010.

Chapter 9
Local and Regional Flaps

Raman Mehrzad, Daniel Kwan, Scott Schmidt, and Paul Y. Liu

Introduction

The field of reconstructive surgery is rapidly advancing. Major advances in wound care have resulted in the ability to heal small- and medium-sized defects without significant sequela. However, secondary intention is not adequate for large, complex wounds. Anatomical and functional considerations along with scar stability require a more sophisticated treatment strategy. In addition, the skin envelope is our first line of defense against microorganisms. Complex defects involving bones, joint, and tendon could lead to major complications if management and coverage are delayed. Consequently, rapid wound coverage may be may be favored over healing by secondary intention.

Finally, wound healing in a medically compromised patient remains a challenge. Polytrauma or medical comorbidities such as coronary artery disease, atherosclerosis, renal insufficiency, or diabetes will play a role in wound coverage. Wound healing becomes more challenging as cellular disturbances impair normal healing necessitating more advanced wound coverage techniques.

The first step in any wound management is assessment. One must consider the techniques available to cover the wound. The implementation of the "reconstructive ladder" provides a basis for decision-making. Technical means for coverage of complex defects include flaps or grafts. A flap is tissue that is transferred from a donor site to a recipient site with its included blood supply. This differs from a graft, which involves tissue transfer without consideration for its native perfusion. Flaps are used

---

Disclosures: None
Conflict of interest: None

R. Mehrzad, MD, MHL • D. Kwan, MD • S. Schmidt, MD • P.Y. Liu, MD, FACS (✉)
Department of Plastic and Reconstructive Surgery, Rhode Island Hospital, The Warren Alpert Medical School of Brown University, Providence, RI, USA
e-mail: pliu@lifespan.org

D.P. Orgill (ed.), *Interventional Treatment of Wounds*,
https://doi.org/10.1007/978-3-319-66990-8_9

in situations where wounds are more complicated and secondary healing is not a sustainable treatment modality. Flaps may provide optimal stable coverage in complicated wounds. As noted, flaps always include a blood supply. Orientation of this blood supply defines the flap type. In addition, flaps vary based on distance to the recipient site. Local, regional, and distant are descriptions of where the flap is located. Flaps may also differ based on anatomical composition such as the bone, muscle, fascia, or skin.

Anatomy

The skin is the human body's first line of defense against microorganisms. It is divided into the epidermis, the dermis, and the subcutaneous tissue. There are mainly two networks of blood vessels, a superficial and a deep network that supplies the skin with blood. The superficial network is located within the papillary layers of the dermis, while the deep network lies between the subcutaneous tissue and the dermis. The epidermis is supplied by the superficial network, collaterals through diffusion, and by perforating arteries that bring blood from the deeper networks [1]. Regional areas that are supplied by individual named blood vessels are termed angiosomes. These areas can encompass the skin, bone, and other soft tissues. Neighboring angiosomes can connect by small capillaries to provide a larger anatomic construct [2]. This concept regarding the angiosome as a composite unit of tissue supplied by a source artery has been well established. This has improved our ability to define smaller and more specialized flaps based on individual "perforators" in which the primary zone of perfusion is limited to the branches of an individual perforator. These perforators then anastomose with adjacent perforator territories. These isolated perforators derived from a deep vascular system through intermuscular septa or underlying muscles supply blood to the flap. Perforators can be classified into direct and indirect perforators as per the origin of the vascular supply. If they only pierce to the deep fascia, they are direct perforators since they do not transverse in any other structural tissues. Indirect perforators, however, first run through other structures before piercing the deep fascia [3].

Flap surgery requires an understanding of the native perfusion network of each individual flap. Flap elevation requires that initial flap survival be based on the defined flap blood supply until incorporation of the flap into the recipient site. Knowledge of angiosomes and flap perfusion will allow for tailoring of the surgical approach and flap design (size, shape, and location) in order to provide the best fit for the defect [2].

Blood Supply

Blood supply to a flap can be characterized as axial or random. In an axial vascular pattern flap, a particular (named) artery or group of arteries provides the axial blood supply. Flaps of this design include the axial vessel and angiosomes of the surrounding vascular areas. In contrast, random flaps do not include an axial vessel. Blood supply is based on a network of many small (unamed) vessels of the subdermal plexus [3–5].

Flaps

Flaps are tissues lifted from a donor site and moved to a recipient site based on a blood supply. As they contain perfused tissue, they can aid in the healing of the recipient site because they are not dependent upon the blood supply within the recipient site Consequently, the quality of the wound bed at the recipient site is not as critical in comparison to the use of grafts. Grafts do not carry their own blood supply and is therefore dependent on the recipient's wound bed vascularization. With this foundation, flaps offer an opportunity to use thicker or larger tissue, and the volume of transferred tissue can be greater than that of a graft. Further, flaps can also contain many types of tissue, including the muscle, bone, fascia, skin, and nerve. However, a continuous vascular supply is required for successful flap transfer, and if the blood supply is compromised, the flap will not survive.

Indications for Flap Coverage

There are several indications for flap coverage. In general, flap surgery has broad applicability with nearly limitless array of flaps available to cover very complex defects. The most typical scenario to perform flap surgery to wounds is when primary repair is unattainable without undue tension and grafts are not sufficient. Flap reconstruction is an excellent choice in the setting of exposed tendon or the bone. Flap surgery is also a great option when large or composite defects exist. Breast reconstruction would be a typical example of this where flaps would be favored over grafting due to the tissue required and cosmetic nature of reconstruction [6].

Wound factors that need to be considered when performing flap surgery include the size of the defect, functional requirements, and location. The patient's medical history, the donor site morbidity, as well as the cosmetic and functional results need to all be taken into account. Furthermore the wound bed needs to be evaluated for what is missing and cofactors that may play a role such as infection and radiation.

Since there are different types of flaps and designs, the flap choice is a selective process based on what is available and what is required.

- **Defects on the face:** these are best closed with local flaps, using the same tissue move as a random pattern transposition or rotational flap, e.g., V-Y advancement flaps and rhomboid flaps [6, 7].
- **Defects on the trunk:** these are less contingent on aesthetics and typically require a bigger tissue volume.
- **Defects on limbs:** areas of the feet and hand could be difficult to replace and require special consideration when choosing flaps closure. Most areas of the hands for instance require thin flaps in order to obtain the optimal functional results.

Preparation for Flaps

In contrast to grafts, the wound bed does not need to be vascularized. However, the wound needs to be clean and free from infectious, necrotic, or ischemic tissue, and edema should be minimized.

Classification

Commonly, flaps are categorized as local, regional, and distant flaps. This chapter will focus on the first two mentioned. In general, if possible, simple local flaps are used. However, if local options are not available or if aesthetic and functional results are better achieved, a distant or regional flap is used.

Local Flaps

Local flaps utilize tissue that abuts the defect that requires coverage. Local flaps are subdivided in skin flaps or fasciocutaneous flaps. A non-individualized network of blood supply connecting from muscle perforators supply the skin flaps, consisting of subcutaneous fat and skin. Fasciocutaneous flaps differ in the way that they also include underlying fascia with additional blood supply. Local flaps are used to cover defects in areas without sufficient tissue laxity to achieve primary closure. Local or sedation anesthesias are typically enough for most local flap transfers.

To allow for primary repair in addition to providing tissue to the recipient site for coverage of the defect, the donor side for a local flap should ideally have enough laxity. However, a skin graft can be used if primary repair of the donor site cannot be accomplished. The head and neck are common areas where local flaps are used after removal of cutaneous carcinomas. Most local flaps use random pattern blood supply with no specific named vascular supply. V-Y flaps, rhomboid flaps, Z-plasty, and bilobed flaps are example of local flaps, V-Y flaps, and Z-plasty.

Two layers are typically used to close the donor site for a local flap: (1) a layer of an absorbable deep dermal fine sutures followed by closure of the skin with intradermal absorbable transcutaneous permanent suture. Due to the decreased reactivity component, absorbable or permanent monofilament sutures are recommended. It is important to not tie the sutures too tightly or leave them to long as suture marks will be visible, decreasing the cosmetic results. Moreover, permanent sutures usually result in less inflammation as long as they are removed in an early state; for facial reconstruction, suture should typically be removed between 3 and 7 days [8].

Another important aspect of local flaps is the length and width ratio. To warrant adequate vascular supply, this ratio should be aimed to be 1:1 in most cases. However, depending on the underlying vascular pattern, this ratio is somewhat variable. A good rule of thumb is to assess the vascularity of the location. Locations with poorly vascularized areas such as the lower extremities require the flap length to be equal to flap width. Richer vascular areas such as the face or flaps with axial vascular patterns can be longer with a narrower base [8].

Notably, local flaps may not take their final form for up to 6 months and may remain erythematous and edematous for many weeks. Thus it is important to delay any revision procedures until flap maturity [8].

Regional Flaps

Regional flaps utilize tissue in the vicinity of the defect without abutting the defect. Most regional flaps are musculocutaneous. Thus, the morbidity of muscle harvest of the donor site must be considered. A forehead flap for nasal tip reconstruction is a classical example. The skin similar in color and quality of the recipient site is used, and regional flaps are typically preferred in cosmetic sensitive areas such as the face for the long-term aesthetic outcome [8].

Angiosome territories are used in regional flaps, and they require identification of the source vessel upon which the tissue transfer will be based, including the arc of rotation of a flap based on that specific vessel. The skin island that is required is typically centered over the vessel, and a handheld Doppler could be used to follow the vessel in most cases [8].

Flap Composition

A variety of tissues could be included in local and regional flaps, and the nature of the defect that is being repaired decides which flap type to use [9]. For example, deep or large tissue defects can be repaired with musculocutaneous flaps, while defects that include the bone can be repaired with osteocutaneous flaps.

Various Types of Flaps

Skin Flaps

The most common utilized local flaps are skin flaps. These cover surgical or traumatic defects and are used to afford primary closure and cover skin defects in areas without sufficient tissue laxity. Local flaps are preferred over skin grafts since it is a simpler and more cosmetically enhanced method of primary closure, and it offers the benefit to avoid a surgery at a second site.

Muscle Flaps

The nerve and associated vascular pedicles of the muscle is used as a muscle flap for defect coverage [10]. The blood supply of the muscle is carried with the muscle and includes the overlying tissue. Since muscle flaps are intensely vascularized, a split-thickness skin graft can be placed if enough skin coverage is not available, to complete wound closure. Attention must be given to the donor site deformity from the muscle sacrifice, since muscle flaps harvest some or all of a particular muscle. Typically, muscle flaps are used for trauma-induced defects, functional purposes, or for large ablative purposes. A common example of a muscle flap for defect coverage is the medical gastrocnemius flap to cover compound fractures of the proximal leg or after total knee replacement complicated with anterior tissue loss [10].

Musculocutaneous Flaps

As the name proposes, a musculocutaneous flap includes the overlying skin, its subcutaneous tissue, and the muscle [10]. These flaps are used, for example, in breast reconstruction or other deep or large defects, such as the latissimus dorsi musculocutaneous flap or the transverse rectus abdominis musculocutaneous (TRAM) [11].

Fasciocutaneous Flaps

Fasciocutaneous flaps include underlying the fascia, the skin, and the subcutaneous tissue and are typically less bulky than musculocutaneous flaps. Thus, they do not include any muscle but instead are based on vessels arising in fascial planes in between or over the muscles. They are utilized to cover large superficial defects when skin flaps are not sufficient to provide optimal coverage. The anterolateral thigh flap used for perineal and genital skin defect is a common example of a fasciocutaneous flap [12].

Osteocutaneous Flaps

When needed to replace missing bone in the head and neck area or the long bones of the extremities, an osteocutaneous flap, which contains a bony component, is used. The fibular free flap is an example of an osteocutaneous flap.

Complications

There are a series of complications that could appear with flap surgery including seroma, hematoma, vascular compromise, surgical site infection, hematoma, and complications specific to the donor site.

The most feared complication is vascular compromise that leads to flaps failure. Failure to follow the angiosome concept of blood supply and poor flap design can lead to partial flap loss. This is typically seen when the flap extends beyond the anatomic boundary of the flap's vascularity, i.e., when there is too much tissue involved. Kinking or torsion of the vascular pedicle during transfer of the flap to the recipient site can also lead to vascular compromise. Thrombosis of the artery or vein is typically the cause of vascular compromise in free flaps. The blood supply is monitored by clinically evaluate the color, capillary refill, bleeding, temperature, edema, and appearance of the flap. A Doppler ultrasound is used to evaluate the arterial and venous signals and can assist in improving the flap salvages rates [13–16].

Recent studies show that tissue oximetry can detect vascular compromise before clinical signs appear. Tissue oximetry has shown to decrease the rate of flap loss from 2.9 to 0.4% [15]. In fact, using tissue oximetry can also reduce time spent in an intensive monitoring setting from 24 to 15 h with significant cost savings and minimal risk of missing a failing free flap [17–19]. Therefore, as a general rule, the first 3 days postsurgery, both Doppler ultrasound and tissue oximetry can be used as initial assessments to monitor flaps for vascular compromise. The frequency of Doppler ultrasound monitoring is every 15 min for the first hour, every 30 min for the second hour, every hour for the next 10 h, and subsequently with routine vital signs every 4 h [15]. If vascular compromise is suspected, the patient should be taken to the operating room for evaluation of the cause and consideration of revision of the flap for salvage. Future technology is currently being assessed and studied to discover new strategies for early recognition and intervention of vascular compromise. These include near-infrared spectroscopy and smartphone and mobile application including multimedia technology which in limited studies have shown to be effective [20, 21]. However, randomized control trials are needed to establish the utility and effectives of these methods in larger populations. If total flap necrosis is detected, the flap needs to be removed. However, debridement and local wound care can be sufficient for partial flap loss if the components of the wound with poor vasculature remains covered.Intraoperative vasospasm is a complication seen in flap surgery. A common treatment modality to treat intraoperative vasospasm is with papaverine; however, shortage of this medication has frequently been seen and may occur in the future. A recent study showed that substituting lidocaine or nicardipine for papaverine to treat vasospasm did not demonstrate an increased rate of flap loss or return to the operating room and thus making these two drugs safe and efficacious alternatives to papaverine [22].

Predicting future viability of tissue while still in the operating room would have major impact on patient's healthcare outcomes since surgeons will be able to intervene perioperatively. To date, no studies have demonstrated a sufficient and accurate method to evaluate tissue perfusion. However, recent studies performed on rats with reverse McFarlane dorsal skin flaps showed that two 750-msec intraoperative near-infrared (NIR) fluorescence images obtained at time 0 and at 5 min after injection of indocyanine green accurately predicted skin flap viability 7 days postsurgery [23]. HyperView™ is a technology that uses proprietary spectrometer to measure light absorption in blood molecules to determine levels of oxyhemoglobin and deoxyhemoglobin and oxygen saturation in superficial tissue. It is a handheld, portable diagnostic imaging device that can assess tissue oxygenation without contacting the patient. The product is intended for use by doctors and healthcare professionals as a noninvasive tissue oxygenation measurement system that reports an approximate value of oxygen saturation, oxyhemoglobin level, and deoxyhemoglobin level in superficial tissue [24].

Flap loss with associated morbidity could be a result of anastomotic thrombosis if not identified and intervened on rapidly. NIR fluorescence imagery was studied in Yorkshire pigs and was able to successfully evaluate flap perfusion and anastomotic thrombosis intraoperatively. It identified large decreases in perfusion in the tissue of the thrombosed flap within 2 min [25]. The use of an intraoperative, NIR fluorescence imaging system for evaluation of perforator location and flap perfusion was first tried in human in 2010 in six subjects. Three dose levels of indocyanine green were assessed using the fluorescence-assisted resection and exploration (FLARE) imaging system. Here they used light-emitting diodes for fluorescence excitation, a different system than the current commercially available ones. The operating surgeons were blinded to the imaging results. The trial was successful; however, due to the of small sample size, the authors did not have sufficient power to detect statistical significance. Nevertheless, this trial demonstrated that NIR assessment of perforator flap for breast reconstruction is reasonable with a light-emitting diode-based system. The dose that yields the best observed contrast-to-background ratio for assessment of flap perfusion was 4 mg of indocyanine green per injection [26].

Spatial frequency domain imaging (SFDI) is a wide-field optical diagnostic technique that is intended to do a large area interrogation of the target tissue and could measure and map absorption coefficients (μa) and reduced scattering coefficients (μ's) in thick tissue such as the skin. SFDI presents a noncontact, objective method of tissue oxygenation over a large field of view. A study done on hemifacial composite flap compromise on Yorkshire pigs demonstrated that SFDI successfully captured changes in oxygenation parameters in all composite tissue flaps. Significant changes in total hemoglobin, oxyhemoglobin, and deoxyhemoglobin were observed relative to controls. The results of this study suggest that this technology could be a favorable tool in providing intraoperative guidance to pedicle vessel integrity. Although further research on this essential topic is warranted, near-infrared fluorescence images and SFDI could be viable tools to predict future viability of tissue [27]. In fact, a human pilot study was performed where three female patients undergoing unilateral breast reconstruction after mastectomy were enrolled to assess the use of SFDI in perforator flap breast reconstruction. Tissue oxyhemoglobin concentration, tissue deoxyhemoglobin concentration, and tissue oxygen saturation were able to be detected with SFDI and suggest that SFDI has the potential to give intraoperative oxygenation images during surgery in real time and potentially improve clinical outcomes by preventing complications [28].

Perforator selection is critical for some surgical indication, such as bilateral deep inferior epigastric perforator (DIEP) flap breast reconstruction, to minimize perfusion-related flap complications. Kamali and colleagues showed that lateral row-based perforators result in significantly less fat necrosis than medial row-based perforators in bilateral DIEP flaps [29]. Moreover, recent data suggest that when a lateral row perforator is added to a dominant medial row perforator, the risk of fat necrosis decreases [29].

References

1. Clark JM, Wang TD. Local flaps in scar revision. Facial Plast Surg. 2001 Nov;17(4):295–308.
2. Guyuron B, Eriksson E, Persing J, Chung K, et al. Plastic surgery: indications and practice, 2-Volume set, 1e. Chapter 8. 2009. Elsiver: Amsterdam, Netherlands.
3. Blondeel PN, Van Landuyt KH, Monstrey SJ, Hamdi M, Matton GE, Allen RJ, Dupin C, Feller AM, Koshima I, Kostakoglu N, Wei FC. "Gent" consensus on perforator flap terminology: preliminary definitions. Plast Reconstr Surg. 2003 Oct;112(5):1378–83.
4. Taylor GI, Corlett RJ, Dhar SC, Ashton MW. The anatomical (angiosome) and clinical territories of cutaneous perforating arteries: development of the concept and designing safe flaps. Plast Reconstr Surg. 2011;127:1447.
5. Taylor GI, Pan WR. Angiosomes of the leg: anatomic study and clinical implications. Plast Reconstr Surg. 1998;102:599.
6. Pribaz JJ, Chester CH, Barrall DT. The extended V-Y flap. Plast Reconstr Surg. 1992;90:275.
7. Guo L, Pribaz JR, Pribaz JJ. Nasal reconstruction with local flaps: a simple algorithm for management of small defects. Plast Reconstr Surg. 2008;122:130e.
8. Morris D, Butler C, Collins K. Principles of grafts and flaps for reconstructive surgery. UpToDate. 2016 May
9. Yao ST. Vascular implantation into skin flap: experimental study and clinical application: a preliminary report. Plast Reconstr Surg. 1981;68:404.
10. Mathes SJ, Alpert BS. Advances in muscle and musculocutaneous flaps. Clin Plast Surg. 1980;7:15.
11. Hartrampf CR, Scheflan M, Black PW. Breast reconstruction with a transverse abdominal island flap. Plast Reconstr Surg. 1982;69:216.
12. Luo S, Raffoul W, Piaget F, Egloff DV. Anterolateral thigh fasciocutaneous flap in the difficult perineogenital reconstruction. Plast Reconstr Surg. 2000;105:171.
13. Salgado CJ, Moran SL, Mardini S. Flap monitoring and patient management. Plast Reconstr Surg. 2009;124:e295.

14. Paydar KZ, Hansen SL, Chang DS, et al. Implantable venous Doppler monitoring in head and neck free flap reconstruction increases the salvage rate. Plast Reconstr Surg. 2010;125:1129.
15. Lin SJ, Nguyen MD, Chen C, et al. Tissue oximetry monitoring in microsurgical breast reconstruction decreases flap loss and improves rate of flap salvage. Plast Reconstr Surg. 2011;127:1080.
16. Rozen WM, Chubb D, Whitaker IS, Acosta R. The efficacy of postoperative monitoring: a single surgeon comparison of clinical monitoring and the implantable Doppler probe in 547 consecutive free flaps. Microsurgery. 2010;30:105.
17. Ricci JA, Vargas CR, Ho OA, Lin SJ, Tobias AM, Lee BT. Evaluating the use of tissue oximetry to decrease intensive unit monitoring for free flap breast reconstruction. Ann Plast Surg. 2017 Mar;79(1):42–6.
18. Ricci JA, Vargas CR, Lin SJ, Tobias AM, Taghinia AH, Lee BT. A novel free flap monitoring system using tissue oximetry with text message alerts. J Reconstr Microsurg. 2016 Jun;32(5):415–20.
19. Koolen PG, Vargas CR, Ho OA, Ibrahim AM, Ricci JA, Tobias AM, Winters HA, Lin SJ, Lee BT. Does increased experience with tissue oximetry monitoring in microsurgical breast reconstruction lead to decreased flap loss? Learn Eff Plast Reconstr Surg. 2016 Apr;137(4):1093–101.
20. Lohman RF, Langevin CJ, Bozkurt M, et al. A prospective analysis of free flap monitoring techniques: physical examination, external Doppler, implantable Doppler, and tissue oximetry. J Reconstr Microsurg. 2013;29:51.
21. Hwang JH, Mun GH. An evolution of communication in postoperative free flap monitoring: using a smartphone and mobile messenger application. Plast Reconstr Surg. 2012;130:125.
22. Ricci JA, Koolen PG, Shah J, Tobias AM, Lee BT, Lin SJ. Comparing the outcomes of different agents to treat vasospasm at microsurgical anastomosis during the Papaverine shortage. Plast Reconstr Surg. 2016 Sep;138(3):401e–8e.
23. Wada H, Vargas CR, Angelo J, Faulkner-Jones B, Paul MA, Ho OA, Lee BT, Frangioni JV. Accurate prediction of tissue viability at postoperative day 7 using only two intraoperative subsecond near-infrared fluorescence images. Plast Reconstr Surg. 2017 Feb;139(2):354–63.
24. HyperMed. Available at: https://hypermed.com/products
25. Vargas CR, Nguyen JT, Ashitate Y, Silvestre J, Venugopal V, Neacsu F, Kettenring F, Frangioni JV, Gioux S, Lee BT. Near-infrared imaging for the assessment of anastomotic patency, thrombosis, and reperfusion in microsurgery: a pilot study in a porcine model. Microsurgery. 2015 May;35(4):309–14.
26. Lee BT, Hutteman M, Gioux S, Stockdale A, Lin SJ, Ngo LH, Frangioni JV. The FLARE intraoperative near-infrared fluorescence imaging system: a first-in-human clinical trial in perforator flap breast reconstruction. Plast Reconstr Surg. 2010 Nov;126(5):1472–81.
27. Vargas CR, Nguyen JT, Ashitate Y, Angelo J, Venugopal V, Kettenring F, Neacsu F, Frangioni JV, Gioux S, Lee BT. Intraoperative Hemifacial composite flap perfusion assessment using spatial frequency domain imaging: a pilot study in preparation for facial transplantation. Ann Plast Surg. 2016 Feb;76(2):249–55.
28. Nguyen JT, Lin SJ, Tobias AM, Gioux S, Mazhar A, Cuccia DJ, Ashitate Y, Stockdale A, Oketokoun R, Durr NJ, Moffitt LA, Durkin AJ, Tromberg BJ, Frangioni JV, Lee BT. A novel pilot study using spatial frequency domain imaging to assess oxygenation of perforator flaps during reconstructive breast surgery. Ann Plast Surg. 2013 Sep;71(3):308–15.
29. Kamali P, Lee M, Becherer BE, Wu W, Curiel D, Tran BN, Tobias AM, Lin SJ, Lee BT. Medial row perforators are associated with higher rates of fat necrosis in bilateral DIEP flap breast reconstruction. Plast Reconstr Surg. 2017 Jul;140(1):19–24.

Chapter 10
Perforator Flaps

Joon Pio (Jp) Hong, Donghoon Choi, and Hyunsuk (Peter) Suh

Evolution to Perforator Flap

Since the first flap from the days of Sushruta onto the middle ages and into the modern wars, evolution of the flaps continues [1]. From using various random pattern skin flaps based on width and length ratio, surgeons slowly began to challenge this idea and understood the function and importance of vascularization [2, 3]. This led to the use of axial pattern flaps such as groin flaps [4, 5]. As skin flaps were being accepted, the use of muscle flaps and musculocutaneous flaps for reconstruction gained wider acceptance. These two new concepts in reconstructive surgery naturally led to recognizing various different types of circulation to the skin entering the deep fascia [6]. With the accumulated knowledge of the source of skin circulation and the territory it supplies, this leads to an era of skin flaps [7]. Based on the anatomical findings, elevation of the skin with its deep fascia represented a new vascular basis for flap design.

A fasciocutaneous flap includes the skin, subcutaneous tissue, and the underlying deep fascia. The vascular supply is derived at the base of the flap from musculocutaneous perforators or direct septocutaneous branches of major arteries. Cormack and Lamberty classified fasciocutaneous flaps based on vascular anatomy [8]. They are classified into the following: Type A flap is supplied by multiple fasciocutaneous perforators that enter at the base of the flap and extend throughout the longitudinal length; Type B flap has a single fasciocutaneous perforator; Type C flap is based on multiple small perforators that run along a fascial septum; and Type D flap is an osteomusculofasciocutaneous flap and is based on multiple small perforators

J.P. Hong, MD, PhD, MMM (✉) • D. Choi, MD • H. Suh, MD, PhD
Department of Plastic Surgery, Asan Medical Center University of Ulsan, Seoul, South Korea
e-mail: joonphong@amc.seoul.kr

D.P. Orgill (ed.), *Interventional Treatment of Wounds*,
https://doi.org/10.1007/978-3-319-66990-8_10

similar to the Type C flap but also includes a portion of adjacent muscle and bone. This classification basically recognizes the arteries which pass along intermuscular and inter-compartmental fascial septa to reach the overlying deep fascia and in turn the superficial fascia and skin. Thus, the concept of "perforator" is actually being clinically used.

Nakajima et al. further expanded the types of fasciocutaneous flaps, in addition to arteries which passed along intermuscular and inter-compartmental fascial septa, into six different types of perforators piercing the deep fascia feeding to the plexus of the skin [9]. This finding shows that any reasonable-sized artery piercing the deep fascia can be used as a fasciocutaneous flap.

Although the actual "perforators" were being used since the fasciocutaneous flaps, further refinements in application have led to the concept of perforator flaps. Perforator flaps have evolved from musculocutaneous and fasciocutaneous flaps without the muscle or fascial carrier. In 1989, Koshima and Soeda first used the term "perforator flaps" in their harvest for the paraumblical skin and fat island flap based on a muscular perforator [10]. Since then, perforator-based flaps using the lower abdomen skin flaps were being applied for breast reconstruction [11, 12]. It was a natural evolution as reconstruction needed fine-tuning while aiming to minimize donor morbidities [13]. A good example of this evolution would be the change from transverse rectus abdominis muscle (TRAM) flap to muscle sparing TRAM to deep inferior epigastric perforator (DIEP) flaps. Slowly other perforator-based flaps were being introduced from various parts of the skin.

Transformation of these flaps has shown that neither a passive muscle carrier nor the underlying fascial plexus of vessels is necessary for flap survival [10]. Thus, a perforator flap, although nomenclature is still under debate, can be generally accepted as a skin flap (with or without fascia) based on a single perforator [14].

Nomenclature

The nomenclature of perforator flaps deserves a separate section as it is confusing and oftentimes misstated. Perforator flaps have been named based on their location (e.g., anterolateral thigh, ALT, flap), arterial supply (e.g., superficial circumflex iliac artery perforator, SCIP, flap and deep inferior epigastric artery perforator, DIEP, flap), or the muscle of origin (e.g., gastrocnemius perforator flap). While Hallock simply defines a perforator as any vessel that pierces through the fenestration in the deep fascia regardless of origin, Wei et al. promote the concept of a true perforator flap which is only a perforator passing through a muscle segment [14, 15]. Thus, a clear definition and classification for perforator flap were needed. Despite the debate and confusion, a consensus document for perforator flaps terminology was reached. It stated a perforator that pierces through the deep fascia without traversing any other structural tissues were called direct perforators while indirect perforators run through deeper structures such as the muscles, septum, and perimysium [16].

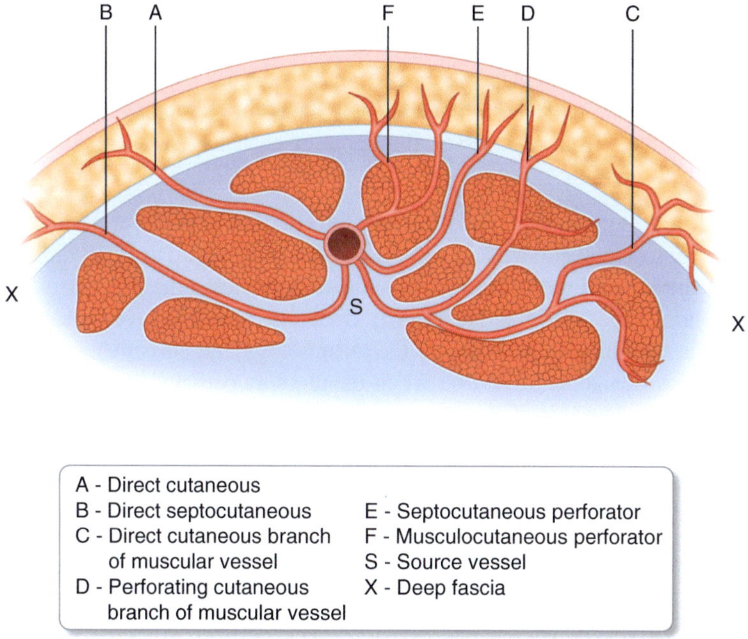

Fig. 10.1 The gent consensus paper simplified it into five types of perforator based on the surgical approach for dissection of the perforators

Evolved from the six patterns of fascial perforators of Nakakima et al., the consensus paper simplified it into five types of perforator based on the surgical approach for dissection of the perforators (Fig. 10.1): Type 1, direct perforators perforate the deep fascia only; Type 2, indirect muscle perforators predominantly supply the subcutaneous tissues; Type 3, indirect muscle perforators predominantly supply the muscle but have secondary braches to the subcutaneous tissues; Type 4, indirect perimysial perforators travel within the perimysium between muscle fibers before piercing the deep fascia; and Type 5, indirect septal perforators travel through the intermuscular septum before piercing the deep fascia. Based on this distinction of different perforators, the consensus paper gives definitions and classification for perforator flap as the following:

Definition 1. A perforator flap is a flap consisting of the skin and/or subcutaneous fat. The vessels that supply the blood to the flap are isolated perforator(s). These perforators may pass either through or in between deep tissues (mostly muscle).

Definition 2. A muscle perforator is a blood vessel that traverses through the septum to supply the overlying skin.

Definition 3. A septal perforator is a blood vessel that traverses only through the septum to supply the overlying skin.

Definition 4. A flap that is vascularized by a muscle perforator is called a muscle perforator flap.

Definition 5. A flap vascularized by a septal perforator is called a septal perforator flap.

Definition 6. A perforator flap should be named after the nutrient artery or vessels and not after the underlying muscle. If there is a potential to harvest multiple perforator flaps from one vessel, the name of each flap should be based on its anatomical region or muscle.

This terminology and the classification into indirect and direct perforator flaps and further into septal and muscle perforator flaps were set up to clearly identify the course of these small terminal branches before they pierce the deep fascia and the technical implications during the surgical procedure [16]. However, recent innovations in this field have made some of the terminology and classification somewhat misleading. An example would be when using short pedicled flaps where source vessel cannot be determined. As with all evolution, new classification and terminology need to be updated.

Perforasome Concept

Like the angiosome concept showing the vascular territory of a source vessel, one must understand the anatomy and physiology of a single perforator territory to obtain the ideal design of the perforator flap [7]. The perforasome theory by Saint-Cyr reported four major characteristics of a perforator flap: (1) Each perforasome is linked with adjacent perforasomes by means of direct and indirect linking vessels; (2) flap design and skin paddle oriental should be based on the direction of the linking vessels, which is axial in the extremities and perpendicular to the midline in the trunk; (3) filling of the perforasomes occurs within perforasome of the same source artery first followed by perforators of the other adjacent source arteries; and (4) mass vascularity of a perforator found adjacent to an articulation is directed away from that same articulation [17].

This theory provides insights to perforator flap vascularity and can clinically guide to harvest a safer free or pedicle perforator flap.

Clinical Application

Preoperative Evaluation

When secondary intension healing is not enough, then plans for reconstruction are prepared. The initial evaluation of the wound involves visual and manual examination. An examination on the location, size, depth, and character of the wound is made. When vital structures such as the bone, tendons, joints, viscera, and majors vessels are exposed, timely coverage is essential. Frequently, negative wound pressure therapy with or without skin grafts may not be enough to prevent secondary complications such as osteomyelitis, desiccation and loss of tendon function, contracture of joint region, bowel perforation, and rupture of vessels. These cases will warrant coverage with a well-vascularized tissue to prevent further complications and to obtain healing. Detailed evaluation of neurological deficit as well as vascular and skeletal status has to be performed to develop a plan for reconstruction. Also, the presence of comorbidities including smoking, diabetes, obesity, and peripheral vascular disease should be accounted for. Through the detailed evaluation, it will allow to address the local wound, formulate a feasible reconstructive plan, and foresee the final outcome. One must also take the socioeconomic status, rehabilitative potential, patient's motivation, and compliance into consideration as the whole process prior and after reconstruction may be complex and time-consuming for the patient.

The first and the foremost important evaluation when considering not only perforator flap but any reconstruction is to examine the vascular status. Any flap used will require a stable vascularity to the flap and also will require a recipient vessel when planning a free flap. If the wound is in the extremity, physical examination of palpable pulse, color, capillary refill, and turgor of the extremity allows assessing initial status. Acoustic Doppler and duplex scans can be used to obtain additional information. The use of preoperative arteriography is considered when physical/Doppler exam reveals inconclusive vascular status, chronic vascular disease is suspected, and/or previous history of trauma is noted. The use of computed tomographic angiography may especially be useful not only to obtain vascular information of the recipient region but can provide perforator information of the donor flap facilitating the planning and the surgical procedure [18, 19].

The perforator flap can be harvested on three planes. The first plane of elevation is subfascial (under and including the deep fascia, same as fasciocutaneous flap), second plane is suprafascial (above the deep fascia without including the deep fascia), and the third plane is a relatively recently identified plane which is on the superficial fascia located between the deep and the superficial fat. Each plane provides unique properties to the flap allowing tailored harvest according to the character of the defect. The subfascially elevated flap with its deep fascia can be used to reconstruct tendon defects, and the suprafacially elevated flap can provide extra fat bulk for a deeper defect [20]. When the flap is elevated on the superficial fascia, it can be thin and pliable adequate for resurfacing skin only defects [21]. Although elevation on different planes can be technically demanding, it will provide tailored approach for each defect.

Debridement and Wound Preparation

The importance of debridement can never be overstated. It is undoubtedly the most important step in the whole process during reconstruction. Debridement must cover the devitalized soft tissue and bone and be performed until fresh bleeding is noted.

Table 10.1 Widely used perforator flaps

Abbreviation	Full name of flap	Nutrient artery
ALT	Anterolateral thigh perforator	Descending branch of lateral femoral circumflex vessels
DIEP	Deep inferior epigastric perforator	Deep inferior epigastric vessels
TAP	Thoracodorsal artery perforator	Thoracodorsal artery vessels
SCIP	Superficial circumflex iliac artery perforator	Superficial circumflex iliac vessels
SGAP	Superior gluteal artery perforator	Superior gluteal vessels
IGAP	Inferior gluteal artery perforator	Inferior gluteal vessels
ICAP	Intercostal perforator	Intercostal vessels
SAP	Sural artery perforator	Sural vessels
AMT	Anteromedial thigh perforator	Innominate branch of descending branch of lateral femoral circumflex vessels
IMAP	Intercostal mammary artery perforator	Intercostal mammary vessels
PAP	Profunda femoris artery perforator	Profunda femoris vessels

Multiple stages of debridement may be needed to achieve adequate wound bed prior to soft tissue coverage. The details of debridement have been discussed in the previous chapter.

When the wound is not sufficient enough to undergo reconstruction, the vacuum-assisted closure can be used to optimize the wound bed and minimize dressing changes until definitive reconstruction. It must be used with caution and in conjunction with serial debridement. It does not replace surgical debridement and should not be used in heavily contaminated wound with necrotic tissues.

Selection of Flap

Perforator flaps can be used both as a local and free flap depending on the defect's location, size, composition, and the availability of the perforator around the defect. Some of the popular perforator flaps are listed in Table 10.1.

Perforator Flap as a Local Flap

The perforator flap concept overcomes the limits of classical local flaps and further widens the application. The planning for the local perforator flap begins with a handheld Doppler marking the potential perforators as a pedicle for the flap. The freestyle approach identifying the perforator and further dissecting toward the source vessel allows improved movement and better flap outcome [22, 23]. The propeller flap is one of the most commonly used pedicled island perforator flap which reaches the recipient site through an axial rotation [24]. When a perforator propeller flap is being elevated, the perforator is dissected free from the fascial and fat adhesions to minimize the chance of kinking. Although less rotation less the chance for kinking, the skin island may be safely rotated up to 180 degrees.

An example of perforator flap overcoming the limitations of classical flaps can be shown with reconstructing the sacral sore. A classical approach would be to use a fasciocutaneous or a musculocutaneous V-Y advancement flap for reconstruction. However, there are many limitations in this approach. The insertion of the gluteus maximus muscle may be divided leading to further muscle dysfunction, high tension on the midline of the sacrum is often noted after setting the flap leading to dehiscence, and when the defect is large, bilateral V-Y flaps have to be used. On the contrary, the local perforator flap will allow multiple flap designs based on various perforators around the defect, minimizes muscle sacrifice, increased arc of rotation, and superior aesthetic outcome. The similar can be said about thigh defects. Using the perforator flaps allows having increased ranges of motion of flaps with good aesthetic outcome. Figure 10.2 shows a patient with a 14 × 8 cm defect after cancer resection on the middle and lower thigh. A perforator flap is designed based on the preoperative Doppler findings. If a CT angiogram is used, multiple perforators leading to the gluteal skin can be noted, and this may facilitate the selection for perforators. After exploring the perforator and confirming a strong pulse, the rest of the flap is designed. An 18 × 8 cm flap is designed. The length of the flap is determined based on the measurement from the perforator to the edge of the defect. The same length is then marked from the perforator to the distal edge of the flap (A). The width is designed as the size of the defect while considering the shape of the defect as well as the closure of the donor site. The next step is to identify a viable perforator. If the perforator is near, a subfascial elevation of the flap can be made to identify the perforator. If this is not feasible, a small exploratory incision can be made along the anticipated design. When there are multiple perforators, several factors can be considered to choose the optimal perforator: perforator allowing flap design with tension-free closure of the donor site, one nearer to the defect to minimize the extent of the design, and visual inspection of the perforator with the greatest pulse and large caliber. Among these factors, I personally consider the perforator pulse and caliber to be the most important. After choosing the perforator, final modification of the flap design can be made. The flap can be elevated subfascially (as a fasciocutaneous flap) or suprafacially based on this perforator and then rotated to cover the defect. In this case, a suprafascial approach was made based on a single perforator (B). Prior to rotation or if reduction in perfusion is suspected after rotation, dissection around the pedicle should be performed while ligating the branches and fascial tissues that may cause kinking of the perforator when rotated. A meticulous dissection toward the source vessel often requires skeletonizing the muscular portion of the perforator, and this

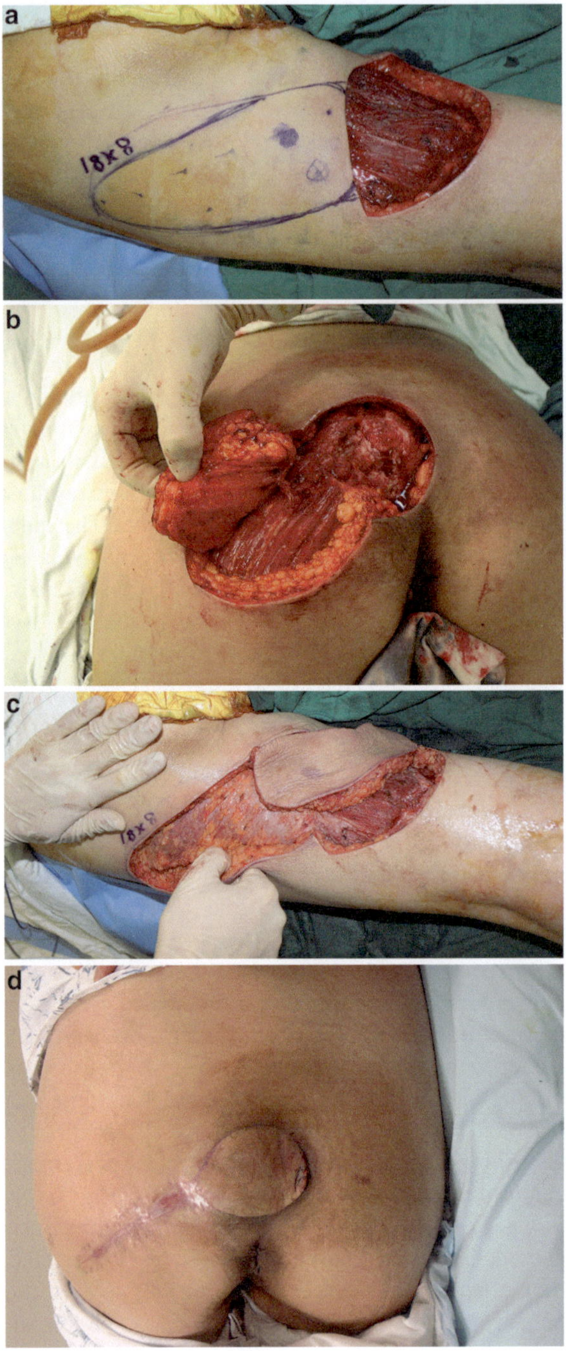

Fig. 10.2 An 18 × 8 cm perforator flap is designed after cancer resection. The length of the flap is determined based on the measurement from the perforator to the edge of the defect. The same length is then marked from the perforator to the distal edge of the flap (**a**). After the identification of a reliable perforator, the rest of the flap design is made and elevated (**b**). After rotation of the perforator flap, the flap is secured on the desired location and the donor closed primarily (**c**). Further follow-up at 6 months reveals a well-maintained reconstruction (**d**)

may be easily performed under a microscope. Although a local perforator flap is a non-microsurgical procedure, the use of microsurgery in certain stage of elevation helps to achieve a finer result. The rotation angle can be maximum of 180°, but choosing the right perforator may spare the flap from maximal rotation to reduce the chance for vascular complication. It is imperative that the perforator is tension free. If the reach of the flap is not enough after the rotation, one can dissect further to include the source vessel to increase the mobility of the flap. This will allow not only to rotate but to achieve advancement as well. After rotation of the perforator flap, the flap is secured on the desired location and drains are used if necessary (C). The donor site is then closed primarily. Further follow-up at 6 months reveals a well-maintained reconstruction (D).

The local perforator flaps can be used to cover wounds throughout the body. There are more than 400 perforators that can be used to cover defects locally [25, 26]. This approach provides alternative solutions especially for the posterior and anterior trunk wounds [17, 27–29]. When large defects involving the midline of the trunk are seen, it becomes very difficult to reconstruct. Using the muscle flaps in the posterior trunk achieves adequate coverage after debridement in majority of the wounds, but it may be difficult to cover wounds located medially and risks deterioration of function of the back. If one perforator flap is not enough to cover the defect, using multiple propeller flaps in conjunction with random pattern flaps in a freestyle approach can achieve tension-free closure by distributing the tension to multiple flaps [28, 29]. The same approach can be used for extremity as well. Most of the thigh defects can be covered with one or two perforator local flaps. However, in sizable defects of the lower leg and foot, primary closure of the donor site is difficult to obtain and frequently requires skin grafts. One must also be prudent when planning a perforator flap on the leg as patients with chronic disease such as diabetes or peripheral vascular disease may have calcified vessels and thus poor supply to the perforator. In these cases, duplex can be used to visualize the actual function of the perforator and can give accurate information compared to the handheld Doppler. Nevertheless, when there is adequate vascular supply, local perforator flaps are a quick and simple solution to difficult problems. Figure 10.3 shows a 75-year-old patient with a diabetic foot ulcer of 4 × 4.3 cm defect of the medial aspect of the foot (A). Preoperative Doppler was used to trace possible perforators around the defect. After complete debridement including part of the bone, a perforator flap was designed with an 8 × 4 cm dimension (B). An exploratory incision is made first to confirm the viability of the marked perforator. If the perforator is deemed feasible based on the caliber and the pulsation of the pedicle, final modification of the design is made based on the location of the perforator. The flap is then elevated and rotated. Usually in the foot when using perforator flaps, it becomes very difficult to close the donor defect primarily. A small skin graft can be used. The patient at 12 months follow-up shows good contour and viability of the flap (C).

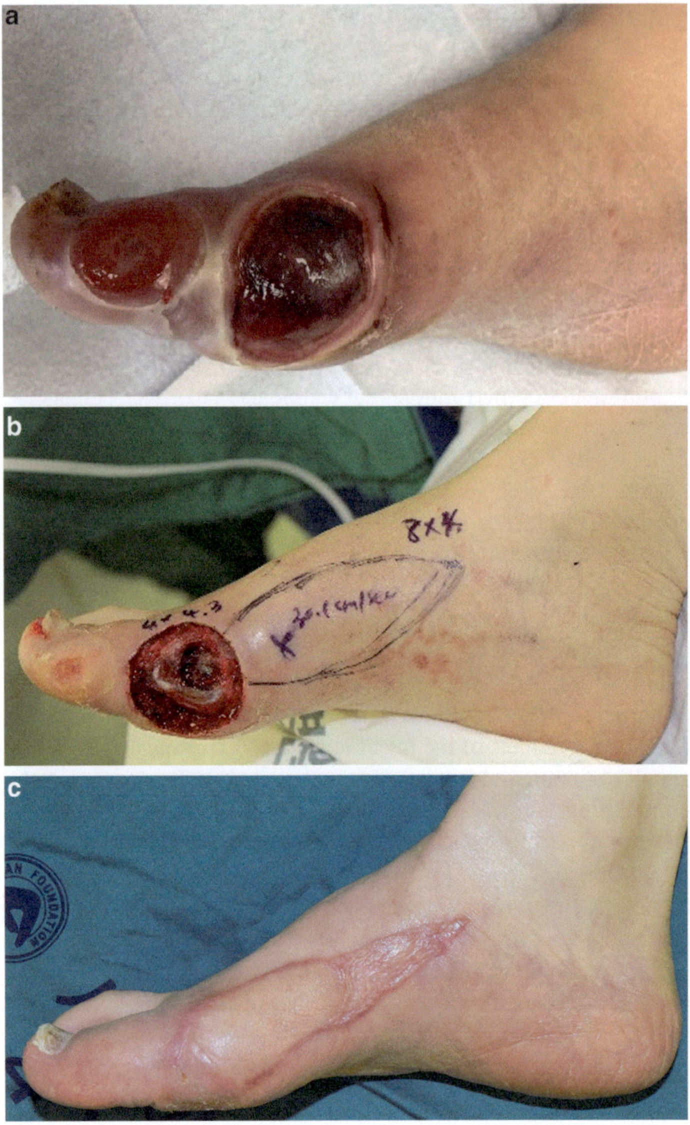

Fig. 10.3 A 75-year-old patient with a diabetic foot ulcer of 4 × 4.3 cm defect of the medial aspect of the foot is presented (**a**). Preoperative Doppler was used to trace possible perforators around the defect. After complete debridement including part of the bone, a perforator flap was designed with an 8 × 4 cm dimension (**b**). If the perforator is deemed feasible based on the caliber and the pulsation of the pedicle, final modification of the design is made based on the location of the perforator. The flap is then elevated and rotated. A small skin graft can be used to assist closure on the donor site. The patient at 12 months follow-up shows good contour and viability of the flap (**c**)

Perforator Flap as a Free Flap

When defects are large, extensive, vital structures or implants exposed and require composition of multiple tissues, perforator flaps can be used as free flaps. Based on the idea of freestyle flap, a perforator can supply a corresponding region of the skin and be used as a flap [23]. Thus any perforator can be used as a perforator flap especially as a free flap. In order to obtain adequate pedicle length, the perforator may be dissected toward the source vessel and frequently harvested with the source vessel. When the perforator is passing through a muscle, the dissection can be tedious and time-consuming. Nevertheless, the advantage of harvesting a thin skin, long pedicle, and minimizing muscle function deficit makes this flap very useful.

Again, one of the most critical steps after debridement is vascular status of the defect and selecting the recipient vessel. In wounds with ischemia or wide zone of injury, this can be a challenging task. The zone of injury, thrombogenic zone, is known to extend beyond what is macroscopically evident, and failure to recognize the true extent of this zone is cited as a leading cause of microsurgical anastomotic failure. It is difficult to find an adequate recipient vessel due to perivascular changes such as increased friability of vessels and increased perivascular scar tissue. This may lead to difficult dissection of recipient vessels and higher incidence of thrombosis after anastomosis [30]. But in clinical situations, determining the actual zone of injury becomes difficult not just the area but also the depth. Isenberg and Sherman demonstrated that clinical presentation of recipient vessel (vessel wall pliability and the quality of blood from transected end of vessel) was more important than the distance from the wound [31]. This idea was further supported by successful anastomosis of perforator to perforator adjacent to or within zone of injury [32]. Based on these findings, one of the most important factors in selecting the recipient vessel may be the vascular quality itself.

Figure 10.4 present a 53-year-old patient with diabetic foot ulcer on the left lateral ankle. The patient's habit of sitting on the floor with cross leg created and aggravated the wound on the nonsensate ankle. Initially with joint capsule exposed and a dirty large dead space, the ulcer underwent multiple debridement with application of negative pressure wound therapy to prepare the wound for reconstruction. The wound was presented with relatively good granulation with a size of 7 × 8 cm defect prior to reconstruction. The preoperative vascular exam which warranted CT angiogram showed some proximal artery segments with calcification but relatively well-preserved foot arteries (B). The anterior artery and vein being proximal to the defect were chosen as recipient vessels. After complete debridement, the anterior tibial artery and vein were exposed and checked with good pulsation. The final defect became slightly larger, but the recipient vessel being near the defect did not require a long pedicle flap. Thus SCIP (superficial circumflex iliac artery perforator) flap was chosen as the flap of choice. A 6 × 9 cm SCIP flap was designed on the ipsilateral groin (C). The SCIP flap is elevated as described in literature.[33]. The flap is elevated along the inferior and lateral borders under 3.5X loupe magnification. The dissection plane, which is identified most clearly inferolaterally, lies on the superficial plane, in between the superficial and deep fat [34]. There is a distinct

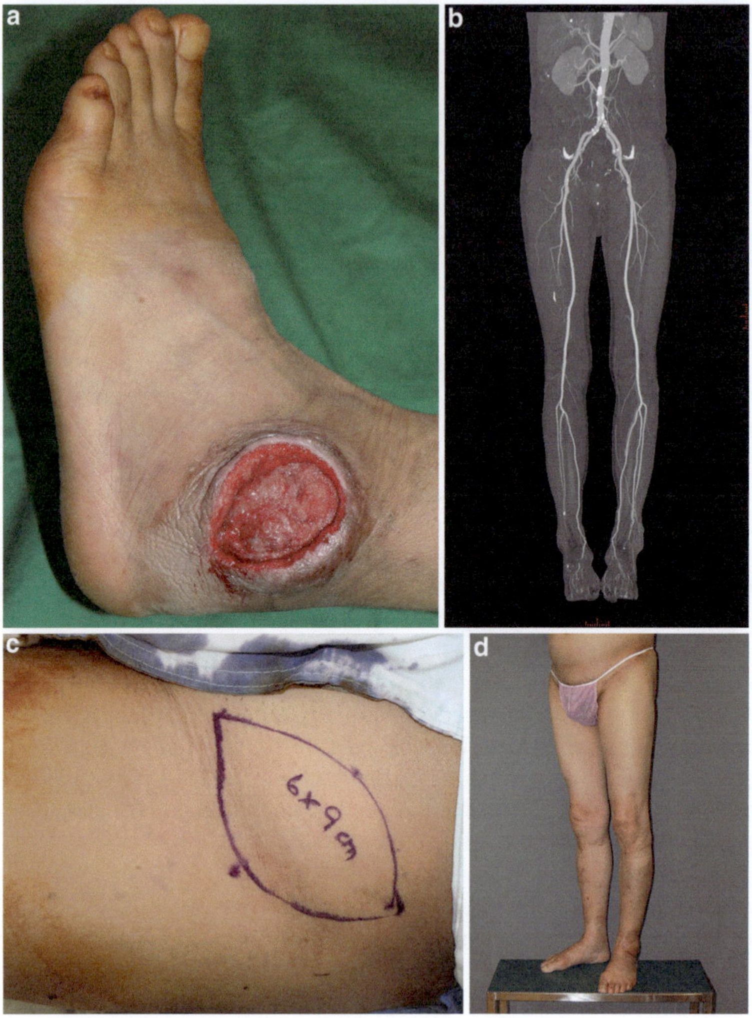

Fig. 10.4 A 53-year-old patient with diabetic foot ulcer of 7 × 8 cm defect on the left lateral ankle is presented after multiple debridements (**a**). The preoperative CT angiogram showed some proximal artery segments with calcification but relatively well-preserved foot arteries (**b**). A 6 × 9 cm SCIP (superficial circumflex iliac artery perforator) flap was designed elevated from the ipsilateral groin (**c**). The patient at 3 years follow-up shows a flap with good contour and donor site with acceptable scar (**d**)

white fascial layer separating the smaller fat lobules from the deeper, larger fat lobules. This is much clearer in a patient with a higher BMI. Superficial lymphatics and lymph nodes are spared as they are found in the deeper adipose tissue. A bloodless field, essential so that staining of the tissue does not interfere with the identification of the perforators, is achieved through diathermy needle dissection. Elevation progresses from lateral to medial, and the deep (and more lateral) branch from the superficial circumflex iliac artery (SCIA) is identified first followed by the superficial (and more medial) branch. Perforators are skeletonized toward the deep fascia and examined for their suitability. The deep branch is clamped to assess for sufficiency of the corresponding superficial branches. If the perfusion of the flap continues to be sufficient, the deep branch is ligated and the flap is raised on the superficial branch. Pedicle dissection is performed in freestyle retrogradely toward the SCIA. The deep fascia can be incised to obtain a longer pedicle length and larger vessel diameter. A superficial vein running from the ASIS toward the pubis is normally identified, and this is preserved. It is often that the accompanying venae drain into the superficial vein. In cases where there is a small or absent superficial vein, the commitante vein is usually of a larger caliber. In cases where the donor vessels are small, dissection is done under the microscope. The average time for flap harvest is 45 min (range, 30–60 min). After elevation, the SCIP flap is taken to the recipient site for anastomosis to the recipient vessels. The artery of the SCIA was anastomosed in end to side to the anterior tibial artery and the superficial vein end to end to the accompanying vein. The flap is then secured with a small drain underneath the flap. During the postoperative period, not only the flap but the patient should be monitored as a whole. It is especially important to monitor hemodynamic and pulmonary function as adequate hydration and oxygenation are critical to flap survival. Input and output of fluid should be monitored closely as distal perfusion is primarily affected by hypotensive episodes. Patients who have chronic renal failures and require assistance of dialysis often remove large volumes and can make fluid maintenance difficult. Limiting range of motion may be needed for flaps covering the joints as extension or flexion may increase the tension of the pedicle. Monitoring flaps, especially free flaps in the first 72 h, is essential due to the high chance of salvage when the flap falls into vascular compromise [35]. There is no ideal method of flap monitoring, but recent techniques such as tissue oxygen measurement, implantable Doppler device, laser Doppler flowmetry, and fluorescent dye injections may assist the judgment made from clinical evaluation which remains as the golden standard of monitoring. The patient at 3 years follow-up shows a flap with good contour and donor site with acceptable scar (D).

There are few special circumstances where debridement and coverage may warrant different approach. The first case is wounds with exposed hardware. Traditional method to manage exposed hardware includes irrigation, debridement, antibiotics, and likely removal of hardware. However, several factors should be taken into account to manage exposed hardware before considering for removal which may set back the treatment plan. Factors such as location of the hardware, infection (type of bacteria and duration of infection), duration of exposure of hardware, and hardware loosening should be considered as important prognostic factors for successful management of exposed hardware [36]. In this retrospective review by Viol et al., they have concluded if hardware is clinically stable, time of exposure is less than 2 weeks, infection is controlled, and the location of the hardware is for bony consolidation, then it may increase the likelihood of salvage of hardware using surgical soft tissue coverage [36].

Perforator flaps are now being widely used to cover various defects that involve skin defect from trauma, cancer resection, diabetic foot ulcers, and others. Perforator flap, like with like, coverage provides the following advantages:

1. Reduced donor site morbidity
2. Versatility in flap design
3. Muscle sparing (less functional deficit)
4. Improved postoperative recovery of the patient

Disadvantages of perforator flaps may include:

1. Meticulous dissection needed to isolate the perforator vessels
2. Increased operative time especially in muscle perforators
3. The variability in the position and size of the perforator vessels
4. Steep learning curve

References

1. Ben-Hur N, Converse JM. The impact of plastic surgery on transplantation from skin graft to microsurgery. Transplant Proc. 1980;12(4):616–20.
2. Allen RJ, Heitmann C. Perforator flaps – the history of evolution. Handchir Mikrochir Plast Chir. 2002;34(4):216–8.
3. Milton SH. Pedicled skin-flaps: the fallacy of the length: width ratio. Br J Surg. 1970;57(7):502–8.
4. McGregor IA, Morgan G. Axial and random pattern flaps. Br J Plast Surg. 1973;26(3):202–13.
5. McGregor IA, Jackson IT. The groin flap. Br J Plast Surg. 1972;25(1):3–16.
6. Mathes SJ, Nahai F. Classification of the vascular anatomy of muscles: experimental and clinical correlation. Plast Reconstr Surg. 1981;67(2):177–87.
7. Taylor GI, Palmer JH. The vascular territories (angiosomes) of the body: experimental study and clinical applications. Br J Plast Surg. 1987;40(2):113–41.
8. Cormack GC, Lamberty BG. A classification of fascio-cutaneous flaps according to their patterns of vascularisation. Br J Plast Surg. 1984;37(1):80–7.
9. Nakajima H, Fujino T, Adachi S. A new concept of vascular supply to the skin and classification of skin flaps according to their vascularization. Ann Plast Surg. 1986;16(1):1–19.
10. Koshima I, Soeda S. Inferior epigastric artery skin flaps without rectus abdominis muscle. Br J Plast Surg. 1989;42(6):645–8.
11. Allen RJ, Treece P. Deep inferior epigastric perforator flap for breast reconstruction. Ann Plast Surg. 1994;32(1):32–8.
12. Blondeel PN. One hundred free DIEP flap breast reconstructions: a personal experience. Br J Plast Surg. 1999;52(2):104–11.
13. Blondeel N, Vanderstraeten GG, Monstrey SJ, Van Landuyt K, Tonnard P, Lysens R, et al. The donor site morbidity of free DIEP flaps and free TRAM flaps for breast reconstruction. Br J Plast Surg. 1997;50(5):322–30.
14. Hallock GG. Direct and indirect perforator flaps: the history and the controversy. Plast Reconstr Surg. 2003;111(2):855–65. quiz 66
15. Wei FC, Jain V, Suominen S, Chen HC. Confusion among perforator flaps: what is a true perforator flap? Plast Reconstr Surg. 2001;107(3):874–6.
16. Blondeel PN, Van Landuyt KH, Monstrey SJ, Hamdi M, Matton GE, Allen RJ, et al. The "gent" consensus on perforator flap terminology: preliminary definitions. Plast Reconstr Surg. 2003;112(5):1378–83. quiz 83, 516; discussion 84–7

17. Saint-Cyr M, Wong C, Schaverien M, Mojallal A, Rohrich RJ. The perforasome theory: vascular anatomy and clinical implications. Plast Reconstr Surg. 2009;124(5):1529–44.
18. Duymaz A, Karabekmez FE, Vrtiska TJ, Mardini S, Moran SL. Free tissue transfer for lower extremity reconstruction: a study of the role of computed angiography in the planning of free tissue transfer in the posttraumatic setting. Plast Reconstr Surg. 2009;124(2):523–9.
19. Masia J, Larranaga J, Clavero JA, Vives L, Pons G, Pons JM. The value of the multidetector row computed tomography for the preoperative planning of deep inferior epigastric artery perforator flap: our experience in 162 cases. Ann Plast Surg. 2008;60(1):29–36.
20. Kuo YR, Kuo MH, Chou WC, Liu YT, Lutz BS, Jeng SF. One-stage reconstruction of soft tissue and Achilles tendon defects using a composite free anterolateral thigh flap with vascularized fascia lata: clinical experience and functional assessment. Ann Plast Surg. 2003;50(2):149–55.
21. Hong JP, Chung IW. The superficial fascia as a new plane of elevation for anterolateral thigh flaps. Ann Plast Surg. 2013;70(2):192–5.
22. Wallace CG, Kao HK, Jeng SF, Wei FC. Free-style flaps: a further step forward for perforator flap surgery. Plast Reconstr Surg. 2009;124(6 Suppl):e419–26.
23. Wei FC, Mardini S. Free-style free flaps. Plast Reconstr Surg. 2004;114(4):910–6.
24. Pignatti M, Ogawa R, Hallock GG, Mateev M, Georgescu AV, Balakrishnan G, et al. The "Tokyo" consensus on propeller flaps. Plast Reconstr Surg. 2011;127(2):716–22.
25. Morris S. Perforator flaps: a microsurgical innovation. Medscape J Med. 2008;10(11):266.
26. Morris SF, Tang M, Almutari K, Geddes C, Yang D. The anatomic basis of perforator flaps. Clin Plast Surg. 2010;37(4):553–70. xi
27. Eom JS, Hong JP. Lower back defect coverage using a free-style gluteal perforator flap. Ann Plast Surg. 2011;67(5):516–9.
28. Oh TS, Hallock G, Hong JP. Freestyle propeller flaps to reconstruct defects of the posterior trunk: a simple approach to a difficult problem. Ann Plast Surg. 2012;68(1):79–82.
29. Park SW, Oh TS, Eom JS, Sun YC, Suh HS, Hong JP. Freestyle multiple propeller flap reconstruction (Jigsaw puzzle approach) for complicated back defects. J Reconstr Microsurg. 2015;31(4):261–7.
30. Arnez ZM. Immediate reconstruction of the lower extremity – an update. Clin Plast Surg. 1991;18(3):449–57.
31. Isenberg JS, Sherman R. Zone of injury: a valid concept in microvascular reconstruction of the traumatized lower limb? Ann Plast Surg. 1996;36(3):270–2.
32. Hong JP. The use of supermicrosurgery in lower extremity reconstruction: the next step in evolution. Plast Reconstr Surg. 2009;123(1):230–5.
33. Goh TL, Park SW, Cho JY, Choi JW, Hong JP. The search for the ideal thin skin flap: superficial circumflex iliac artery perforator flap – a review of 210 cases. Plast Reconstr Surg. 2015;135(2):592–601.
34. Hong JP, Choi DH, Suh H, Mukarramah DA, Tashti T, Lee K, et al. A new plane of elevation: the superficial fascial plane for perforator flap elevation. J Reconstr Microsurg. 2014;30(7):491–6.
35. Chen KT, Mardini S, Chuang DC, Lin CH, Cheng MH, Lin YT, et al. Timing of presentation of the first signs of vascular compromise dictates the salvage outcome of free flap transfers. Plast Reconstr Surg. 2007;120(1):187–95.
36. Viol A, Pradka SP, Baumeister SP, Wang D, Moyer KE, Zura RD, et al. Soft-tissue defects and exposed hardware: a review of indications for soft-tissue reconstruction and hardware preservation. Plast Reconstr Surg. 2009;123(4):1256–63.

Chapter 11
Free Tissue Transfer

Benjamin J. Mitchell, Michael V. DeFazio, and Karen Kim Evans

Introduction

Free tissue transfer (FTT) has emerged as the workhorse for reconstructing complex wounds of various etiologies throughout the body. Microvascular FTT is the autotransplantation of isolated tissue on a vascular supply that is initially dependent on the anastomosis of the feeding artery and draining vein to the corresponding recipient-site vessels. Free flaps may contain numerous tissue components (i.e., skin, subcutaneous fat, fascia, muscle, bone, or any combination thereof) and may be supplied by one or more distinct vascular pedicles. The composition of such flaps is determined by a number of factors, notably donor- and recipient-site characteristics, as well as aesthetic and functional requirements, among others. Given their versatility, free tissue constructs often provide the most complete solution to meet the unique reconstructive demands, capacity, and goals of each patient. FTT should be considered as an early management option for coverage of complex wounds.

The first experimental free flaps based on superficial epigastric vessels were performed on dogs and reported by Krizek et al. in 1965 [1]. Daniel and Taylor introduced the first well-described free flap in 1972 when they published on the groin flap [2]. Over the ensuing decades, new flaps emerged and indications for their use were developed. During this progressive period, the primary focus of microvascular surgery evolved from anatomical classification and flap survival to include a more patient-centric focus on functional and aesthetic outcomes, donor-site morbidity, and microsurgical technique.

B.J. Mitchell, BS • M.V. DeFazio, MD • K.K. Evans, MD (✉)
Department of Plastic Surgery, Center for Wound Healing, Medstar Georgetown University Hospital, Washington, DC, USA
e-mail: karen.k.evans@gunet.georgetown.edu

D.P. Orgill (ed.), *Interventional Treatment of Wounds*,
https://doi.org/10.1007/978-3-319-66990-8_11

The introduction of the angiosome concept by Taylor and Palmer in 1987 significantly enhanced our understanding of tissue perfusion by source vessels throughout the body [3]. However, with the popularization of perforator flaps and supermicrosurgery techniques, the impetus of vascular knowledge has migrated from the source artery to the perforator itself. A perforator is a vascular branch that penetrates the deep fascia to supply the overlying skin territory. Perforator flaps differ from conventional fasciocutaneous flaps in that they are harvested above the deep fascial plane using a retrograde "freestyle" dissection technique that permits the elevation of ultrathin, (i.e., suprafascial) skin flaps for precise contour resurfacing [4]. In general, nearly any perforator in the body may serve as the source vessel for a local pedicled (propeller) or free flap. The use of perforators as source vessels allows for increased flexibility in flap design, greater accuracy of flap harvest, decreased concern over anatomic variability of source vessels, and decreased donor-site morbidity [5]. In 2009, Saint-Cyr et al. introduced the "perforasome theory" in which anatomical and perfusion characteristics were detailed for clinically relevant perforators throughout the body [4].

Over the past several decades, increasing emphasis placed on function, aesthetics, and quality of life has shifted the expectations of patients with debilitating physical deformities. This change in paradigm has redefined the role of FTT as a primary solution for complex congenital, traumatic, metabolic, and/or oncologic defects involving the head and neck, trunk, and extremities. Further application of microsurgical principles and techniques has significantly improved the treatment of lymphedema and enabled advancements in facial reanimation, limb salvage, and composite tissue allotransplantation alike. Advances in technology, experience, and knowledge of vascular anatomy over time have generated free flap success rates in the range of 95.9–99% at high-volume centers [6, 7]. With the ever-expanding indications for microsurgery and evolving standards for success, specialized training in the evaluation and management of microsurgical candidates, operative planning, and execution of advanced microvascular techniques have become critical to the provision of state-of-the-art care for reconstructive patients.

This chapter will focus on the factors that guide successful microvascular reconstruction including preoperative evaluation, patient selection, the relevant anatomic and intraoperative considerations for commonly utilized flaps, as well as postoperative monitoring and care of the free flap patient.

Indications for Free Tissue Transfer

Free flap reconstruction has proven to be a safe and effective method for achieving wound closure and multifaceted structural repair. FTT is indicated for the reconstruction of complex, composite defects and wounds with exposed vital structures (i.e., vessels, nerves, tendons, bones, joint space, etc.) when simpler or local options for coverage are either unavailable or inadequate to achieve structural and/or functional restoration [5]. In many cases, local or regional tissue may be unsuitable due to infection, inflammation, trauma, irradiation, insufficient volume or surface area, insufficient vascular pedicle length, and/or unsuitable morbidity at the donor site [8]. Free flaps are favored because they have greater versatility in tissue composition and orientation (i.e., no restrictions on the distance of flap transfer as with pedicled flaps) and may allow for more complex reconstructions to be performed in single operations. Other indications include hand and digit replantation, functional muscle transfer (i.e., such as in the case of facial nerve paralysis), vascularized bone and/or lymph node transfers, and irradiated wounds.

Traditionally, reconstructive surgery has followed the concept of the "reconstructive ladder." This algorithm promotes the progression of increasingly complex reconstructive modalities to address wounds. As technology and technique have improved, this idea has given way to the "reconstructive elevator" which asserts that the most appropriate option to meet the reconstructive demands for a given wound should be chosen [9]. Simply put, FTT is now considered a first-line solution for select complex and/or composite defects and is no longer reserved as measures of last resort. This early implementation of more sophisticated techniques has contributed to the overall higher success rates and superior reconstructive results that are currently being reported. The more recent idea of the "reconstructive matrix" adds another dimension to the reconstructive algorithm by taking into account surgical complexity, sophistication of available technology, and the individual patient's surgical risk and medical comorbidities [9].

FTT holds various advantages over other reconstructive options. Wound healing by secondary intention is lengthy, often leaves significant scarring, and has a high revision rate. Skin grafts and dermal regenerate templates require well-vascularized wound beds and may be complicated by scar adhesions and contracture development. Advantages over pedicled or local flaps include avoiding donor-site morbidity or surgical trauma to a region with an existing burden; preserving local blood flow through both major and collateral vessels; and providing well-vascularized tissue that will promote healing, reduce infectious risk, and enable coverage of large wounds [6]. Pedicle flaps may also be limited by arc of rotation and may require prolonged immobilization postoperatively. Further, most composite reconstructions are more appropriately designed as free flaps. FTT should always be evaluated and considered early in the treatment assessment if it may increase the chances for a better outcome.

There are no consistently established absolute contraindications to microsurgical reconstruction. Microsurgery practice is typically driven by observational studies and conventional wisdom passed from surgeon to surgeon due to various factors that limit the statistical power for generating level 1 evidence [10]. Based on the trends of lower-level evidence, however, one can ascertain that several factors of preoperative patient selection that were previously believed to be absolute contraindications in microvascular surgery may be compatible with FTT. Age, smoking, obesity, and peripheral vascular disease are several conditions that should not rule patients out for FTT. Rather, control over these conditions should be optimized to reduce rates of flap failure. As an example, smoking does not influence anastomotic patency rates but does negatively impact the healing of the wound and flap interface [10]. Patients should be counseled to stop smoking 4 weeks prior to reconstruction to decrease the incidence of perioperative complications compared with active smokers [10]. Comorbidities that are uncorrected and impede wound healing tip the balance away from the high success rates that FTT enjoys today. Thus, it is important to counsel patients to appropriately address these issues prior to reconstruction.

Recent introduction of supermicrosurgery principles and techniques has further expanded the indications for microvascular reconstruction in patients with severe peripheral arterial disease [11]. Masia et al. defined supermicrosurgery as microsurgery with application to vessels under 0.8 mm in size [12]. As such, supermicrosurgery targets the use of appropriately selected collateral perforators as potential recipient vessels, thereby permitting perforator-to-perforator anastomosis in the absence of available major vessels. The use of small vessels or perforators from well-vascularized adjacent angiosomes will provide sufficient perfusion to facilitate coverage of moderately sized defects in regions of localized ischemia [11]. In diabetic patients with advanced peripheral arterial disease, the implementation of supermicrosurgical techniques has improved rates of flap success to 90.5% and overall limb salvage rate during follow-up to 93.7% [13].

Preoperative Considerations

When assessing patients' candidacy for FTT, there are many factors and considerations that should be addressed in the preoperative period that will determine whether a free flap is an appropriate option and, if so, the course of treatment. Central to this process is addressing wound etiology and comorbidities, wound optimization and infection control (i.e., debridement, culture-directed antibiotic therapy, etc.), evaluation and/or establishment of adequate blood supply, proper nutrition, and lifestyle modifications (i.e., smoking status, hygiene, etc.).

Patient Selection

Considerations must be made for comorbidities that may influence wound healing. Pertinent comorbid diseases include cardiac disease, renal disease, infection, vasculopathy, diabetes, neuropathy, venous hypertension, lymphatic obstruction, immunological deficiency, hypercoagulability, connective tissue disease, malnutrition, autoimmune disease, vasospasm, neoplasm, and psychiatric illness [14]. Often times, multiple comorbidities must be accounted for. Discovery of some of these comorbidities relies on thorough history taking and patient evaluation. The presence of autoimmune conditions such as rheumatoid arthritis, pyoderma gangrenosum, systemic lupus erythematosus, and scleroderma is frequently associated with inflammatory wounds that initially necessitate medical management [14]. In the same way, managing coagulopathies in patients with vasculitic wounds is important for proper flap integration and wound healing. Furthermore, thorough preoperative evaluation by an anesthesiologist is necessary to ensure that patients are healthy enough to withstand a prolonged operation under general anesthesia.

Effective assessment for FTT also necessitates a thorough history and examination of the wound site. Previous treatment (including failed reconstructive attempts), origin, and age of the wound should be determined. An example of the importance of such is the use of prior topical therapy (i.e., hydrogen peroxide, 10% iodine, Dakin's solution, etc.), which can be caustic and contribute to wound chronicity and evolution [14]. Furthermore, a complete list of medications should be obtained as certain medications (i.e., steroids, chemotherapeutic agents, anticoagulants, etc.) may impede wound healing and/or cause excessive hemorrhage. Nutritional status should be improved to promote healing (albumin >3.5 g/dL and/or total lymphocyte count >1500) [14]. Glucose levels should ideally be <200 mg/dL perioperatively, and HgbA1c should be less than 8.0 prior to any elective reconstruction [14]. Smoking significantly decreases local cutaneous blood flow, and patients should be counseled on its deleterious effects toward wound healing. Given the complexity of various disease processes, multiple specialties are often called upon to assist in optimizing the patient's medical condition for wound healing. The multidisciplinary approach to preoperative evaluation of free flap candidates must be appreciated.

Physical examination of the wound should include consideration of the wound's etiology, dimensions, location, and determination of exposed or damaged structures [5]. The various tissue types involved in the wound should be noted (i.e., epidermis, dermis, subcutaneous tissue, fascia, muscle, tendon, joint capsule, bone, etc.). Any infection needs to be clinically noted for character and extent so the progress of the infection, response to treatment, or resulting tissue death can be followed.

For limb reconstruction, functional assessment of the extremity, including the patient's current and anticipated level of activity, must also be considered. This will aid in both the determination of whether a free flap is warranted and appropriate for flap selection. In these cases, a sensorimotor examination should be conducted to evaluate protective sensation in the areas surrounding the wound as well as to gauge the strength and range of motion of the affected limb. Sensibility impairments are helpful in determining wound etiology and assessing the need for offloading, postoperatively [15].

Differences in patient characteristics also influence preoperative evaluation and planning. For example, trauma patients are typically younger and healthier compared to the highly comorbid diabetic limb salvage or cancer patient. These differences influence decision-making on issues such as timing of reconstruction, flap selection, and postoperative management.

Vascular Workup

Ensuring adequate perfusion to the wound bed is essential for facilitating wound healing and planning successful FTT. Bipedal pulse examination and detection of a biphasic or triphasic audible Doppler signal, using a handheld device, signals the adequacy of blood flow to support proper healing. Doppler studies may be used in conjunction with other modalities such as pulse volume recordings (PVRs), segmental pressures, tissue oxygenation pressure, and duplex imaging in order to characterize the vascular network with more accuracy. If these noninvasive tests suggest ischemia, an arterial imaging study should be performed to determine if vascular intervention is necessary. Newer endovascular techniques allow for direct and indirect revascularization with dilatation, recanalization, and arthrectomy of stenosed or obstructed arteries in patients who are poor candidates for open vascular bypass [16].

DeFazio et al. suggested that all patients with non-palpable pulses and absent or monophasic Doppler sounds (i.e., suggestive for ischemia) should obtain a diagnostic angiogram in preparation for microvascular reconstruction [16]. This provides an accurate anatomical representation of blood flow. In scenarios where intervention is needed, targeted percutaneous transluminal angioplasty (PTA), with or without stent placement, can be performed in the same setting to restore both direct and peripheral inflow [14]. Such a strategy eliminates the need for separate diagnostic (i.e., computed tomographic angiography) and therapeutic procedures. PTA can also be used in a targeted fashion to improve recipient vessel caliber in locations where calcifications, occlusions, and stenosis complicate microvascular anastomosis [14]. The success of this protocol in patients with multivessel disease may indicate a role for the use of targeted endovascular therapy as an adjunct to FTT in areas of diminished distal blood flow [16].

In cases of perforator flap reconstruction, most surgeons use the handheld Doppler to identify viable perforators; however, other preoperative imaging techniques may also be useful. Preoperative perforator mapping with duplex ultrasound confirms the velocity of arterial flow near the recipient site and enhances the safety and efficiency of flap harvest through precise identification of relevant donor perforators. In general, a peak systolic velocity greater than 15–20 cm/s defines the minimum criterion threshold for donor and/or recipient artery selection [13]. Other modalities popular in some institutions include the routine use of CTA to identify the largest perforators prior to surgery. Although cost may be prohibitive, noninvasive computed tomographic angiography provides additional information regarding general vascular anatomy, as well as the presence of atherosclerotic disease, and can be used to map the precise location of potential donor and recipient perforators relative to key anatomic locations. Final determination of perforator viability, however, is confirmed through direct visualization of a pulsatile artery during intraoperative dissection.

Wound Debridement and Infection Control

When attempting FTT, it is imperative to perform an early, thorough debridement in order to remove any infected and/or nonviable tissue [5]. A definitive decision for salvage or amputation should only be made after an adequate debridement is performed. Necrotic tissue, biofilm, and bacteria, as well as any foreign material in the wound, may impede the body's attempt to heal due to the production of proteases, collagenases, and elastases that overwhelm the local healing process [17]. Debridement is especially important if the wound is acutely infected with purulent drainage, malodor, or any overlying erythema. Immediate and aggressive debridement lessens the chance for infectious spread, sepsis, and amputation. Even in the absence of infection, debridement turns a subacute or chronic contaminated wound into an acute clean wound, which enhances the healing potential and allows thorough assessment for reconstruction [18].

For noninfected wounds, single-stage debridement is preferred over traditional serial debridement, as the latter may make evaluation of tissue viability difficult, delay final wound closure, and cause additional tissue loss from desiccation due to prolonged dressing changes [5]. Furthermore, the removal of devitalized bone and soft tissue during this process is crucial for preventing late osteomyelitis and flap deterioration as popularized by Gustilo and Cierny in the trauma population [19, 20]. Early debridement and reconstruction are also associated with earlier return to mobility and functionality.

Adequate debridement may be determined by tissue color in conjunction with post-debridement culture results. Normal tissue colors (i.e., red, white, and yellow) must be recognized by the surgeon in order to adequately remove grossly infected tissue as well as recognize an endpoint for debridement [21]. Traditionally, debridement to negative cultures has been the standard before reconstruction. Recently, however, culture-guided debridement to negative cultures and its role in determining timing of reconstruction have been examined in greater detail. This practice often requires multiple trips to the operating room until negative cultures can be achieved, which may unnecessarily postpone definitive wound closure, prolong hospital stays, and delay rehabilitation and recovery. Our institution examined debridement to negative cultures vs. cultures that remained positive at closure (or exhibited delayed growth after culture) in both local flaps and free flaps. Negative cultures prior to FTT resulted in a 14% flap failure rate compared to the 28% failure rate in the local flap cohort [22]. Approximately 35% of each cohort had positive post-debridement cultures [22]. Univariate and multivariate analysis reveals that positive post-debridement cultures were significantly associated with failure in only the local flap cohort. This included even the most virulent organisms such as MRSA, pseudomonas, and VRE. These results may suggest that the most important factors determining timing of closure are signs of healthy wound healing rather than positive vs. negative cultures.

When used as an adjunct in wound reconstruction, negative pressure wound therapy (NPWT) potentiates healing through increased local blood flow and granulation, reduced tissue edema, and control of bacterial proliferation [14, 20, 23]. NPWT with instillation (NPWTi) is a further modified wound management method for acute/chronically infected wounds, osteomyelitis, and exposed orthopedic hardware [24]. NPWTi combines negative pressure with automated, intermittent instillation of a topical wound solution (antimicrobial or normal saline) [14]. Surprisingly, antimicrobial solutions and normal saline have been found to have similar effects on healing outcomes—highlighting the mechanical advantage of cyclical irrigation and its importance in eradicating bacteria from the wound. NPWTi was shown to reduce the total number of operative procedures, accelerate the time to wound closure, and shorten the length of hospital stay when compared to NPWT alone [24]. In addition, NPWTi increases the percentage of wounds closed by discharge and demonstrates qualitative improvement in gram-positive cultures [25].

In infected wounds, tissue cultures should be taken during debridement and are obtained deep to the surface of the infected tissue and purulence. Deep bone cultures and other relevant pathologies should be sent prior to flap reconstruction. Broad spectrum antibiotics should be started after deep tissue cultures are collected and later adjusted based on culture results and sensitivities. Deep cultures may miss two-thirds of the bacterial species present; thus, any continuing signs of infection after 48 h of antibiotic therapy may point to the need for a change in antibiotics or further debridement. Utilizing a multidisciplinary approach that includes early consultation with infectious disease specialists is key to optimizing success of the healing wound bed.

Timing of Free Tissue Transfer

Timing of FTT reconstruction is dependent on the establishment of a healthy, vascularized wound bed with clinical signs of healing (i.e., granulation tissue, neo-epithelialization). Many authors agree that reconstruction should be attempted as early as tolerable following an adequate debridement and recipient-site optimization. This may include serial debridement and techniques such as NPWT before definitive closure with a free flap can be achieved. The time course may further vary depending on wound etiology. Some wounds require adjunctive measures, such as revascularization procedures, or other medical management to optimize healing potential at the recipient site prior to FTT. There is broad consensus for immediate flap coverage in the setting of exposed vital structures or the need for FTT to salvage a devascularized limb.

Flap Selection and Classification

Classification

Many classifications for FTT have been proposed based on tissue composition, vascular anatomy, and harvest technique. For the purposes of clarity, however, a description of flap type according to its structural components is most frequently employed in the clinical setting and has implications with regard to certain recipient-site requirements.

Muscle flaps are commonly used in reconstruction of composite three-dimensional defects where significant bulk is required to fill a large dead space. However, muscle flaps may also provide a thin, pliable, and well-contoured coverage based on the amount of muscle initially dissected with the flap. The initial bulky appearance of muscle flaps is often diminished over time due to muscular atrophy from denervation [26]. In such a case, appropriately sized muscle flaps may actually lead to a thin and well-contoured flap. Debulking can be performed at a later time if necessary. These flaps also offer enhanced vascularity that is capable of suppressing bacterial inoculation by aiding in the delivery of neutrophils and parenteral antibiotics to the site [27–29]. Thus, muscle flaps are often employed for largely contaminated wounds and chronically infected wounds with large amounts of dead space. Mathes and Nahai have classically divided muscle flaps into five distinct categories based on the pattern of vascular supply (Table 11.1). Muscle flaps are also used for innervated functional restoration such as the innervated gracilis flap in cases of facial reanimation.

Table 11.1 Mathes and Nahai classification of muscle flaps

Type	Definition	Clinical examples
I	Single dominant vascular pedicle	Tensor fascia lata Gastrocnemius Abductor digiti minimi (hand) Abductor pollicis brevis Genioglossus Hyoglossus
II	Dominant pedicle(s) and minor vascular pedicle(s)	Gracilis Rectus femoris[a] Adductor digiti minimi Flexor digitorum brevis Abductor halluces Brachioradialis Platysma Trapezius
III	Two dominant pedicles	Gluteus maximus Rectus abdominis Semimembranosus Rectus femoris[a] Serratus anterior
IV	Segmental vascular pedicles	Sartorius External oblique Extensor halluces longus Flexor halluces longus Extensor digitorum longus Flexor digitorum longus Tibialis anterior
V	One dominant pedicle and secondary segmental pedicles	Latissimus dorsi Pectoralis major

[a]Rectus femoris may be classified as a type II (54%) or a type III (46%) muscle flap based on the presence of a codominant oblique branch from the lateral circumflex femoral artery

Fasciocutaneous flaps are ideal for wound resurfacing and are capable of restoring contour and facilitating adequate tendon glide along the flap-native wound interface [5]. These flaps are also useful for staged reconstruction of underlying tissue components (i.e., joint prosthesis), as they can be rapidly reevaluated. Some fasciocutaneous flaps may be bulky due to large amounts of subcutaneous fat if the patient has a high BMI or excessive fatty collection at the donor site. Surgical debulking procedures and liposuction may be required at a later time to improve contour. Mathes and Nahai have classified fasciocutaneous flaps as types A, B, and C (Table 11.2) [27].

Perforator flaps are flaps that receive their blood supply from branches of named vessels that "perforate" through the muscle or fascial septum to supply the overlying skin and subcutaneous tissues. Unlike fasciocutaneous flaps, however, these flaps are harvested above the level of deep fascia using retrograde "freestyle" perforator dissection techniques until adequate pedicle length is achieved. This technique facilitates wound resurfacing with ultrathin adipocutaneous flaps, enhances the freedom of flap design, and minimizes the need for secondary debulking [30]. However, the learning curve associated with suprafascial dissection is high, and detailed preoperative mapping is essential to avoid inadvertent injury to perforators at this level. With increased knowledge of perforator anatomy and flow characteristics (i.e., perforasome theory), nearly any perforator in the body can be chosen as a source of vascular supply for a local (i.e., propeller) or free flap. Primary disadvantages of perforator flap harvest include variability in perforator size and location, greater complexity of dissection, and a slightly higher risk of fat necrosis and partial flap loss due to their more tenuous vascular supply [31–33]. For these reasons, perforator flaps are ideal for coverage of moderately sized defects and require detailed preoperative planning (i.e., perforator mapping) to enhance the safety and efficiency of flap harvest.

Table 11.2 Mathes and Nahai classification of fasciocutaneous flaps

Type	Definition	Clinical examples
A	Direct cutaneous pedicle	Superficial circumflex iliac artery perforator flap Temporoparietal fascia flap Sural flap
B	Septocutaneous pedicle	Anterolateral thigh flap[a] Dorsalis pedis flap Radial forearm flap Lateral arm lap Scapular flap
C	Musculocutaneous pedicle	Anterolateral thigh flap[a] Lateral thigh Superior gluteal artery perforator flap Inferior gluteal artery perforator flap Deep inferior epigastric artery perforator flap

[a]Anterolateral thigh flap can be classified as a type B or type C fasciocutaneous flap based on whether the perforating vessel to the skin passes within the intermuscular septum located between the rectus femoris and vastus lateralis or through the vastus lateralis, respectively

Flap Selection

Flap selection is largely dependent on the defect dimension (i.e., dead space), required pedicle length, presence of infection and/or exposed vital structures, aesthetic and functional demands of both the donor and recipient site, potential to restore sensation, patient positioning in the operating room, and the patient's body habitus [5]. Suh et al. defined an algorithm for selecting perforator free flaps for the lower extremity after cancer resection [34]. The components of this algorithm include three-dimensional defect characterization, composition of the defect, condition of the recipient vessel, pedicle length of the flap, and the position of the patient [34]. Based on these important characteristics, flap selection can be streamlined and optimized. This process of assessing relevant characteristics for reconstruction not only applies to lower extremity resections but also to wounds in various anatomical areas. In regions where aesthetics and function play a major role, additional algorithmic consideration may be made on such grounds.

Intraoperative Considerations

After thorough debridement of the recipient site, the resulting defect should be evaluated, and a final decision about the type and technique of reconstruction should be made. Surgical templates assist in accurately defining the dimensions of the wound and are especially helpful in complex three-dimensional wounds. It is critical to obtain adequate pedicle and flap length in order to anastomose to viable recipient vessels and provide coverage to the wound site. Precise reconstruction is necessary to optimize functional and aesthetic outcomes. Computer-aided design and manufacturing (CAD-CAM) and CT have been utilized in some reconstructive settings to create three-dimensional representations of defects. Virtual surgery planning utilizing CAD-CAM provides increased efficiency, precision, and accuracy during reconstruction. Studies and data on various anatomical areas of the body are limited given its novelty. However, in mandibular reconstruction, virtual planning reduces time for intraoperative measurement, decreases traumatic graft manipulation and ischemia time, and improves bone-to-bone contact [35]. This technology may hold promise in other complex anatomic regions.

A variety of factors regarding recipient vessels should be evaluated prior to free flap harvest. These include assessment of vessel pulsatility, distance from the defect (i.e., the pedicle length), caliber, patency, flow, and condition [8]. Vessels may suffer from atherosclerotic disease including calcification, radiation damage, trauma, or infection. Recipient vessels should be thoroughly inspected for the ability to undergo microvascular anastomosis. If the vessels are not appropriate, the adjacent angiosomes/perforasomes should be explored and alternative vasculature identified. At the donor site, Doppler ultrasonography has proven to be a reliable tool for identifying perforating vessels that supply cutaneous flaps. The flap's vascular pedicle is dissected under magnification to a length determined from preoperative planning and intraoperative measurement.

Relevant considerations regarding donor- and recipient-site anatomy such as major arterial and venous supply, variations in vascular anatomy, important associated structures, as well as nerve supply must be well understood. Vessels at the donor and recipient sites should be compatible in caliber in order to facilitate successful end-to-end anastomosis. End-to-side anastomosis should be considered for extremity flaps if there is a sizeable mismatch in the donor and recipient artery caliber. In some situations, vein grafts may be utilized to bridge gaps between donor and recipient vessels [8].

After microsurgical anastomosis, it is crucial to ensure that the flap has adequate flow and that the anastomosis is patent. In some cases, there may be elements of twisting, torque, or tension on the pedicle during the flap inset. Constant scrutiny of flap perfusion should be as assessed prior to leaving the operating room setting to ensure that any avoidable technical mishap may be corrected.

Common Free Flap Constructs

Common "workhorse" free flaps used in a variety of reconstructive settings are listed in Table 11.3. Clinical examples of several of these flaps are also provided in Figs. 11.1, 11.2, 11.3, 11.4, and 11.5.

Postoperative Management

Postoperative monitoring serves to accurately and continuously assess vessel patency and in turn flap success. Clinical examination is the main source of monitoring flap progress in the early postoperative setting. There are a variety of clinical signs and symptoms that are suggestive of arterial insufficiency including pale flap color, reduction in flap temperature, loss of capillary refill, and loss of flap turgor [8]. Venous insufficiency or congestion may manifest as a dark purple hue, swelling, abrupt capillary refill, and dark brisk bleeding on pin prick [8]. In the early postoperative period, venous insufficiency and occlusion is a more common complication than arterial thrombosis.

Clinical examination may be accompanied by handheld Doppler monitoring. An experienced and knowledgeable staff is key to obtaining flap retention rates above 95%, as reported at high-volume centers. Standardized flap monitoring protocols are utilized to enhance early detection of thrombotic complications and/or impending flap failure. At our institution, serial Doppler assessments are performed by trained staff every 15 min for the first 4 h postoperatively, followed by every 30 min for the subsequent 8 h, and then hourly until the second postoperative day. For patients with uncomplicated recoveries, the interval between flap checks increases to every 2–4 h

Table 11.3 Commonly used workhorse flaps

Body region	Flap	Dominant vascular pedicle or source	Components	Mathes /Nahai classification	Typical max. size for primary closure	Pedicle length	Pedicle size	Relevant nerve (N.) supply	Advantages	Disadvantages	Technical notes
Thigh											
	Anterolateral thigh (ALT)	Perforators from the descending branch of the lateral circumflex femoral artery	Muscle, myocutaneous, fasciocutaneous	B/C	35 × 10 cm	12 cm	1.0–2.5 mm	S: Lateral femoral cutaneous n. (L2–L3) M: N. to VL	Durable, long pedicle, thin	Pedicle may be variable, lack of suitable perforators	
	Vastus lateralis (VL)	Muscular branch from the descending branch of the lateral circumflex femoral artery	Muscle, myocutaneous	II	30 × 10 cm	8 cm	1.0–2.5 mm	M: N. to VL	Pliable, safe and quick dissection, large volume, possible muscle-sparing dissection	Bulk (if not harvested as muscle sparing)	
	Rectus femoris (RF)	Descending branch of lateral circumflex femora artery	Muscle, myocutaneous	II	35 × 9 cm	2–3 cm	1.0 mm	S: Inter mediate AFCN (L2–L3) M: N. to RF	Large-caliber pedicle, safe and quick dissection	Not primary option in ambulatory patient because RF is powerful hip flexor/knee extensor, postoperative knee immobilizer for 2 weeks	
	Gracilis	Medial circumflex femoral artery	Muscle, myocutaneous, fasciocutaneous	II	20 × 6 cm	6 cm	1.0–2.0 mm	S: Anterior femoral cutaneous n. M: Obturator N.	Thin and pliable, easy harvest	Small, skin paddle distally unreliable, short pedicle	
Gluteal region											
	Superior gluteal artery perforator (SGAP)	Superior gluteal artery perforators	Fasciocutaneous	III	22 × 8 cm	5–7 cm	3–4 mm	S: Cluneal nerves, direct spinal (L1–L3) branches	Thick flap adequate pedicle for breast reconstruction	Contour defects, visible scar, asymmetry	

(continued)

Table 11.3 (continued)

Body region	Flap	Dominant vascular pedicle or source	Components	Mathes /Nahai classification	Typical max. size for primary closure	Pedicle length	Pedicle size	Relevant nerve (N.) supply	Advantages	Disadvantages	Technical notes
	Inferior gluteal artery perforator (IGAP)	Inferior gluteal artery perforators	Fasciocutaneous	III	30 × 12 cm	7–10 cm	3–4 mm	S: Cluneal nerves, direct spinal (L1–L3) branches	Thick flap, longer pedicle for breast reconstruction, scar coverage, less contour defect than SGAP, long pedicle may anastomose to throracodorsal system	Pain and discomfort more common, traction may be seen with injury to posterior femoral cutaneous nerve	
Trunk											
	Latissimus dorsi [TDAP]	Thoracodorsal artery [thoracodorsal artery]	Muscle, myocutaneous, osteocutaneous [perforator paddle]	V	25 × 15 cm [25 × 15 cm]	15 cm	2.0–3.0 mm	S: Posterior branches of lateral cutaneous branches of intercostal n. M: Thoracodorsal n.	Both: Reliable, large area, reliable flap in pediatric reconstruction	Positioning, muscular donor-site morbidity	
	TRAM [DIEP]	Superior epigastric [1] and deep inferior epigastric [2] [deep inferior epigastric]	Muscle, myocutaneous, fasciocutaneous [perforator paddle]	III	40 × 20 cm	6–8 cm [4–7 cm]	2.5–3.5 mm [0.75–3.5 mm]	S: Intercostal N. T7–12 [intercostal N. T7–12]	Both: Ease of dissection, improved body contour at donor site, stable pedicles	TRAM: Hernia, functional impairment risk, longer length of stay DIEP: Longer OR time, less functional impairment	

	Scapular	Horizontal branch of superficial circumflex scapular artery	Adipofascial, myocutaneous, fasciocutaneous, osseous (see "bone" section below)	B	25 × 10 cm	10–12 cm	3.5–4 mm	S: Intercostal N.	No functional morbidity, long pedicle, large-caliber pedicles, thin and pliable	Tight closure can restrict thoracic expansion, flap cannot be neurotized with single nerve, hairless but not good color match for head and neck	
	Parascapular	Vertical branch of the superficial circumflex scapular artery	Adipofascial, myocutaneous, fasciocutaneous	B	25 × 10 cm	10–12 cm	3.5–4 mm	S: Intercostal N.	No functional morbidity, long pedicle, large-caliber pedicles, thin and pliable	Tight closure can restrict thoracic expansion, flap cannot be neurotized with single nerve	
	Serratus	Lateral thoracic artery [1] and serratus branches of the thoracodorsal artery [2]	Myocutaneous, fasciocutaneous, myooseous	III	20 × 15 cm	6–8 cm [1, 2]	2–2.5 cm [1] 2–3 cm [2]	M: Long thoracic N. S: T2–C4 segmental intercostal n.	Reliable blood supply, useful when prior thoracotomy has transected viable latissimus muscle	Risk of scapular winging with long thoracic nerve injury	
	Groin flap [SCIP]	Superficial circumflex iliac artery	Fascia, adipose tissue, iliac bone, lateral femoral cutaneous nerve, sartorius muscle, [perforator]	A	25 × 10 cm [25 × 10 cm]	2.5–7 cm [2.5–7 cm]	0.8–2 mm [0.4–1.2 mm]	S: Lateral cutaneous N., intercostal T12	Both: Minimal donor-site morbidity, reliable blood supply SCIP flap only: Shorter flap elevation time	Both: Bulky in medial aspect, short pedicle and small vessel, pubic hair possible SCIP: Supermicrosurgery for small and short vessels, anatomic variation of SCIA system	

(continued)

Table 11.3 (continued)

Body region	Flap	Dominant vascular pedicle or source	Components	Mathes /Nahai classification	Typical max. size for primary closure	Pedicle length	Pedicle size	Relevant nerve (N.) supply	Advantages	Disadvantages	Technical notes
Upper extremity											
	Radial forearm (RF)	Radial artery	Fasciocutaneous, osteocutaneous, musculocutaneous, fascial flap	B	35 × 15 cm	15–22 cm	2.5–3.5 mm	S: M. and L. antebrachial cutaneous	Thin, pliable, durable, very long pedicle, can harvest under regional anesthesia	Sacrifice radial artery, not possible if palmar arch incomplete	Preoperative Allen's test, palmaris longus tendon may be used in tendon reconstruction
	Ulnar forearm flap (UFF)	Ulnar artery	Fasciocutaneous, myocutaneous, osteomyocutaneous	B	12 × 8 cm	4 cm	2.5–3.0 mm	S: M. and L. antebrachial cutaneous	Thin, pliable, durable, less hair than radial graft	Sacrifice ulnar artery, harvest of ulnar bone makes prone to fracture, ulnar nerve vulnerable to injury with dissection	Preoperative Allen's test
	Posterior interosseus (PI)	Posterior interosseus artery	Fasciocutaneous, osteocutaneous	B	15 × 7 cm	5 cm	1.5 mm	S: Lower branch of dorsal antebrachial N., medial antebrachial cutaneous N.	Versatile with long pedicle, able to cover the dorsal or volar aspect of the hand, forearm, and elbow, as well as harvested for FTT	Small pedicle length, risk of flap necrosis due to precarious blood supply to the skin paddle, 7 cm width for primary closure	

Intra-abdominal											
	Jejunal	Branches of superior mesenteric arterial arcades	Jejunum, mesentery	I	7–25 cm × 4 cm	4–6 cm	3–4 mm diameter	M: Mesenteric plexus	Functional benefits in esophageal/pharyngeal reconstruction, simple harvest	Ischemic susceptibility, relevant mortality with esophageal reconstruction, fistulization potential, inherent laparotomy/laparoscopy risk	
	Omental	Right gastroepiploic artery (a), left gastroepiploic artery (b)	Fat	III	30 × 60 cm	6 cm (a), 4 cm (b)	2–3 mm (a), 2 mm (b)	Autonomic: Splanchnic nerve plexus	Large area of coverage, rich blood supply	Required skin grafting when used on surface defects	Regional use: Chest, trunk scalp, extremity Specialized use: Cheek (Romberg's hemifacial atrophy)
Bone											
	Free fibula	Peroneal artery	Osseous, regional musculature, overlying fascia, skin		Skin: 12 × 6 cm Bone length: 6–26 cm (adult); 6–20 cm (child)	2–4 cm	1.0–2.5 mm	S: Lateral sural N.	Axial skeleton reconstruction, well-defined vasculature	Decreased ankle function, prominent donor-site scarring, must preserve 6 cm proximal fibula preserved for knee stability, 6 cm distal fibula preserved for ankle stability	

(continued)

Table 11.3 (continued)

Body region	Flap	Dominant vascular pedicle or source	Components	Mathes /Nahai classifi cation	Typical max. size for primary closure	Pedicle length	Pedicle size	Relevant nerve (N.) supply	Advantages	Disadvantages	Technical notes
	Scapular	Angular scapular artery (branch of thoracodorsal or serratus) and branches of circumflex scapular system	Osseous		Bone: 2 × 10 cm	Variable based on tissue harvested	3.5–4 mm	S: Intercostal N.	Compared with other osteocutaneous flaps (i.e., fibula and iliac crest), skin paddle and osseous segment can be manipulated separately for greater flexibility of inset		
	Iliac crest	Deep circumflex iliac artery	Bone + muscle, fascia, subcutaneous fat, skin		Skin: 20 × 16 cm; bone: 16 × 4 cm (1–1.5 cm thick)	9 cm	2–3 mm	S: T12	Donor site easily concealed, natural contour ideal for lateral mandibular reconstruction	Curvature may be limiting, skin paddle thick and bulky due to location, donor-site neuropathy	

[ ] Notates perforator variant of the corresponding flap listed; *M* motor, *S* sensory

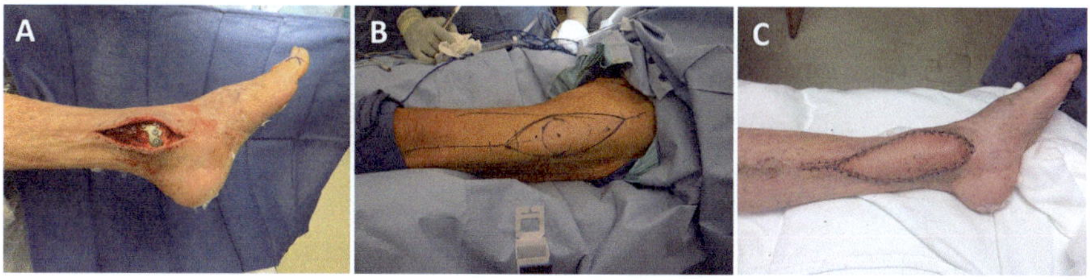

Fig. 11.1 Anterolateral thigh flap. (**a**) Complex medial malleolar defect with exposed bone and hardware. (**b**) Skin paddle design is shown. Relevant perforators are identified near the midpoint of an axis that extends from the anterior superior iliac spine and the superolateral border of the patella. (**c**) Follow-up at 3 weeks demonstrating a well-healed flap with satisfactory aesthetic contour of the medial ankle

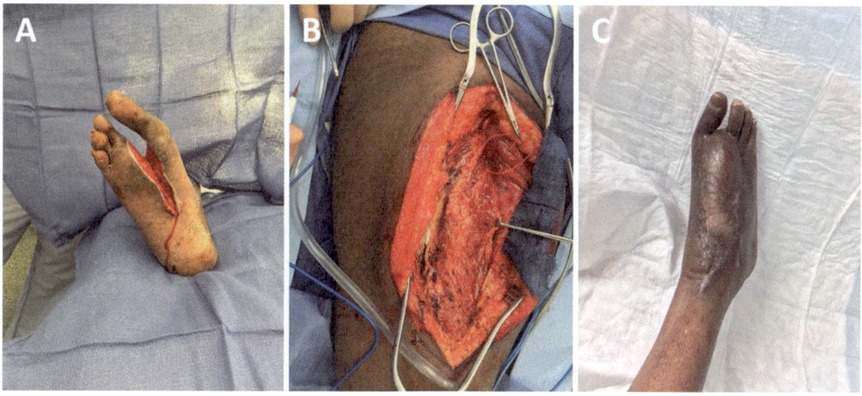

Fig. 11.2 Vastus lateralis free flap. (**a**) Composite intermetatarsal defect of the right foot following second ray amputation and soft tissue debridement. (**b**) Reconstruction was performed utilizing a split vastus lateralis muscle flap with end-to-side anastomosis between the anterior tibial artery and the descending branch of the lateral circumflex femoral artery. A split-thickness skin graft was harvested from the ipsilateral thigh for protective coverage of the exposed muscle. (**c**) Postoperative follow-up at 1 year showing stable, contoured soft tissue resurfacing

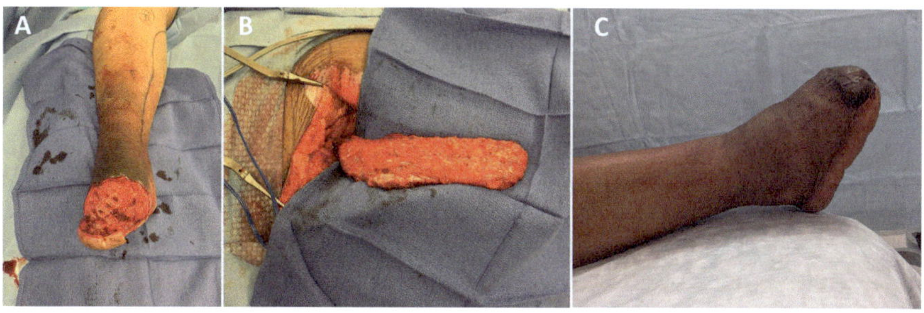

Fig. 11.3 Free gracilis muscle flap used to preserve length and maintain ambulation capacity in a patient with prior transmetatarsal amputation (TMA) complicated by infection. (**a**) Open right TMA with exposed bone and soft tissue loss. (**b**) Flap dissection and isolation of the vascular pedicle. (**c**) Postoperative result at 2 years is shown. Note the adequate contour that results from atrophy of the denervated muscle flap over time

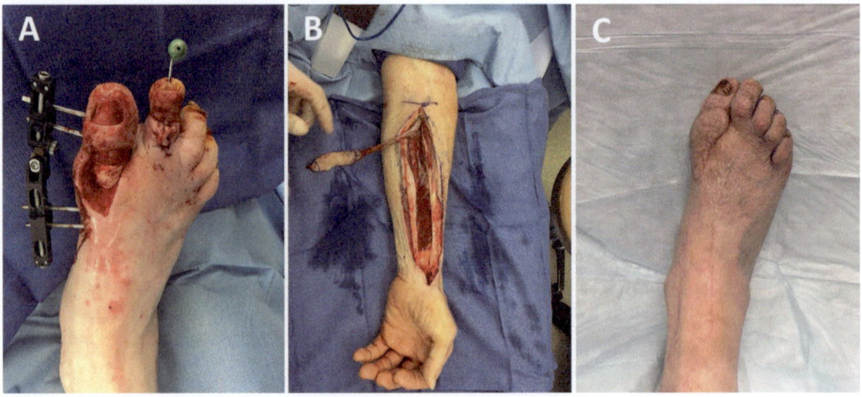

Fig. 11.4 Radial forearm free flap used in conjunction with an antibiotic spacer for reconstruction of an ablative defect involving the first metatarsophalangeal (MTP) joint. (**a**) Right dorsal hallux defect with exposed bone and antibiotic spacer. (**b**) Harvest of the radial forearm fasciocutaneous flap. A long pedicle length can be achieved by dissecting the radial artery to its proximal takeoff from the brachial artery. (**c**) Postoperative follow-up at 1 year demonstrating a well-healed and adequately contoured flap without excessive bulk

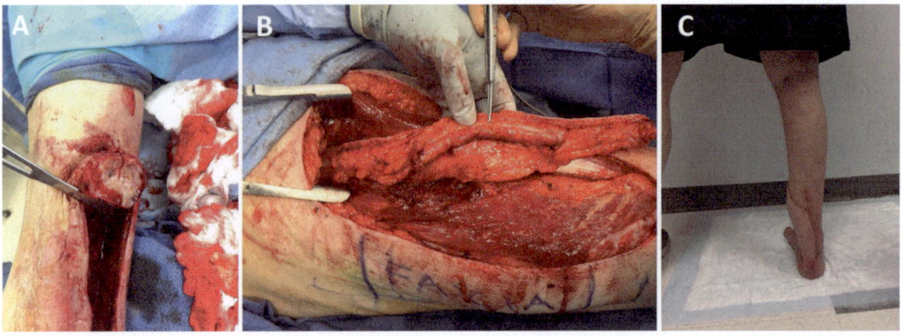

Fig. 11.5 Composite anterolateral thigh/vascularized fascia lata reconstruction of a combined tendocutaneous defect of the Achilles. (**a**) Segmental loss of the Achilles tendon with large overlying soft tissue deficit. (**b**) Harvest of the free anterolateral thigh flap with associated strip of fascia lata. The fascial strip is then rolled to form a neo-tendon construct, which is secured to the proximal and distal remnants of the native Achilles tendon. (**c**) Follow-up evaluation at 6 months demonstrating the aesthetic contour of the reconstructed Achilles

until postoperative day 5 or when the patient is transferred to the floor. The threshold for surgical take-back should be very low, as microvascular compromise may be devastating. Early identification and re-exploration of a compromised flap dramatically increase salvage rate. Kroll et al. report that the majority (80%) of pedicle thrombosis occurs within the first two postoperative days [36]. Mirzabeigi et al. found that arterial thrombosis was correctable by surgical take-back at much high rates than venous take-back within the first 48 h; specifically, there is a 77% arterial salvage rate versus 50% venous salvage rate [37]. Salvage rates decrease as time from the operation passes and approach 0% beyond postoperative day 4 (i.e., greater than 96 h).

One of the most effective advanced methods of monitoring flap viability is the implantable Doppler. With the implantable Doppler device, probes are placed circumferential on the venous segment due to the fact that arterial signals may persist for a time after venous thrombosis. Rozen et al. in a series of 547 breast flaps were able to report that implantable Doppler increased salvage rates 1.4 times compared to clinical monitoring, without increasing false-positive detection and reoperations [38]. This data allows implantable Doppler probe to be used as a safe and effective stand-alone monitoring technique in the postoperative setting [38].

Currently, there is no consensus regarding the optimal anticoagulation protocol following FTT, with the majority of recommendations being anecdotal and/or based on surgeon preference. In some instances, patients with uncomplicated flap procedures may use a generic protocol consisting of 325 mg aspirin daily along with prophylactic subcutaneous heparin. Patients in whom therapeutic levels of anticoagulants should be considered include those with thrombophilia, small-caliber anastomoses, poor-quality and/or friable vessels, and irradiated tissue and heavy smokers [8].

Complications

Advances in microsurgical technique have contributed to significantly reduced rates of postoperative complications and ultimate flap failure at high-volume centers. Complications after FTT are variable and may include seroma, hematoma, superficial epidermolysis, wound separation, inadequate coverage of defect, infection, and partial or complete flap loss [30]. Flap loss can be due to intrinsic factors that compromise blood supply (i.e., thrombosis, kinking) or extrinsic factors such as infection, hypotension, compression, and/or the use of vasoconstricting agents [30]. Other complications include functional limitations, sensory impairment, donor-site scar, and the need for revision/debulking. Complications and failures may often be attributed to poor planning, choice of donor- or recipient-site vasculature, timing, or technique [30]. The surgeon should be knowledgeable in all areas of the decision-making process in order to reduce such adverse events.

Lakhiani et al. described donor-site morbidities from commonly utilized thigh-based flaps. They proposed that flap selection is highly individualized, and the implications of aesthetic, perioperative, and/or functional morbidities should not be underestimated [39]. Patients should be counseled on potential risks specific to each flap type in order to optimize outcomes and overall satisfaction.

Conclusions

In the appropriate setting, FTT has proven to be an effective primary solution for complex wound reconstruction. Advances in our knowledge of vascular anatomy, surgical technique, and postoperative patient care have enabled substantial improvements in microvascular success rates over time. As prior data have shown, vigilance in all stages of preoperative patient selection, operative planning, technical execution, and postoperative rehabilitation is essential to optimize reconstructive outcomes, satisfaction, and complication profiles for microsurgical candidates.

References

1. Krizek TJ, Tani T, Desprez JD, et al. Experimental transplantation of composite grafts by microsurgical vascular anastomoses. Plast Reconstr Surg. 1965;36(5):538–46.
2. Choi DH, Goh T, Cho JY, Hong JP. Thin superficial circumflex iliac artery perforator flap and supermicrosurgery for face reconstruction. J Craniofac Surg. 2014;25(6):2130–3.
3. Taylor GI, Palmer JH. The vascular territories (angiosomes) of the body: experimental study and clinical applications. Br J Plast Surg. 1987;40(2):113–41.
4. Saint-Cyr M, Wong C, Schaverien M, Mojallal A, Rohrich RJ. The perforasome theory: vascular anatomy and clinical implications. Plast Reconstr Surg. 2009;124(5):1529–44.
5. Saint-Cyr M, Wong C, Buchel EW, Colohan S, Pederson WC. Free tissue transfers and replantation. Plast Reconstr Surg. 2012;130(6):858e–78e.
6. Serletti JM, Deuber MA, Guidera PM, et al. Comparison of the operating microscope and loupes for free microvascular tissue transfer. Plast Reconstr Surg. 1995;95:270–6.
7. Oliva A, Lineaweaver WC, Buncke HJ, et al. Salvage of wounds following failed tissue transplantation. J Reconstr Mircosurg. 1993;9:257–63.
8. Butler CE, Adelman DM. Grabb and Smith's plastic surgery. 7th ed. Philadelphia: Wolters Kluwer/Lippincott Williams & Wilkins Health; 2014. Part I, Chapter 8, Principles of Microsurgery
9. Buchanan PJ, Kung TA, Cederna PS. Evidence-based medicine: wound closure. Plast Reconstr Surg. 2016;138:257S.
10. Fan KL, Patel KM, Mardini S, Attinger C, Levin LS, Evans KK. Evidence to support controversy in microsurgery. Plast Reconstr Surg. 2015;135:595e.
11. Suh HS, Oh TS, Hong JP. Innovations in diabetic foot reconstruction using supermicrosurgery. Diabetes Metab Res Rev. 2016;32:275–80.
12. Masia J, Olivares I, Koshima I, et al. Barcelona consensus on supermicrosurgery. J Reconstr Microsurg. 2015;30:53–8.
13. Suh HS, Oh TS, Lee HS, Lee SH, Cho YP, Park JR, Hong JP. A new approach for reconstruction of diabetic foot wounds using the angiosomes and supermicrosurgery. Plast Reonstr Surg. 2016;148(4):702e–9e.
14. DeFazio MV, Han KD, Attinger CE. Volume 4: chapter 8: foot reconstruction. In: Neligan PC, editor Plastic surgery. 4th ed. Atlanta, GA: Elsevier. in press; 2017.
15. Boulton AJ. What you can't feel can hurt you. J Vasc Surg. 2010;52(3):28S–30S.
16. DeFazio MV, Han KD, Akbari CM, Evans KK. Free tissue transfer after targeted endovascular reperfusion for complex lower extremity reconstruction: setting the stage for success in the presence of multivessel disease. Ann Vasc Surg. 2015;29:1316.e7–e15. df
17. Falanga V. Growth factors and chronic wounds: the need to understand the microenvironment. J Dermatol. 1992;19:667–72.
18. Greene TL, Beauy ME. Soft tissue coverage for lower-extremity trauma: current practice and techniques. J Orthop Trauma. 1988;2:158–73.
19. Gustilo RB, Merkow RI, Templeman D. The management of open fractures. J Bone Joint Surg. 1990;72:299–304.
20. Argenta LC, Morykwas MJ. Vacuum-assisted closure: a new method for wound control and treatment: clinical experience. Ann Plast Surg. 1997;38:563–76.
21. Endara M, Attinger C. Using color to guide debridement. Adv Skin Wound Care. 2012;25:549–55.

22. Kanuri A, DeFazio MV, Anghel E, Kumar A, Evans KK, Attinger CE. Examining the use of post-debridement cultures to optimize debridgement and improve outcomes in lower extremity reconstruction. Continuing medical education resident conference, Georgetown University School of Medicine. Lecture Given 2016.
23. Armstrong DG, Lavery LA, Consortium DFS. Negative pressure wound therapy after partial diabetic foot amputation: a multicenter, randomized controlled trial. Lancet. 2005;366:1704–10.
24. Kim PJ, Attinger CE, Steinberg JS, et al. Negative-pressure wound therapy with instillation: international consensus guidelines. Plast Reconstr Surg. 2013;132:1569–79.
25. Kim PJ, Attinger CE, Steinberg JS, et al. The impact of negative-pressure wound therapy with instillation compared with standard negative-pressure wound therapy: a retrospective, historical, cohort, controlled study. Plast Reconstr Surg. 2014;133:709–16.
26. Lakhiani C, Evans KK, Attinger CE. Chapter 16: free flap reconstruction for soft tissue coverage of the diabetic lower extremity. In: Zgonis T, editor. Surgical reconstruction of the diabetic foot. In Press, 2017.
27. Heller L, Kronowitz SJ. Lower extremity reconstruction. J Surg Oncol. 2006;94:479–89.
28. Mathes SJ, Alpert BS, Chang N. Use of the muscle flap in chronic osteomyelitis: experimental and clinical correlation. Plast Reconstr Surg. 1982;69:815–29.
29. Mathes SJ, Feng LG, Hunt TK. Coverage of the infected wound. Ann Surg. 1983;198:420–9.
30. Hansen SL, Young DM, Lang P, Sbitany H. Plastic surgery: principles volume 1. 3rd ed. London: Elsevier Health Sciences; 2013. Chapter 24, Flap classification and applications
31. Hallock GG. Anatomic basis of the gastrocnemius perforator-based flap. Ann Plast Surg. 2001;47:517.
32. Blondeel N, Vanderstraeten GG, Monstrey SJ, et al. The donor site morbidity of free DIEP flaps and free TRAM flaps for breast reconstruction. Br J Plast Surg. 1997;50:322–30.
33. Kimura N. A microdissected thin tensor fasciae latae perforator flap. Plast Reconstr Surg. 2002;109:69.
34. Hyun SS, Lee JS, Jooh PH. Consideration in lower extremity reconstruction following oncologic surgery: patient selection, surgical techniques, and outcomes. J Surg Oncol. 2016;113:955–61.
35. Sink J, Hmlar D, Kademani D, Khariwala SS. Computer-aided stereolithography for presurgical planning in fibula free tissue reconstruction of the mandible. J Reconstr Microsurg. 2012;28(6):395–403.
36. Kroll SS, Schusterman MA, Reece GP, et al. Timing of pedicle thrombosis and flap loss after free-tissue transfer. Plast Reconstr Surg. 1996;98:1230–3.
37. Mirzabeigi MN, Wang T, Kovach SJ, Taylor JA, Serletti JM, Wu LC. Free flap take-back following postoperative microvascular compromise: predicting salvage versus failure. Plast Reconstr Surg. 2012;130:579–89.
38. Rozen WM, Chubb D, Whitaker IS, Acosta R. The efficacy of postoperative monitoring: a single surgeon comparison of clinical monitoring and the implantable Doppler probe in 547 consecutive free flaps. Microsurgery. 2010;30:105–10.
39. Lakhiani C, DeFazio MV, Han K, Falola R, Evans KK. Donor-site morbidity following free tissue harvest from the thigh: a systemic review and pooled analysis of complications. J Reconstr Microsurg. 2016;32(05):342–57.

Chapter 12
Negative-Pressure Wound Therapy

Lauren R. Bayer

Introduction

When Louis Argenta and Michael Morykwas published their seminal research on vacuum-assisted closure in 1997 [1], they likely could not have imagined that the technology would become one of the most revolutionary wound treatments of the late twentieth century. Basic treatment of acute, chronic, and surgical wounds is generally limited to normal saline-dampened gauze or other moist dressings based on work by Winter [2], who illustrated the importance of keeping the wound bed moist to avoid tissue desiccation. More advanced wound dressings include dressings impregnated with silver, collagens, alginates, and foams, but they may not be as effective or practical for large wounds or those with a large amount of exudate. Dermal substitutes and bioengineered skin have shown promise in several types of wounds [3].

Suction, irrigation, and drainage of infected internal cavities and large wounds have been employed in medical settings for decades [4]. Argenta and Morykwas showed that subatmospheric pressure applied to an open wound filled with an open-cell foam sealed with an adhesive drape could not only evacuate fluid but also induce granulation tissue formation and facilitate wound contracture [1].

Eventually marketed as vacuum-assisted closure (V.A.C.®) by Kinetic Concepts Incorporated (KCI) in 1997, the treatment has become ubiquitous and the subject of vast research. Because the KCI V.A.C. ® was the only marketed device for over 15 years, most published research has used the V.A.C.®. There are now dozens of

Electronic Supplementary Material: The online version of this chapter (https://doi.org/10.1007/978-3-319-66990-8_12) contains supplementary material, which is available to authorized users.

L.R. Bayer, PA-C (✉)
Wound Care Center, Department of Surgery, Division of Plastic Surgery,
Brigham and Women's Hospital – Harvard Medical School, Boston, MA, USA
e-mail: lbayer@partners.org

D.P. Orgill (ed.), *Interventional Treatment of Wounds*,
https://doi.org/10.1007/978-3-319-66990-8_12

negative-pressure wound therapy (NPWT) devices. Generic to most of the devices is an interface material ranging from standard gauze to open-pore foam, a semiocclusive adhesive dressing, suction tubing, and a suction device. Disposable, one-time devices are available for smaller wounds or those without much drainage. Some in vivo animal [5] and clinical studies [6] have compared gauze filler with open-cell foam and showed no difference in tissue growth and wound contraction. Nevertheless, open-cell, polyurethane foam interface is preferred by many users. Recently, the technology has been combined with instillation of a variety of fluids [7].

Mechanisms of Action

The primary and secondary mechanisms of action of NPWT systems have been studied extensively in preclinical models and in humans. Proposed primary mechanisms include macrodeformation when the wound edges are drawn together, microdeformation at the wound-foam interface, fluid removal, and maintenance of a stable wound environment (Fig. 12.1). Resultant granulation tissue formation, angiogenesis, neurogenesis, and cell proliferation are secondary mechanisms of action that enhance the wound-healing cascade [8].

NPWT depends on differential pressure applied to tissues. Based on cell culture work showing that cells that are stretched from their spherical shape tend to divide and proliferate [9, 10], Lu et al. [11] designed a model in which vacuum pressure is applied to tissue cells via incompressible foam in vitro. In vivo, different pressures and pore sizes were studied and surface deformations of the cells resulted. The deformations predicted by the model were similar to the undulations noted on the wound surface when an NPWT device was applied. The cells are stretched, allowing them to divide and proliferate. Thus, application of vacuum to tissues causes microdeformations in the tissues, inducing angiogenesis and cellular proliferation and explaining an important mechanism of action of NPWT [12].

The open-pore foam used in most NPWT systems transmits a vacuum quite efficiently and has been shown to decrease in size by about 80% when exposed to 125 mmHg suction [13, 14]. The wound collapses due to the centripetal forces placed on the wound surface and the degree of wound contraction will depend on the deformability of the tissues. Packing the wound with a piece of foam cut to fit inside will facilitate wound contracture as vacuum pressure is applied.

Excess fluid in a wound or in the extracellular space can adversely affect wound healing. Suction applied to the foam dressing evacuates the excess fluid in the wound and has been observed to decrease soft tissue edema, as in the case of fasciotomy wounds and large open abdominal wounds. Fluid removal decreases compression on the microvasculature, which in turn can increase tissue perfusion [8]. Toxins, bacteria, and harmful exudate are also removed, potentially improving wound healing.

The foam and semiocclusive polyurethane drape that make up most NPWT systems has limited permeability to gases and vapor and is therefore effective in keeping

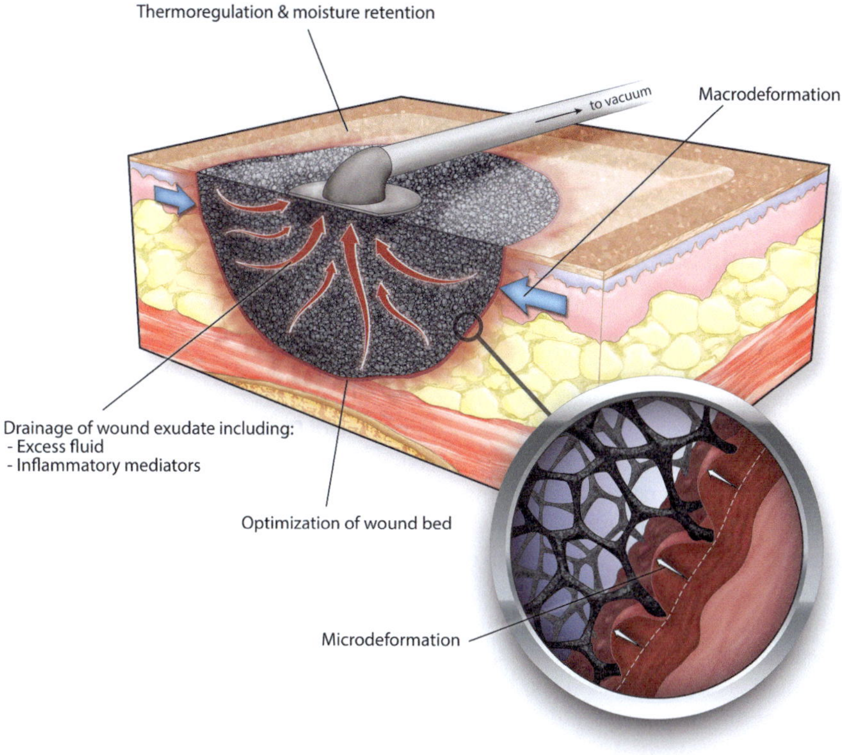

Fig. 12.1 The primary mechanisms of action of NPWT (From Huang et al. [8]. With permission from Elsevier)

the wound moist and normalizing the wound temperature, thus stabilizing the wound environment. In addition, the drape is impermeable to proteins and microorganisms, reducing the risk of infection transmission from the environment [8].

Induced microvascular blood flow has been reported in wounds treated with NPWT and is dependent on the amount of pressure, distance from the wound edges, and the type of tissue. Combined with increased partial pressure of oxygen and lactate levels, more robust wound healing has been noted [15].

Clinical Applications

NPWT has been used for a variety of acute and chronic wounds, anatomic locations, and wound etiologies. Common wound types include surgical and traumatic wounds, orthopedic wounds, diabetic and vascular ulcers, and pressure injuries. NPWT has been shown to heal complex wounds with less invasive surgical intervention [16, 17]. The reconstructive ladder is well known to surgeons and begins at the bottom with primary closure of a wound and progresses upward in complexity through the rungs from skin grafts, local flaps, regional flaps to the most complex, and free flaps at the top [16, 17]. Using NPWT at the outset to treat a wound that would otherwise require surgical closure with a flap, for example, facilitates a shift down the reconstructive ladder, decreasing the need for a complex closure [18].

Basic Application of NPWT in an Open Wound

NPWT is most commonly used in an open wound. In order to be most affective, the open-cell foam packing is placed in direct contact with the wound bed. The exception being direct foam contact with visceral organs, large nerves, tendons, the heart, or large blood vessels where an intervening nonadherent layer, viable tissue, or tissue-engineered construct should be placed to avoid erosion. The foam is cut to fit the wound size and packed loosely into the wound. Ideally, only one piece of foam should be placed in the wound. The use of more than one piece of foam should be documented and checked at the time of removal when dressing is changed.

A semipermeable adhesive drape is placed over the wound, overlapping the surrounding skin 3–5 centimeters. Suction tubing is attached to the dressing and connected to the vacuum device. Vacuum settings range from 50 to 150 mmHg depending on the device and can be set as low or high as necessary to achieve adequate suction. The adhesive drape must be generally free of leaks or else suction cannot be maintained. A small amount of air that transits the system can help avoid a vapor lock. In the setting of large amounts of drainage, suction may need to be adjusted to maintain a seal and to fully evacuate the wound. Small, drier wounds may have little drainage (Fig. 12.2).

Dressings should be changed every 2–3 days, depending on drainage amount, wound etiology, and goal of therapy. For granulating a large wound with a large amount of drainage, more frequent dressing changes may be necessary. In the event of a device malfunction, the dressing should be removed within 2 h if suction cannot be maintained [19].

Optimal cycling of NPWT has been debated. Most manufacturers recommend the device be set on a continuous cycle, delivering a constant rate of vacuum suction. Intermittent suction has been shown in experimental settings to yield a greater biological effect and may be advantageous over continuous suction, but it can often be unpleasant for the patient. Too rapid cycling can also be deleterious [20, 21].

During dressing changes, care must be taken to avoid damage to the tissues, bleeding, and pain. Irrigating the foam with saline can loosen the foam from the tissues. Adding lidocaine to the saline or injecting the foam directly with a large bore needle can help reduce the pain sometimes associated with dressing removal. Once the dressing is removed, the wound should be inspected for residual foam adhered to the tissue, necrosis, and bleeding. Wounds should be cleaned and debrided if necessary prior to reapplying the dressing.

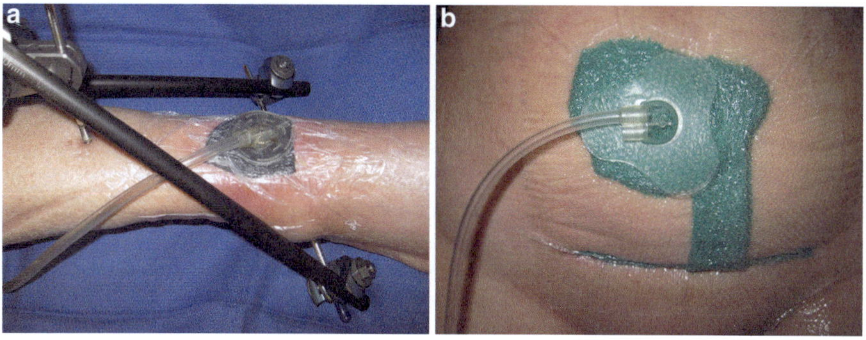

Fig. 12.2 (**a**) NPWT dressing on a traumatic wound after tib fib fracture, debridement, and external fixator (**b**) NPWT dressing on a cesarean section wound using the bridging technique

While there are few limits to the anatomic location or wound type for NPWT use, not all applications have been studied. The following section reviews common uses of NPWT and supportive data when available.

Diabetic Foot Ulcers

Diabetic foot ulcers (DFU) affect more than 25% of diabetics over their lifetime [22] and are the source of severe morbidity and mortality. Treatment of DFU includes debridement, moist dressings, and offloading with a goal toward avoiding amputation. Prevalence of lower extremity amputation in diabetics was 1.8 between 2006 and 2008, tripling in patients with concomitant peripheral artery disease [23]. DFU requiring advanced therapy include primary deep ulcerations and postsurgical wounds and may be amenable NPWT.

Randomized control studies with Level I–II evidence comparing NPWT with standard of care (moist wound therapy with alginates, hydrocolloids, foams, or hydrogels) [24, 25] on DFU showed increased granulation tissue, wound area reduction [26], reduction in operative intervention [27] including reamputation [24], and decreased infections [28]. Dumville et al. [29] reported some evidence that NPWT is clinically effective in reducing time to healing and risk of amputation in chronic DFU and postsurgical wounds.

DFU should be debrided prior to application of NPWT as the necrotic bone, connective tissue, or subcutaneous tissue will prevent healing [30] and may worsen with NPWT. Radiologic studies may be necessary to rule out underlying osteomyelitis before beginning therapy. Patients should be adequately offloaded [31] and blood glucose optimized to ensure maximum benefit.

Dressing application to the foot can be challenging and toe and heel contours may make keeping a seal difficult. Applying skin prep, a thin hydrocolloid or pieces of adhesive drape around the wound add an extra surface on which the wound-covering drape can adhere. Using the bridging technique if the wound is on the heel or plantar foot moves the tubing away from the walking surface and can be more comfortable. The dressing foam cut slightly smaller than the wound size is packed into the wound. A piece of adhesive drape or hydrocolloid is applied from the wound to a relocation area on the dorsal foot or lower leg to protect the skin. A thin piece of foam is applied (bridged) from the wound to the relocation area over the drape or hydrocolloid. An additional piece of adhesive drape is applied to cover all pieces of foam, and the tubing connection is placed on the end of foam bridge. As long as the bridged foam and wound packing foam are contiguous, the vacuum will reach the wound (Fig. 12.3). Dressings should be changed two to three times per week, and wounds should be carefully monitored for necrosis and infection.

Deep Pressure Injuries

Wounds caused by pressure can be a devastating complication of prolonged hospital or nursing home stay, immobility, or debilitation. NPWT for stage 3 or 4 pressure injuries aids in fluid evacuation, granulation tissue proliferation, and wound contraction to optimize wounds for secondary closure or preparation for surgical closure [32]. There are few randomized control studies using NPWT in pressure wounds, and none compare NPWT with advanced therapies [33]. Despite the dearth of data, clinical use is ubiquitous as pressure injuries become more prevalent, especially in our aging population.

Wounds should be free of necrotic tissue prior to commencing therapy, facilitated by serial sharp debridements augmented by mechanical debridement with saline or ¼ strength Dakin's (sodium hypochlorite) dampened gauze packing. Imaging studies to rule out osteomyelitis and abscess should be obtained. Large, deep wounds should ideally be packed with only one piece of foam to avoid multiple pieces of foam that could be lost in the wound with subsequent dressing changes. Dead spaces, undermined areas, and tracks should be packed, using caution in areas of narrow tracking. Applying the foam just at the base of a narrow track to prevent tissue from walling off the area can often suffice. The foam should be trimmed to a size slightly smaller than the wound to facilitate wound contraction and the wound should never be overpacked. The device tubing can be "bridged" away from the wound to avoid the patient lying or sitting on the tubing (Fig. 12.4). Suction can be set at the lowest setting that maintains a seal and evacuates fluid; 100–125 mm Hg is recommended. Sensate patients may have pain with higher suction so the setting can be reduced.

Minimizing pressure on the wound with complete offloading with limited or no sitting, boots for extremity pressure injuries and use of a pressure relieving mattress can ensure effective treatment. Optimizing nutritional status, managing incontinence and cessation of nicotine products will also aid in healing. NPWT is not recommended in the setting of malnutrition, dermatitis, incontinence affecting the dressing seal, persistent tissue necrosis, bleeding, and pain.

After prolonged use, the wound, dressing, and/or canister can become malodorous. NPWT can be discontinued for 2–3 days while the wound is packed with gauze

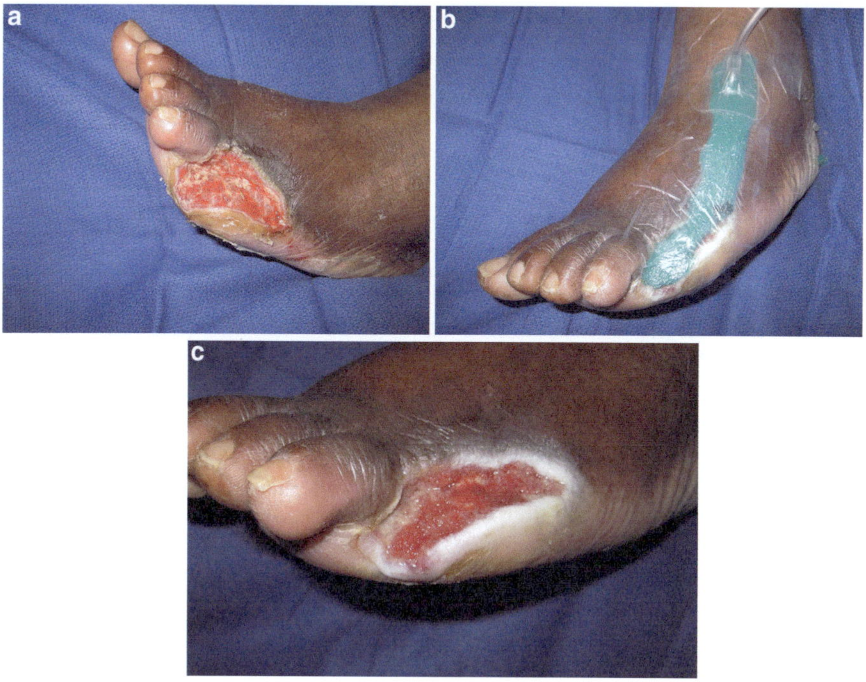

Fig. 12.3 (**a**) Diabetic foot ulcer before NPWT. (**b**) NPWT dressing with bridge. (**c**) Two weeks after NPWT treatment

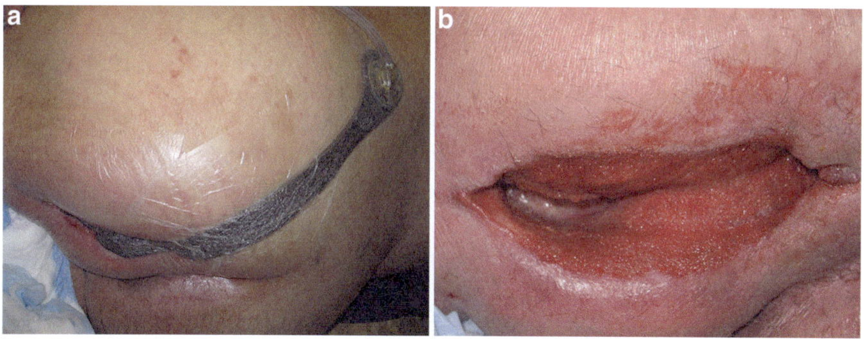

Fig. 12.4 (**a**) Bridged NPWT dressing. (**b**) Resultant granulating stage 4 left ischial pressure injury

dampened with saline or quarter strength Dakin's to treat bacterial colonization and odor. NPWT can then be resumed. Wound measurements should be obtained weekly, and once the wound is no longer decreasing in size, other treatments should be investigated, including flap closure for surgical candidates. Indolent infection, including osteomyelitis or abscess, may be a cause of a stalled wound, and should be ruled out with cultures or imaging studies.

Vascular Lower Extremity Ulcers (Venous/Arterial)

Chronic lower extremity ulcers are generally caused by either venous stasis or arterial insufficiency. The hallmark of venous stasis ulcer treatment is compression, and there are many advanced wound therapies also available. NPWT, while not commonly used, can optimize the wound bed for application of a skin graft or dermal substitute, aid in fluid management, decrease matrix metalloproteinases, and decrease bioburden in select cases [34]. NPWT has also been used in the treatment of lymphocele and lymph fistulas as a complication from vascular procedures. Case studies reported decreased lymphorrhea which led to eventual wound healing [35].

The use of NPWT in the setting of arterial disease is most commonly necessary after wound debridement, groin wound complications [36, 37], or amputations. NPWT should only be considered if the extremity has been adequately revascularized and debrided of all devitalized tissue. Complications of using NPWT dressings in open groin wounds include infection and bleeding. Exposed vital structures must be covered with fascia or a nonadherent dressing under the NPWT foam and should be carefully monitored during treatment. NPWT can be used to assist in secondary healing or preparation for skin graft or flap in open or dehisced amputation wounds. Wounds left open because of infection or edema can be optimized with NPWT and surgically closed at a later date.

Traumatic Wounds

Traumatic injuries of lower extremities, which often include both complex bone fractures (Gustilo Grade IIIA and B) [38] and soft tissue damage can be managed with NPWT. Early coverage of the exposed bone is important to prevent infection, and often the wounds require frequent washouts and debridements in the operating room before definitive fracture fixation and soft tissue closure [16]. Reduced morbidity and time of healing using NPWT compared to standard gauze dressings has been shown [39]. Sealing the wound in the sterile dressing serves to decrease wound infection [40–42] as it can decrease dressing changes and provide protection from nosocomial contamination [43]. Sinha et al. [44] saw significantly reduced wound size in open musculoskeletal injuries treated with NPWT, reduced bacterial growth by day 8, significant angiogenesis, and granulation tissue formation. When immediate primary closure is not possible, delayed closure with skin grafts or flaps may be required. When NPWT is used on lower extremity traumatic wounds, researchers have noted fewer free flaps were used for closure, trending toward the ability for delayed closures with local flaps and skin grafts [16, 18, 45].

After thorough debridement, irrigation, hemostasis, fracture stabilization, and coverage of exposed vessels and nerves with a nonadherent dressing, NPWT is applied in the operating room. The dressing foam can be placed directly on exposed tendon to prevent desiccation and promote ingrowth of granulation tissue (Fig. 12.5).

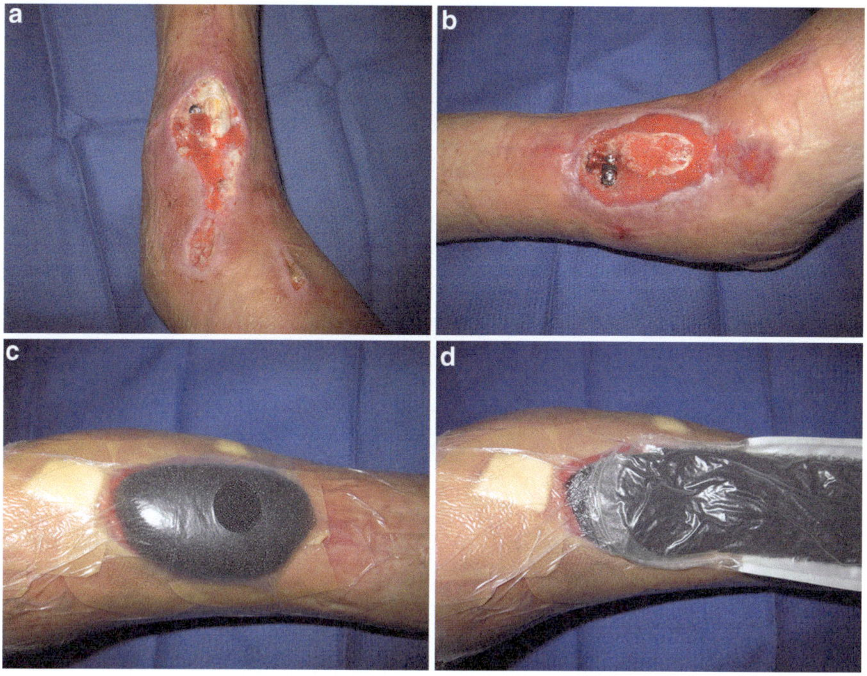

Fig. 12.5 (**a**) Traumatic tib fib fracture and wound dehiscence with exposed tendon. (**b**) After NPWT with granulating tendon. (**c**) NPWT dressing in place. (**d**) NPWT bridge dressing in place

Between debridements, wounds should be monitored carefully for bleeding. NPWT devices with the capability of instilling fluid may be beneficial in lower extremity traumatic wounds [7].

Patients with intra-abdominal trauma may require massive amounts of fluid resuscitation resulting in severe edema of the abdominal cavity and making closure of large abdominal wounds not possible. Applying NPWT for temporary abdominal closure (TAC) of a large open wound to facilitate delayed primary closure while the patient stabilizes has been shown to be successful [46]. A systematic review of NPWT for TAC [47] resulted in several observations and recommendations. The highest rates of primary fascial closure were seen using commercially available NPWT dressings and the "dynamic closure" technique, which includes mesh and retention sutures along with NPWT dressing. Septic patients did not fare as well. Other recommendations include using an interface layer over exposed organs to avoid adhesions between the foam and bowel and the abdominal wall and using a foam-based dressing instead of gauze, use for managing abdominal fluid, and the device should be set on a continuous rather than intermittent setting. Concern for enterocutaneous fistula is warranted but has been found to not be more common when using NPWT over plain gauze packing in open abdominal wounds [47].

Sternal Wounds

Complications from median sternotomy can be fraught with patient morbidity and extremely challenging due to the vital structures within the thorax. Prior to the advent of commercially available NPWT systems, sternal wound infection was routinely treated with antimicrobial irrigation via catheters and gauze packing [48, 49]. Once the infection was eradicated, closure was performed using pectoralis and/or omental flaps, with or without sternectomy. With the advent of NPWT, treatment of open chest wounds improved significantly. Several reports describe use of NPWT versus gauze dressings and showed better sternal stability and reduced need for mechanical ventilation while the chest was open, [50] increased granulation tissue formation, decreased C-reactive protein levels [51] and lower recurrence rate, and increased ability to salvage the sternum [52].

After OR debridement of the infected tissue, muscle, and bone, a fluid-permeable nonadherent dressing or fascia is applied to cover the heart, if exposed, large vessels, and friable bone to eliminate the risk of vital structure rupture. The foam interface is then placed into the wound. The adhesive drape keeps the open mediastinum sterile and maintains a moist wound environment. Vacuum suction pulls the wound edges together, stabilizing the chest, and evacuates fluid accumulation. If the sternum is open, dressings are changed under anesthesia. If the wound is superficial, with an intact sternum, dressings can be changed at bedside every 2–3 days. Superficial wounds can be left to heal by secondary intention. Deep sternal or chest wounds may require a flap. Once the wound is deemed ready for closure, omentum can be brought up to fill in any dead space and flaps, including pectoralis major, latissimus dorsi muscle, rectus abdominus muscle can be raised to cover the mediastinum [53].

Complications from using NPWT in the chest have been reported and should serve as cautionary tales. Bleeding from coronary artery venous bypass grafts, ascending aorta, and the sternum [54] and right ventricular rupture [55] have been reported.

Fasciotomy Wounds

Fasciotomy incisions are created to relieve pressure in the setting of compartment syndrome. Because concurrent edema is common, incisions are difficult to close primarily even after the pressures have normalized. After debridement and hemostasis, NPWT can be applied directly to the open wounds to facilitate edema reduction and splint the wound edges together allowing for either delayed primary closure, skin grafts or healing by secondary intention [18, 56]. If a skin graft is employed, NPWT can continue to be utilized as a bolster to further limit fluid collection under the graft and improve graft take [56].

Burns

Management of large acute burns includes medical stabilization and particular attention to the wounds. NPWT may assist in the goals of burn wound care including preventing infection, preventing burn progression, and providing a moist environment that will facilitate healing and minimize fluid evaporation. NPWT may also be beneficial at preventing burn wound progression [18]. A porcine study of NPWT application within 12 h of burn injury reduced the depth of tissue necrosis, but not after 18 h. Optimum window of time for NPWT to prevent burn progression may be less than 12 h, but there are no robust studies to support its use. Progression of burn depth has been studied in both porcine [57] and human models [58] and shown to decrease progression as well as reduce inflammatory infiltrates [57].

NPWT dressings on large burns can limit the frequency of often painful dressing changes and offer stabilization of the microenvironment during physiological recovery [58]. The dressings can prepare the burn wound beds for skin grafting by stimulating granulation tissue and vascularity and potentially decreasing the surface area and wound depth ultimately needing closure [59]. When used as a bolster, NPWT dressings can secure the skin grafts and improve graft take [60].

Clinical application is similar to that of any large wound, with some modifications. Due to pain and patient instability, dressings may need to be changed under sedation or in an operating room. Silver impregnated foam can be used to potentially decrease bioburden in the wounds and help prevent infection [61]. Keeping a dressing seal can be challenging on large TBSA burns, and methods such as preparing the skin with benzoin, securing the adhesive drapes with staples or sutures, using additional layers of drape, and using multiple pumps have been described [62]. NPWT can be used for residual open wounds after skin grafting, and using silver foam in the event of early graft failure may prevent further graft loss and promote healing [63].

Skin Grafts

Skin graft take is dependent on elimination of fluid accumulation under the graft, immobilization and stabilization of the graft, keeping the graft moist to avoid desiccation, and providing an environment that limits infection risks [64]. For most skin grafts, a cotton or foam bolster is sufficient, but for larger grafts or those at higher risk of failure, using NPWT before and after graft placement is a viable option. Optimizing the wound bed prior to skin graft placement with debridements and NPWT has been shown to increase split- and full-thickness graft take in various wound types such as Achilles [65], lower extremity traumatic wounds [64], burns [66], and fasciotomies [67]. Pretreatment with NPWT is dependent on the severity and depth of the wound. Multiple debridements and several weeks of NPWT treatment may be required before the wound bed is ready for grafting, but often, 5–7 days of NPWT followed by coverage with a spilt-thickness or fenestrated full-thickness skin graft is enough to improve skin graft take substantially [18, 66].

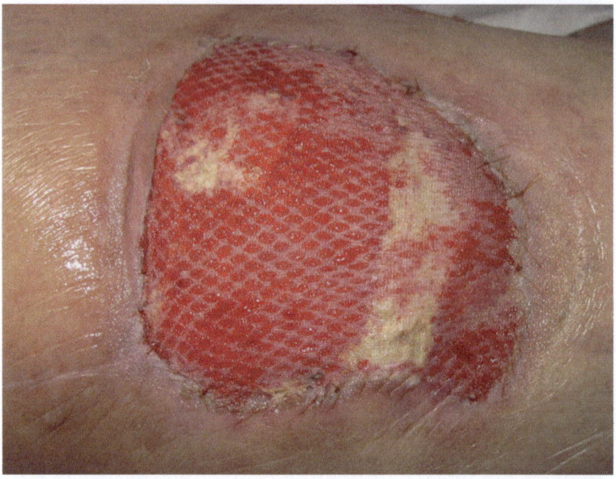

Fig. 12.6 Knee wound after removal of infected hardware, debridement, skin graft, and NPWT

The skin graft can be applied to the wound and anchored with suture or staples per surgeon preference. A nonadherent dressing (petroleum gauze, meshed nonadherent dressing) is usually placed over the skin graft and the NPWT dressing is applied, covered with adherent drape (Video 12.1). The vacuum is set at 75–100 mm Hg, continuous. The dressing is left for 4–5 days and then carefully removed and replaced with a moist dressing according to surgeon preference (Fig. 12.6).

Instillation and Incisional Applications

Surgical site infections (SSI) in acute care facilities are still relatively common, estimated at over 160,000–300,000 per year in the United States with 2–11 times higher mortality rate compared with surgical patients without SSI and a financial cost of $3.5 billion to $10 billion annually in healthcare expenditures (adjusted for 2007 dollars) [68, 69]. Preventative measures have been mandated by the CDC and Healthcare Infection Control Practices Advisory Committee [68]. Applying NPWT to closed incisions and using instillation therapy are both showing promise in further decreasing the risk of SSI [69].

Incisional NPWT

In a meta-analysis of studies comparing incisional NPWT to standard surgical closure, Semsarzadeh et al. [69] found overall SSI rate in the closed incision NPWT group to be 6.61% compared to 9.36% in the control group. Used when patients are at high risk of surgical wound dehiscence, seroma formation, or infection – diabetics, obese, and orthopedic trauma – an incisional dressing may prevent SSI or wound dehiscence by evacuating accumulated serous fluid, reducing wound dead space and keeping the incision splinted under a sterile adherent dressing [70].

Incisional NPWT has been shown to decrease wound complications in hip arthrectomies [71] and in lower extremity fractures at high risk for wound dehiscence and infection [72].

A cost analysis by Australian authors noted incisional NPWT cost-effective for preventing SSI in obese patients undergoing cesarean section [73]. Lewis et al. [74] conducted a cost analysis for laparotomy for gynecologic malignancies in high-risk, obese patients and proposed there would be a cost savings if incisional NPWT reduced wound complications by at least 33%.

NPWT dressings are placed over the sutured or stapled incision, either with a specifically made system (PREVENA®) or using standard NPWT systems with a contact layer over the skin (meshed nonadherent dressing, petroleum gauze). Device setting is recommended at 75–100 mmHg. The dressing remains in place for up to 7 days and is then removed and replaced with a dry dressing.

Instillation Therapy

Chronic or contaminated wounds may harbor high bacterial burden, negatively effecting wound healing. Although Morykwas et al. saw modest success in reducing wound bioburden using NPWT in a porcine model of infected wounds [75], conflicting results have been seen in humans. In 1998, Fleischmann suggested instilling various solutions into wounds to facilitate wound closure [76]. Goss et al. [77] studied a small cohort of 16 chronically infected lower extremity wounds treated with operating room debridement with NPWT and instilled ¼ strength Dakin's solution. They found a statistically significant reduction in absolute bioburden in the wounds treated with NPWT with instillation (NPWTi). In a retrospective historical cohort-controlled trial examining NPWT with and without instillation, Kim et al. noted a reduction in total number of operative debridements, shorter time to wound closure, and shortened length of stay in patients with infected wounds treated with NPWTi [78]. Other types of instillation fluids have been studied including saline, polyhexamine [79], superoxidized water, diluted iodine, and antibiotic solution [80]. Kim et al. randomized 100 patients with infected wounds in a prospective study comparing instillation of saline and 0.1% polyhexanide plus 0.1% betaine and found no statistical difference in the number of operating room visits, length of hospital stay, proportion of wounds closed or covered, and proportion of wounds that remained closed at 30 days of follow-up [80]. Brickert et al. prospectively studied 131 wounds treated with NPWT with saline instillation, and in 98% of the cases, the wounds could be closed after debridement and NPWTi used for 12–19 days [81]. There are no clinical studies comparing different types of instillation solutions and their efficacy on decreasing bioburden in wounds.

Instillation therapy uses a modified NPWT device to add fluid to the wound through the dressing. A separate port is employed to instill fluid directly into the wound (Fig. 12.7). The vacuum suction is shut off, and the fluid remains in the wound for a predetermined dwell time before the vacuum is resumed and the fluid is evacuated [82]. Complete debridement of all devitalized or infected tissue is still required prior to commencing treatment.

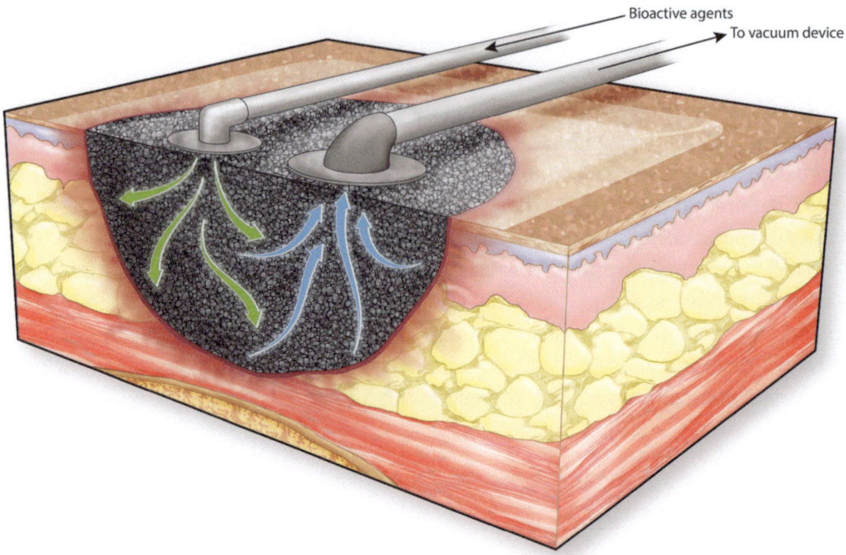

Fig. 12.7 NPWT with instillation (From Huang et al. [8]. With permission from Elsevier)

Contraindications

According to FDA guidelines [83], the use of NPWT is specifically contraindicated in patients with malignancy in the wound, untreated osteomyelitis, non-enteric, and unexplored fistulas and necrotic tissue with eschar in the wound, exposed vasculature, nerves, anastomotic sites, and organs. In addition, the FDA recommends caution in patients at high risk for bleeding and hemorrhage, especially when anticoagulated, patients with friable or infected blood vessels, sharp edges in the wound, and spinal cord injury (may induce stimulation of sympathetic nervous system). An NPWT device should be removed for MRI, hyperbaric oxygen therapy and if defibrillation is required. Care should be taken when the device is used near the vagus nerve, as it may cause bradycardia. Circumferential dressing application should be used with caution.

Risk Factors and Complications

The most common complications from NPWT include bleeding, infection, foam retention, skin irritation, and pain. The most serious complication with NPWT use is bleeding, with 12 deaths reported since 2009 [83]. Most of the bleeding complications were seen in patients who had synthetic bypass grafts with wound infection and were anticoagulated when the foam dressing would become adherent to the underlying vascular structures causing bleeding upon removal. There were 27 reports of retained foam causing worsening infections in open infected wounds and many reports of the foam attaching to the wound tissues requiring hospitalization for removal. Most complications were noted in home care and long-term care facilities. Reported complications with NPWT use in open abdominal wounds include a higher incidence of intestinal leakage and enterocutaneous fistula formation [84, 85]. Skin irritation from the adhesive drape or from the foam placed directly on the skin has been reported.

Given the commonplace use of NPWT by clinicians with varying experience in the technology, the number of complications may increase. Education about the use of NPWT, as well as careful attention to potential complications, vigilant monitoring of the device, and early recognition of adverse events, is paramount. As with any wound care therapy, if there is a complication, the wound is worsening or not progressing, NPWT should be discontinued (Fig. 12.8).

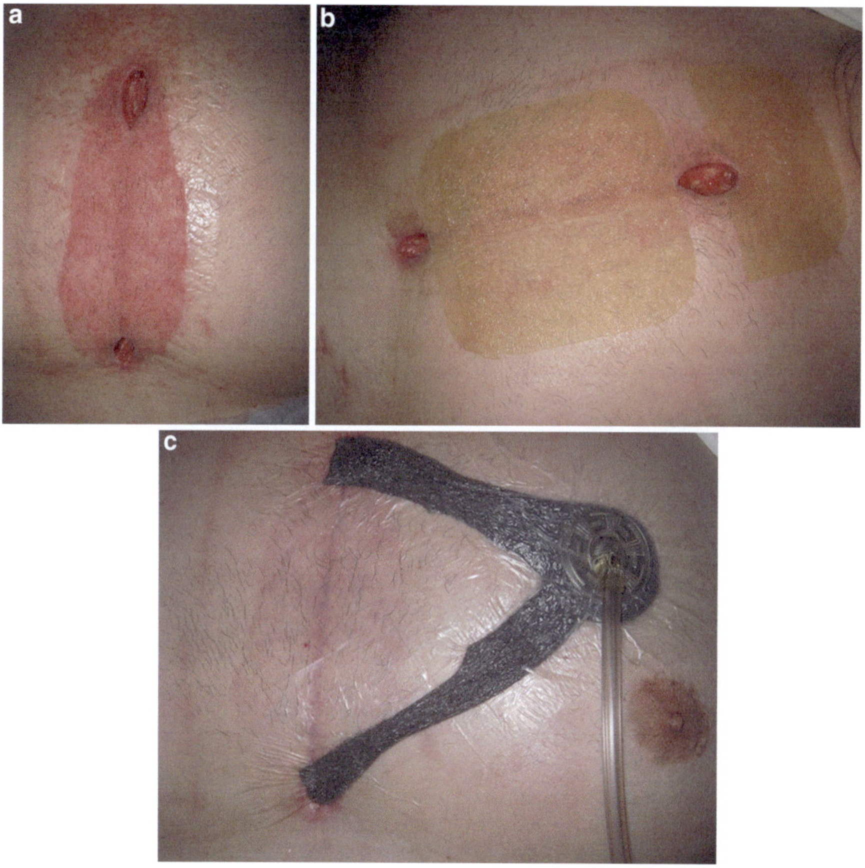

Fig. 12.8 (**a**) Sternotomy incision dehiscence with dermatitis from dressing foam placed directly on the skin. (**b**) Resolved dermatitis with thin hydrocolloid for skin protection. (**c**) Bridged foam dressing

Conclusion

In a short time period, the use of NPWT in the treatment of acute and chronic wounds has become widely accepted and has changed the landscape of wound healing despite few robust prospective randomized trials. Clinicians have experienced improved healing in a variety of wounds that otherwise would have lingered or required complex surgical closure, adding to increased patient morbidity and possibly even mortality. Researchers continue to debate the optimum interface product and level of vacuum applied, the kinetics of application and the use of instillation solutions. New, smaller devices have been developed. There does not seem to be much debate, though, that negative-pressure wound therapy holds an integral place in our wound-healing portfolio.

References

1. Argenta LC, Morykwas MJ. Vacuum-assisted closure: a new method for wound control and treatment: clinical experience. Ann Plast Surg. 1997;38(6):563–76. discussion 577
2. Winter G. Letters to nature. Nature. 1962 Jan;193:293–4.
3. Shores JT, Gabriel A, Gupta S. Skin substitutes and alternatives: a review. Adv Skin Wound Care. 2007;20(9 Pt 1):493–508.
4. Fleischmann W, Strecker W, Bombelli M, Kinzl L. Vacuum sealing as treatment of soft tissue damage in open fractures. Unfallchirurg. 1993;96(9):488–92. German.
5. Borgquist O, Gustafsson L, Ingemansson R, Malmsjö M. Micro- and macromechanical effects on the wound bed of negative pressure wound therapy using gauze and foam. Ann Plast Surg. 2010;64(6):789–93. https://doi.org/10.1097/SAP.0b013e3181ba578a.
6. Lavery LA, Murdoch DP, Kim PJ, Fontaine JL, Thankral G, Davis KE. Negative pressure wound therapy with low pressure and gauze dressings to treat diabetic foot wounds. J Diabetes Sci Technol. 2014;8(2):346–9.
7. Kim PJ, Attinger CE, Steinberg JS, Evans KK, Lehner B, Willy C, Lavery L, Wolvos T, Orgill D, Ennis W, Lantis J, Gabriel A, Schultz G. Negative-pressure wound therapy with instillation: international consensus guidelines. Plast Reconstr Surg. 2013;132(6):1569–79. https://doi.org/10.1097/PRS.0b013e3182a80586.
8. Huang C, Leavitt T, Bayer LR, Orgill DP. Effect of negative pressure wound therapy on wound healing. Curr Probl Surg. 2014;51(7):301–31. https://doi.org/10.1067/j.cpsurg.2014.04.001.
9. Folkman J, Moscona A. Role of cell shape in growth control. Nature. 1978;273(5661):345–9.
10. Huang S, Ingber DE. The structural and mechanical complexity of cell-growth control. Nat Cell Biol. 1999;1(5):E131–7.
11. Lu F, Ogawa R, Nguyen DT, Chen B, Guo D, Helm DL, Zhan Q, Murphy GF, Orgill DP. Microdeformation of three-dimensional cultured fibroblasts induces gene expression and morphological changes. Ann Plast Surg. 2011;66(3):296–300. https://doi.org/10.1097/SAP.0b013e3181ea1e9b.
12. Heit YI, Dastouri P, Helm DL, Pietramaggiori G, Younan G, Erba P, Münster S, Orgill DP, Scherer SS. Foam pore size is a critical interface parameter of suction-based wound healing devices. Plast Reconstr Surg. 2012;129(3):589–97. https://doi.org/10.1097/PRS.0b013e3182402c89.
13. Scherer S, Pietramaggiori G, Mathews J, Prsa MJ, Huang S, Orgill DP. The mechanism of action of the vacuum assisted closure device. Plast Reconstr Surg. 2008 Sep;122(3):786-97. doi: 10.1097/PRS.0b013e31818237ac.

14. Borgquist O, Ingemansson R, Malmsjo M. The influence of low and high pressure levels during negative-pressure wound therapy on wound contraction and fluid evacuation. Plast Reconstr Surg. 2011;127(2):551–9. https://doi.org/10.1097/PRS.0b013e3181fed52a.
15. Wackenfors A, Gustafsson R, Sjogren J, Algotsson L, Ingemansson R, Malmsjo M. Blood flow responses in the peristernal thoracic wall during vacuum-assisted closure therapy. Ann Thorac Surg. 2005;79(5):1724–30; discussion 1730-1.
16. Parrett BM, Matros E, Pribaz, JJ, Orgill DP. Lower extremity trauma: trends in the management of soft-tissue reconstruction of open tibia-fibula fractures. Plast Reconstr Surg. 2006;117(4):1315–22; discussion 1323-4.
17. Janis JE, Kwon RK, Attinger CE. The new reconstructive ladder: modifications to the traditional model. Plast Reconstr Surg. 2011;127(Suppl 1):205S–12S. https://doi.org/10.1097/PRS.0b013e318201271c.
18. Krug E, Berg L, Lee C, Hudson D, Birke-Sorensen H, Depoorter M, Dunn R, Jeffery S, Duteille F, Bruhin A, Caravaggi C, Chariker M, Dowsett C, Ferreira F, Martínez JM, Grudzien G, Ichioka S, Ingemansson R, Malmsjo M, Rome P, Vig S, Runkel N, Martin R, Smith J. Evidence-based recommendations for the use of negative pressure wound therapy in traumatic wounds and reconstructive surgery: steps towards an international consensus. Injury. 2011;42(Suppl 1):S1–12. https://doi.org/10.1016/S0020-1383(11)00041-6.
19. V.A.C.® Therapy Clinical Guidelines. A reference source for clinicians. www.acelity.com. Assessed November 17, 2017.
20. Dastouri P, Helm DL, Scherer SS, Pietramaggoiri G, Younan G, Orgill DP. Waveform modulation of negative-pressure wound therapy in the murine model. Plast Reconstr Surg. 2011;127(4):1460–6. https://doi.org/10.1097/PRS.0b013e31820a63cb.
21. Malmsjo M, Gustafsson L, Lindstedt S, Gesslein B, Ingemansson R. The effects of variable, intermittent, and continuous negative pressure wound therapy, using foam or gauze, on wound contraction, granulation tissue formation and ingrowth into the wound filler. Eplasty. 2012;12:e5.
22. Singh N, Armstrong DG, Lipsky BA. Preventing foot ulcers in patients with diabetes. JAMA. 2005;293(2):217–28.
23. AHRQ. Data Points #1: prevalence of diabetes, diabetic foot ulcer, and lower extremity amputation among Medicare beneficiaries, 2006–2008. https://www.effectivehealthcare.ahrq.gov. Assessed 11 Feb 2017.
24. Armstrong DG, Lavery LA, Diabetic Foot Study Consortium. Negative pressure wound therapy after partial diabetic foot amputation: a multicentre, randomised controlled trial. Lancet. 2005;366(9498):1704–10.
25. Anghel EL, Kim PJ. Negative-pressure wound therapy: a comprehensive review of the evidence. Plast Reconstr Surg. 2016;138(3 Suppl):129S–37S. https://doi.org/10.1097/PRS.0000000000002645.
26. Sajid MT, Mustafa Q, Shaheen N, Hussain SM, Shukr I, Ahmed M. Comparison of negative pressure wound therapy using vacuum-assisted closure with advanced moist wound therapy in the treatment of diabetic foot ulcers. J Coll Physicians Surg Pak. 2015;25(11):789–93. doi: 11.2015/JCPSP.789793
27. Apelqvist J, Armstrong DG, Lavery LA, Boulton AJ. Resource utilization and economic costs of care based on a randomized trial of vacuum-assisted closure therapy in the treatment of diabetic foot wounds. Am J Surg. 2008;195(6):782–8. https://doi.org/10.1016/j.amjsurg.2007.06.023.
28. Blume PA, Walters J, Payne W, Alaya J, Lantis J. Comparison of negative pressure wound therapy using vacuum-assisted closure with advanced moist wound therapy in the treatment of diabetic foot ulcers. Diabetes Care. 2008;31(4):631–6. Epub 2007 Dec 27.
29. Dumville JC, Hinchliffe RJ, Cullum N, Game F, Stubbs N, Sweeting M. Negative pressure wound therapy for treating foot wounds in people with diabetes mellitus (protocol). Cochrane Database of Systematic Reviews 2013, Issue 1. Art. No.: CD010318. 2013. Doi: https://doi.org/10.1002/14651858.CD010318.

30. Steed DL. Clinical evaluation of recombinant human platelet-derived growth factor for the treatment of lower extremity diabetic ulcers. Diabetic ulcer study group. J Vasc Surg. 1995;21(1):71–8; discussion 79-81.
31. Bus SA, van Deursen RW, Armstrong DG, Lewis JEA, Caravaggi CF, Cavanagh PR, International Working Group on the Diabetic Foot. Footwear and offloading interventions to prevent and heal foot ulcers and reduce plantar pressure in patients with diabetes: a systematic review. Diabetes Metab Res Rev. 2016;32(Suppl 1):99–118. https://doi.org/10.1002/dmrr.2702.
32. Niezgoda JA, Mendez-Eastman S. Effective management of pressure ulcers. Adv Skin Wound Care. 2006;19(Suppl 1):3–15.
33. Dumville JC, Webster J, Evans D, Land L. Negative pressure wound therapy for treating pressure ulcers. Cochrane Database of Systematic Reviews 2015, Issue 5. Art. No.: CD011334. 2015. doi:https://doi.org/10.1002/14651858.CD011334.pub2.
34. Vuerstaek JD, Vainas T, Wuite J, Nelemans P, Neumann MH, Veraart JC. State-of-the-art treatment of chronic leg ulcers: a randomized controlled trial comparing vacuum-assisted closure (V.A.C.) with modern wound dressings. J Vasc Surg. 2006;44(5):1029–37; discussion 1038. Epub 2006 Sep 26.
35. Abai B, Zickler RW, Pappas PJ, Lal BK, Padberg FT Jr. Lymphorrhea responds to negative pressure wound therapy. J Vasc Surg. 2007;45(3):610–3.
36. Svensson S, Monsen C, Kölbel T, Acosta S. Predictors for outcome after vacuum assisted closure therapy of peri-vascular surgical site infections in the groin. Eur J Vasc Endovasc Surg. 2008;36(1):84–9. https://doi.org/10.1016/j.ejvs.2007.12.020. Epub 2008 Mar 4
37. Pinocy J, Johannes A, Wicke C, Ruck P, Ziemer G. Treatment of periprosthetic soft tissue infection of the groin. Wound Repair Regen. 2003;11(2):104–9.
38. Gustilo RB, Mendoza RM, Williams DN. Problems in the management of type III (severe) open fractures: a new classification of type III open fractures. J Trauma. 1984;24(8):742–6.
39. Milcheski DA, Ferreira MC, Nakamoto HA, Pereira DD, Batista BN, Tuma P Jr. Subatmospheric pressure therapy in the treatment of traumatic soft tissue injuries. Rev Col Bras Cir. 2013;40(5):392–6.
40. Schlatterer D, Hirshorn K. Negative pressure wound therapy with reticulated open cell foam-adjunctive treatment in the management of traumatic wounds of the leg: a review of the literature. J Orthop Trauma. 2008;22(10 Suppl):S152–60. https://doi.org/10.1097/BOT.0b013e318188e2d7.
41. Stannard JP, Volgas DA, Stewart R, McGwin G Jr, Alonso JE. Negative pressure wound therapy after severe open fractures: a prospective randomized study. J Orthop Trauma. 2009;23(8):552–7. https://doi.org/10.1097/BOT.0b013e3181a2e2b6.
42. Blum ML, Esser M, Richardson M, Paul E, Rosenfeldt FL. Negative pressure wound therapy reduces deep infection rate in open tibial fractures. J Orthop Trauma. 2012;26(9):499–505. https://doi.org/10.1097/BOT.0b013e31824133e3.
43. Putnis S, Khan WS, Wong JM. Negative pressure wound therapy: a review of its uses in orthopaedic trauma. Open Orthop J. 2014;8:142–7. doi:https://doi.org/10.2174/1874325001408010142. eCollection 2014.
44. Sinha K, Chauhan VD, Maheshwari R, Chauhan N, Rajan M, Agrawal A. Vacuum assisted closure therapy versus standard wound therapy for open musculoskeletal injuries. Adv Orthop. 2013;2013:245940. https://doi.org/10.1155/2013/245940. Epub 2013 Jun 26
45. Dedmond BT, Kortesis B, Punger K, et al. The use of negative pressure wound therapy (NPWT) in the temporary treatment of soft-tissue injuries associated with high-energy open tibial shaft fractures. J Orthop Trauma. 2007;21(1):11–7.
46. Stone PA, Hass SM, Flaherty SK, DeLuca JA, Lucente FC, Kusminsky RE. Vacuum-assisted fascial closure for patients with abdominal trauma. J Trauma. 2004;57(5):1082–6.
47. Bruhin A, Ferreira F, Chariker M, Smith J, Runkel N. Systematic review and evidence based recommendations for the use of negative pressure wound therapy in the open abdomen. Int J Surg. 2014;12(10):1105–14. https://doi.org/10.1016/j.ijsu.2014.08.396. Epub 2014 Aug 28

48. Zacharias A, Habib RH. Delayed primary closure of deep sternal wound infections. Tex Heart Inst J. 1996;23(3):211–6.
49. Jones G, Jurkiewicz MJ, Bostwick J, Wood R, Bried JT, Culbertson J, Howell R, Eaves F, Carlson G, Nahai F. Management of the infected median sternotomy wound with muscle flaps. The Emory 20-year experience. Ann Surg. 1997;225(6):766–76. discussion 776-8
50. Hersh RE, Jack JM, Dahman MI, Morgan RF, Drake DB. The vacuum-assisted closure device as a bridge to sternal wound closure. Ann Plast Surg. 2001;46(3):250–4.
51. Gustafsson R, Johnsson P, Algotsson L, Blomquist S, Ingemansson R. Vacuum-assisted closure therapy guided by C-reactive protein level in patients with deep sternal wound infection. J Thorac Cardiovasc Surg. 2002;123(5):895–900.
52. Fleck T, Fleck M. Negative pressure wound therapy for the treatment of sternal wound infections after cardiac surgery. Int Wound J. 2014;11(3):240–5. https://doi.org/10.1111/j.1742-481X.2012.01079.x. Epub 2012 Sep 3
53. Orgill DP, Austen WG, Butler CE, Fine NA, Horvath KA, Mihaljevic T, Song DH, Wolfe WG. Guidelines for treatment of complex chest wounds with negative pressure wound therapy. Wounds. 2004;16(12 SUPPL. B):1–23.
54. Petzina R, Malmsjo M, Stamm C. Major complications due to negative pressure wound therapy in poststernotomy mediastinitis after cardiac surgery. J Thorac Cardiovasc Surg. 2010;140(5):1133–6. https://doi.org/10.1016/j.jtcvs.2010.06.063.
55. Sjögren J, Gustafsson R, Nilsson J, Lindstedt S, Nozohoor S, Ingemansson R. Negative-pressure wound therapy following cardiac surgery: bleeding complications and 30-day mortality in 176 patients with deep sternal wound infection. Interact Cardiovasc Thorac Surg. 2011;12(2):117–20. https://doi.org/10.1510/icvts.2010.252668.
56. Yang C, Chang D, Webb L. Vacuum-assisted closure for fasciotomy wounds following compartment syndrome of the leg. J Surg Orthop Adv. 2006;15(1):19–23.
57. Morykwas MJ, David LR, Schneider AM, Whang C, Jennings DA, Canty C, Parker D, White WL. Use of subatmospheric pressure to prevent progression of partial thickness burns in a swine model. J Burn Care Rehabil. 1999;20(1 Pt 1):15–21.
58. Kamolz LP, Andel H, Haslik W, Winter W, Meissl G, Frey M. Use of subatmospheric pressure therapy to prevent burn progression in human: first experience. Burns. 2004;30(3):253–8.
59. Kantak NA, Mistry R, Halvorson EG. A review of negative-pressure wound therapy in the management of burn wounds. Burns. 2016;42(8):1623–33.
60. Petkar KS, Dhanraj P, Kingsly PM, Sreekar H, Lakshmanarao A, Lamba S, Shetty R, Zachariah JR. A prospective randomized controlled trial comparing negative pressure dressing and conventional dressing methods on split-thickness skin grafts in burned patients. Burns. 2011;37(6):925–9. https://doi.org/10.1016/j.burns.2011.05.013. Epub 2011 Jul 1
61. Bukovcan P, Koller J, Hajská M, Záhorec P. Clinical experience with the use of negative pressure wound therapy combined with a silver-impregnated dressing in mixed wounds: a retrospective study of 50 cases. Wounds. 2016;28(8):255–63.
62. Fischer S, Wall J, Pomahac B, Riviello R, Halvorson EG. Extra-large negative pressure wound therapy dressings for burns – initial experience with technique, fluid management, and outcomes. Burns. 2016;42(2):457–65. https://doi.org/10.1016/j.burns.2015.08.034.
63. Poulakidas S, Kowal-Vern A. Facilitating residual wound closure after partial graft loss with vacuum assisted closure therapy. J Burn Care Res. 2008;29(4):663–5. https://doi.org/10.1097/BCR.0b013e31817db8b6.
64. Stone P, Prigozen J, Hofeldt M, Hass S, DeLuca J, Flaherty S. Bolster versus negative pressure wound therapy for securing split-thickness skin grafts in trauma patients. Wounds. 2004;16(7):219–23.
65. Repta R, Ford R, Hoberman L, Rechner B. The use of negative-pressure therapy and skin grafting in the treatment of soft-tissue defects over the Achilles tendon. Ann Plast Surg. 2005;55(4):367–70.

66. Landau AG, Hudson DA, Adams K, Geldenhuys S, Pienaar C. Full-thickness skin grafts: maximizing graft take using negative pressure dressings to prepare the graft bed. Ann Plast Surg 2008;60(6):661–6. doi:https://doi.org/10.1097/SAP.0b013e318146c288.
67. Scherer LA, Shiver S, Chang M, Meredith JW, Owings JT. The vacuum assisted closure device: a method of securing skin grafts and improving graft survival. Arch Surg. 2002;137(8):930–3. discussion 933-4
68. Anderson DJ, Podgorny K, Berríos-Torres SI, Bratzler DW, Dellinger EP, Greene L, Nyquist AC, Saiman L, Yokoe DS, Maragakis LL, Kaye KS. Strategies to prevent surgical site infections in acute care hospitals: 2014 update. Infect Control Hosp Epidemiol. 2014;35(6):605–27. https://doi.org/10.1086/676022.
69. Semsarzadeh NN, Tadisina KK, Maddox J, Chopra K, Singh DP. Closed incision negative-pressure therapy is associated with decreased surgical-site infections: a meta-analysis. Plast Reconstr Surg. 2015;136(3):592–602. https://doi.org/10.1097/PRS.0000000000001519.
70. Stannard JP, Robinson JT, Anderson ER, McGwin G Jr, Volgas DA, Alonso JE. Negative pressure wound therapy to treat hematomas and surgical incisions following high-energy trauma. J Trauma. 2006;60(6):1301–6.
71. Pachowsky M, Gusinde J, Klein A, Lehrl S, Schulz-Drost S, Schlechtweg P, Pauser J, Gelse K, Brem MH. Negative pressure wound therapy to prevent seromas and treat surgical incisions after total hip arthroplasty. Int Orthop. 2012;36(4):719–22. https://doi.org/10.1007/s00264-011-1321-8.
72. Stannard JP, Volgas DA, McGwin G 3rd, Stewart RL, Obremskey W, Moore T, Anglen JO. Incisional negative pressure wound therapy after high-risk lower extremity fractures. J Orthop Trauma. 2012;26(1):37–42. https://doi.org/10.1097/BOT.0b013e318216b1e5.
73. Tuffaha HW, Gillespie BM, Chaboyer W, Gordon LG, Scuffham PA. Cost-utility analysis of negative pressure wound therapy in high-risk cesarean section wounds. J Surg Res. 2015;195(2):612–22. https://doi.org/10.1016/j.jss.2015.02.008.
74. Lewis LS, Convery PA, Bolac CS, Valea FA, Lowery WJ, Havrilesky LJ. Cost of care using prophylactic negative pressure wound vacuum on closed laparotomy incisions. Gynecol Oncol. 2014;132(3):684–9. https://doi.org/10.1016/j.ygyno.2014.01.014. Epub 2014 Jan 17
75. Morykwas MJ, Argenta LC, Shelton-Brown EI, McGuirt W. Vacuum-assisted closure: a new method for wound control and treatment: animal studies and basic foundation. Ann Plast Surg. 1997;38(6):553–62.
76. Fleischmann W, Russ M, Westhauser A, Stampehl M. Vacuum sealing as carrier system for controlled local drug administration in wound infection Unfallchirurg. 1998 Aug;101(8):649–54. German.
77. Goss SG, Schwartz JA, Facchin F, Avdagic E, Gendics C, Lantis JC 2nd. Negative pressure wound therapy with instillation (NPWTi) better reduces post-debridement bioburden in chronically infected lower extremity wounds than NPWT alone. J Am Coll Clin Wound Spec. 2014;4(4):74–80. https://doi.org/10.1016/j.jccw.2014.02.001. eCollection 2012
78. Kim PJ, Attinger CE, Steinberg JS, Evans KK, Powers KA, Hung RW, Smith JR, Rocha ZM, Lavery L. The impact of negative-pressure wound therapy with instillation compared with standard negative-pressure wound therapy: a retrospective, historical, cohort, controlled study. Plast Reconstr Surg. 2014;133(3):709–16.
79. Timmers MS, Graafland N, Bernards AT, Nelissen RG, van Dissel JT, Jukema GN. Negative pressure wound treatment with polyvinyl alcohol foam and polyhexanide antiseptic solution instillation in post-traumatic osteomyelitis. Wound Repair Regen. 2009;17:278–86.
80. Kim PJ, Attinger CE, Oliver N, Garwood C, Evans KK, Steinberg JS, Lavery LA. Comparison of outcomes for normal saline and an antiseptic solution for negative-pressure wound therapy with instillation. Plast Reconstr Surg. 2015;136(5):657e–64e. https://doi.org/10.1097/PRS.0000000000001709.
81. Brinkert D, Ali M, Naud M, Maire N, Trial C, Téot L. Negative pressure wound therapy with saline instillation: 131 patient case series. Int Wound J. 2013;10:56–60. https://doi.org/10.1111/iwj.12176.

82. V.A.C. ULTA ™ Negative Pressure Wound Therapy System monograph. www.acelity.com. Assessed November 17, 2017.
83. Update on serious complications associated with negative pressure wound therapy systems: FDA safety communication. Issued February 24, 2011. [cited February 11, 2017]. Available from: http://www.fda.gov/MedicalDevices/Safety/AlertsandNotices/ucm244211.htm. Assessed.
84. Rao M, Burke D, Finan PJ, Sagar PM. The use of vacuum-assisted closure of abdominal wounds: a word of caution. Color Dis. 2007;9(3):266–8.
85. Fischer JE. A cautionary note: the use of vacuum-assisted closure systems in the treatment of gastrointestinal cutaneous fistula may be associated with higher mortality from subsequent fistula development. Am J Surg. 2008;196(1):1–2. https://doi.org/10.1016/j.amjsurg.2008.01.001. Epub 2008 Mar 26

Chapter 13
Matrices and Dermal Substitutes for Wound Treatment

Sumanas W. Jordan, Sergey Y. Turin, Eric Robert Zielinski, and Robert D. Galiano

Introduction

Physiologic wound healing is a coordinated progression of inflammation, proliferation, and remodeling, toward the goal of a stable, epithelialized scar. Specific processes of inflammation, macrophage activation, epithelialization, scar contracture, collagen deposition, cellular ingrowth, angiogenesis, and matrix remodeling are closely entwined and may become dysregulated by any number of factors including infection, ischemia, and poor nutrient supply. When wound healing becomes problematic and chronic or in wounds with large areas of full-thickness loss, biofunctional wound matrices may serve to change the healing milieu or accelerate regeneration by reducing substrate needs. As adjuncts to a standard treatment regimen of debridement, dressings, and inflammation and edema control, these advanced wound treatments supplement potential rate-limiting elements such as collagen, glycosaminoglycans, and growth factors. Herein, we review the vast range of skin substitutes and biofunctional wound care matrices, highlighting prototypic products and their specific indications, with a focus on the available evidence for the treatment of wounds.

Financial Disclosure Statement: R. Galiano is a consultant for the Musculoskeletal Transplant Foundation and for Smith & Nephew. He receives research funding through grants to Northwestern University Feinberg School of Medicine. The remaining authors have no relevant disclosures in relation to this article.

S.W. Jordan, MD, PhD • S.Y. Turin, MD • E.R. Zielinski, MD
Division of Plastic and Reconstructive Surgery, Northwestern University Feinberg School of Medicine, Chicago, IL, USA

R.D. Galiano, MD (✉)
Division of Plastic and Reconstructive Surgery, Northwestern University Feinberg School of Medicine, Chicago, IL, USA

Division of Plastic Surgery, Northwestern Memorial Hospital, Chicago, IL, USA
e-mail: Robert.galiano@nm.org

D.P. Orgill (ed.), *Interventional Treatment of Wounds*,
https://doi.org/10.1007/978-3-319-66990-8_13

Table 13.1 Criteria for application of advanced wound care matrices and dermal substitutes. Ulcer measurements should be carefully documented at all stages of treatment. Failure of response is defined as an ulcer that is increasing in size or demonstrates less than 30% closure from baseline. Wound should be free of infection and underlying osteomyelitis

Acute burn injury	Partial- or full-thickness burns Autograft options undesirable due to lack of donor sites or patient condition
Diabetic foot ulcer	Present greater than four (4) weeks of duration *or* failure to respond to standard measures, including off-loading, for greater than one (1) month of duration
Venous stasis ulcer	Present greater than four (4) weeks of duration *or* failure to respond to standard measures for greater than three (3) weeks of duration

Indications and Contraindications

In general, advanced wound care matrices are considered for wounds that have failed to progress toward healing despite optimal, standard wound care measures over a defined period of time (Table 13.1). Failure of response is defined as an ulcer that is increasing in size or demonstrates less than 30% closure from baseline. Sheehan et al. examined the trajectory of successful wound healing of uncomplicated diabetic foot ulcers with a standard regimen of off-loading, sharp debridement, and moist wound dressings and demonstrated that at 4 weeks, those that went on to heal had a mean reduction in ulcer size of 82% compared to non-healers who had a mean reduction of only 25%. They concluded that a 53% reduction in ulcer area within the *first 4 weeks* was predictive of wound closure with a sensitivity of 91% [1]. Similarly, Phillips et al. studied venous ulcers prospectively managed with a consistent, defined system of local wound care with a moisture-retentive dressing and edema control with paste bandage graduated compression. Ulcers with a small baseline area and short-term duration were more likely to progress to complete healing with a shorter time to healing. Progress of 44% reduction in ulcer size by *3 weeks* was predictive of complete healing in 77% of cases [2]. These studies demonstrate that early wound healing may predict the need for adjuncts such as advanced matrices.

In addition to local wound care, the treatment of wounds should include systemic management of inflammation, blood glucose, general nutrition, pain, and underlying infection. Contraindications to advanced wound matrices include irreversible hypoxia, infection, heavy contaminate or bioburden, active Charcot disease, and hypersensitivity to any of the components of the matrices (Table 13.2). Substrates containing growth factors should be avoided in patients with active malignancy within the wound bed [3–5].

Historical Perspective and Types of Biofunctional Matrices

Given the vast number of wound care products on the market, it may be useful to group these biofunctional matrices into some organizational scheme. Some have categorized the products as temporary dressings or devices versus permanent

Table 13.2 Contraindications to biofunctional matrices for wound care

Irreversible ischemia (e.g., arterial occlusive disease with ABI < 0.65)
Infection
Grossly contaminated wound or heavy bioburden
Active Charcot disease
Hypersensitivity to any component

Products have not been studied in patients who are pregnant and lactating, have uncontrolled diabetes, or are taking corticosteroids or immunosuppression

wound coverage or synthetic versus biological [6, 7]. However, these descriptions do not provide insight on the mechanism or utility of the substrate to reverse the wound healing aberrancy, and varying degrees of processing may blur the lines between synthetic and naturally derived materials. From a historical developmental perspective, we chose to categorize the advanced wound matrices by their material components and presumed bioactivity, which roughly correspond to Food and Drug Administration (FDA) regulation processes. In doing so, clinical applications for these substrates may be more selective. These four categories are skin allografts and xenografts, dermal regenerative scaffolds, cellular substrates, and bioactive decellularized ECM-based products (Tables 13.3, 13.4, 13.5, and 13.6).

Acellular Allogenic Dermal Matrices

Skin allografts and xenografts for wound coverage trace back to the sixteenth century with the classical notion of "replacing like with like." However, these dermal substitutes in non-altered form were subject to rejection. Today, allografts take the form of minimally processed human tissues that have had antigenic cellular components removed, such as the prototypic acellular dermal matrix (ADM), AlloDerm (LifeCell Corp., Bridgewater, NJ). One randomized controlled trial (RCT) of AlloDerm versus wound gel and gauze dressings for full-thickness diabetic lower-extremity ulcers (n = 28) demonstrated 86% wound closure in the AlloDerm group versus 29% in the control group at 16 weeks [8]. AlloPatch (MTF, Edison, NJ) is a newer offering and is also an acellular human dermis allograft, harvested from the reticular layer of the dermis. This selective harvest eliminated orientation specificity and is aimed at producing a more uniform and more open ADM. A recent study showed efficacy of the device in the treatment of diabetic foot ulcers and 6 and 12 weeks [9]. However, with respect to wounds, the roles of both allografts and xenografts generally remain limited to temporary wound coverage prior to autografting. Table 13.3 lists dermal allograft and xenograft products for wound healing.

Table 13.3 Skin allograft and xenograft wound care products

Product name	Manufacturer	Description	Storage	FDA indications	Contraindications	Recommended use
AlloDerm	LifeCell, KCI	Cryopreserved acellular human dermal matrix	Room temperature	Repair or replacement of damaged or inadequate integument, other homologous use	Allergy to gentamicin, cefoxitin, lincomycin, polymyxin B, and vancomycin and polysorbate 20	Rehydrate in warm saline up to 4 h prior; place dermal side against wound bed; bolster dressing for 7 days
AlloSkin	AlloSource	Epidermal and dermal allograft	Room temperature	Wound care	Refer to package insert	Refer to package insert
AlloPatch	Musculoskeletal Transplant Foundation	Acellular human dermal matrix harvested from the reticular dermis	Room temperature	Replacement of damaged or inadequate integument or other similar indications	Refer to package insert	Apply and secure as graft, no specific orientation is required
DermACELL	LifeNet Health	Acellular human dermal matrix	Room temperature	Treatment of chronic non-healing wounds	Not specified	Apply and secure as graft with nonadherent dressing
E-Z Derm	AM Scientifics	Porcine skin cross-linked with aldehyde	Room temperature	Temporary coverage of wounds prior to autograft, partial-thickness skin loss	Not available in the USA. Refer to local market specifications	Not available in the USA. Refer to local market specifications
GammaGraft	Promethean LifeSciences	Irradiated human skin	Room temperature	Temporary graft for venous stasis ulcers, diabetic foot ulcers, and full-thickness wounds	Allergy to penicillin/ gentamicin	Apply as graft with nonadherent dressing

GraftJacket	LifeCell, Wright Medical, KCI	Cryopreserved acellular human dermal matrix	Room temperature	Scaffold for wound repair	Allergy to polysorbate 20 or ingredients listed on package	Rehydrate in normal saline until paper backing separates
LTM Wound Dressing	LifeCell	Terminally sterilized, processed porcine dermal matrix	No longer listed on manufacturer website, refer to package insert	Management of wounds	No longer listed on manufacturer website, refer to package insert	No longer listed on manufacturer website, refer to package insert
MatrixHD	RTI Biologics	Acellular human dermal matrix	Room temperature	Reconstructive surgery and treatment of chronic wounds	Refer to package insert	Refer to package insert
MemoDerm	Memometal Inc.	Acellular human dermal matrix	Room temperature	Wound and connective tissue repair in orthopedic applications	Refer to package insert	Refer to package insert
TheraSkin	Soluble Systems	Cryopreserved cellular human skin allograft	Frozen prior to implantation	Treatment of diabetic foot ulcers, venous stasis ulcers, pressure ulcers	Refer to package insert	Thaw and apply as graft, cover with non-stick dressing

Table 13.4 Dermal regenerative scaffolds (primarily collagen and other structural proteins) and semisynthetic wound matrices

Product name	Manufacturer	Description	Storage	FDA indications	Contraindications	Recommended use
Integra Bilayer Matrix	Integra LifeSciences	Bilayered matrix of cross-linked bovine collagen and chondroitin sulfate on a semipermeable silicone layer, creating a scaffold which can provide regenerative capabilities	Refrigerated at 35°–46° F (2–8 °C) for up to 2 years	Management of partial- and full-thickness wounds, pressure ulcers, venous ulcers, diabetic ulcers, chronic and vascular ulcers, surgical wounds, trauma wounds, and draining wounds	Bovine allergy, third-degree burns	Place matrix layer against wound bed, fenestrate silicone, cover with permeable silver dressing, and NPWT dressing; replace silver/ NPWT dressing weekly; autograft may be placed after 3–4 weeks
Biobrane	Mylan Laboratories	Nylon mesh fabric coated with porcine Type I collagen bonded to a silicone layer, acts as dressing to optimize native wound healing	Room temperature	Partial- and full-thickness burns	Allergy to porcine products	Secure under tension
Hyalomatrix, Jaloskin	Anika Therapeutics	Biosynthetic, nonwoven pad of benzyl esters of hyaluronic acid (HYAFF); Hyalomatrix includes a semipermeable silicone layer, acts as dressing to optimize native wound healing	Room temperature	Management of superficial moderately exuding wounds, traumatic wounds, and first- and second-degree burns	Hypersensitivity to hyaluronan and/or its derivatives and silicone; infection	Apply and secure like a graft, cover with nonadherent dressing
Talymed	Marine Polymer Technologies	Matrix of poly-N-acetylglucosamine isolated from microalgae, acts as dressing to optimize native wound healing	Room temperature for up to 3 years	Management of various wounds	None	Apply to wound, wet with saline to conform to contour, cover for nonadherence and semi-permeability, then apply retention dressing

[*]This list does not include a number of collagen sponges marketed as wound dressings

Table 13.5 Cellular substrates and placental-derived wound therapies

Product name	Manufacturer	Description	Storage	FDA indications	Contraindications	Recommended use
AmnioBand	Musculoskeletal Transplant Foundation	Dehydrated human amnion/chorion membrane	Room temperature up to 3 years	Acute and chronic wounds (DFUs, VLUs, pressure and ischemic wounds)	See package insert	Fenestrate and secure to wound bed as needed, secondary dressing to provide moist environment
Apligraf	Organogenesis	Bilayered substitute of epidermal human keratinocytes and dermal human fibroblasts seeded on bovine type I collagen; cells derived from neonatal foreskins	Controlled room temperature 20–23 °C (68–73 °F) until ready to be used	Venous stasis ulcers that have not responded to conventional treatment for >1mo; diabetic ulcers that have not responded to conventional treatment for >3 weeks	Infected wounds, allergy to bovine products or agarose shipping medium	May be meshed; efficacy data supports up to five applications; assess weekly
Dermagraft	No longer available in the USA	Cryopreserved human dermal fibroblasts from neonatal foreskins on a polyglactin mesh	−75 °C until ready to be used	Full-thickness diabetic foot ulcers >6 weeks of duration; treatment of dystrophic epidermolysis bullosa	Irreversible ischemia, infection, sinus tracts, hypersensitivity to bovine products used during processing	Thawed and rinsed according to package insert; up to eight applications weekly for 12 weeks
EpiFix	MiMedx	Dehydrated human amnion/chorion membrane including a single layer of epithelial cells	Room temperature for up to 5 years	Various full- and partial-thickness wounds	Infection	Matrix is imprinted with epithelium side up; secure to wound bed and rehydrate with sterile saline; change every 1–2 weeks
Grafix	Osiris Therapeutics	Cryopreserved placental membrane including mesenchymal stem cells		Acute and chronic wounds, pyoderma gangrenosum, epidermolysis bullosa	Infection	Thaw and rinse; apply every 7–14 days for up to 12 weeks
Neox	Amniox	Cryopreserved human umbilical cord and amniotic membrane				
OrCel	Ortec International	Bilayered substitute of human epidermal keratinocytes and dermal fibroblasts cultured in separate layers of a bovine collagen sponge				
TransCyte	No longer available in the US	Nylon mesh fabric coated with porcine Type I collagen and human fibroblasts bonded to silicone		Temporary wound coverage for deep partial-thickness and full-thickness burns prior to autografting; treatment of indeterminate- or partial-thickness burns expected to heal without autografting		Secure under tension; trim excess as it peels at 7–14 days; remove fabric prior to autograft

Table 13.6 Decellularized ECM-based materials for cutaneous wounds. Classified by the FDA as wound dressings based on collagen, these products additionally claim to contain various growth factors and adhesive molecules, in addition to structural proteins

Product name	Manufacturer	Description	Storage	FDA indications	Contraindications	Recommended use
ACell UBM, MatriStem	ACell, Inc.	Decellularized porcine urinary bladder matrix (UBM)	Room temperate	Single-use management of various wound types	Allergy to porcine products	Rehydrate for >15 mins, then place and secure as graft
EndoForm Dermal Template	Mesynthes	Decellularized ovine forestomach	Room temperature	Single-use treatment of various wound types	Allergy to ovine products	Rehydrate with saline and then place and secure as graft
Oasis, SIS Wound Dressing II, SS Matrix	Cook Biotech	Decellularized porcine small intestinal submucosa (SIS)	Room temperature for up to 2 years	Single-use management of various wound types	Infection, heavy exudate; allergy to porcine products	Secure edges of Oasis sheet beyond the wound edges; rehydrate with sterile saline and covered with a nonadherent dressing; reapply every 7 days or as needed
PriMatrix	TEI Biosciences	Decellularized fetal bovine dermis, primarily type III collagen	Room temperature	Single-use management of various wound types	Allergy to bovine products	Apply to wound and rehydrate

Dermal Regenerative Scaffolds and Semisynthetic Wound Matrices

A major advance in skin engineering came with the study of collagen and other structural matrix protein-based biomaterials. We have classified these materials as dermal regenerative scaffolds and semisynthetic wound matrices (Table 13.4). Collagen-based materials initiate platelet deposition and the inflammatory cascade, stimulate fibroblast proliferation, and may reset the MMP-TIMP imbalance seen in chronic wounds [10]. In the late 1970s and early 1980s, Yannas and Burke recognized the importance of porosity, protein degradation rates, and integrin binding site density on fibroblast migration and proliferation and neovascularization [11, 12]. This led to Integra dermal regenerative template (Integra LifeSciences, Plainsboro, NJ), a bilayered matrix of cross-linked bovine collagen and shark-derived chondroitin sulfate supported by a semipermeable silicone layer, which was introduced in 1980 and received FDA approval in 1996 for use in partial- and full-thickness wounds, pressure ulcers, venous leg ulcers, surgical wounds, second-degree burns, and draining wounds [13]. Dermal template integration occurs similarly to autograft take but with a longer time course. Imbibition and fibroblast migration take place during the first 2 weeks, followed neovascularization by 3 weeks, and matrix remodeling at 4 weeks [14]. The use of Integra for dermal reconstruction of full-thickness scalp wounds and complex trauma have been well-documented [15–19]. In one series, the combination of Integra, negative-pressure wound therapy, and eventual skin graft for combat injuries with exposed tendon or bone had an overall primary success rate of 83% [19]. A recent RCT, the Foot Ulcer New Dermal Replacement (FOUNDER) Study ($n = 307$), demonstrated its efficacy for the treatment of diabetic foot ulcers with complete closure in 51% of Integra patients compared to 32% in the control group at 16 weeks ($p = 0.001$). Mean time to closure was 43 versus 78 days, respectively [20].

Talymed (Marine Polymer Technologies, Inc., Danvers, MA) is a wound care device composed of poly-N-acetylglucosamine derived from microalgae for the management of various full- and partial-thickness wounds including diabetic ulcers, venous ulcers, pressure sores, surgical wounds, and second-degree burns [13]. Talymed provides wound coverage and supplements wound healing with inherent antibacterial properties. Similarly, Biobrane and Hyalomatrix are composed of a biologic construct (porcine Type I collagen in the case of Biobrane and benzyl esters of hyaluronic acid, in case of Hyalomatrix) bonded to a synthetic substrate (nylon mesh fabric and semipermeable silicone layer for Biobrane and Hyalomatrix, respectively). These products, unlike Integra should be expected to function more as a biologically active dressing supporting the wound healing process already occurring in the wound bed, as opposed to a true regenerative matrix that provides a scaffold for tissue ingrowth.

Cellular Substrates: Human Skin Equivalents for Wound Healing

Following these relatively inert biomaterials designed to act as scaffolds for host cell migration, cellularly augmented products were developed, often utilizing fetal or neonatal fibroblasts and keratinocytes. Cellular substrates (Table 13.5) provide temporary wound coverage and are thought to actively secrete and regulate cytokines and other growth factors to stimulate wound healing [21]. The cellular human skin equivalents are eventually replaced by host cells [22]. In a systematic review of 13 RCTs of largely cellular substrates (e.g., Apligraf, EpiFix, Hyalograft 3D) for the treatment of diabetic foot ulcers, Santema et al. found a pooled risk ratio for complete healing of 1.55 (95%CI 1.30–1.85) in favor of advanced wound care matrices with a possible trend toward fewer limb amputations [23].

The prototypic product, Apligraf (Organogenesis, Canton, MA), is a living bilayered composite of bovine type I collagen seeded with human fibroblasts and an outer epidermal layer of human keratinocytes derived from neonatal foreskins. Apligraf received premarket approval (PMA) by the FDA in 1998 for the treatment of recalcitrant venous stasis ulcers of greater than 1-month duration and in 2001 for non-healing diabetic ulcers of greater than 3-week duration which extend through the dermis but without tendon, muscle, capsule, or bone exposure [13]. For diabetic foot ulcers, Veves et al. reported significantly higher rates of complete wound healing by 12 weeks with Apligraf treatment compared to standard wound care (56% vs 38%) with shorter median time to closure (65 vs 90 days) [24]. For venous stasis ulcers, Falanga and colleagues compared Apligraf with compression therapy to compression therapy alone and observed 63% wound closure with Apligraf compared to 49% in the compression only group at 6 months ($p = 0.02$) [4]. Moreover, the group found that Apligraf was more efficacious than standard therapy for difficult-to-heal venous stasis ulcers >1000mm^2 and those present for greater than 1 year (49% Apligraf vs 19% control) [3]. Figure 13.1 shows a case example of Apligraf applied to a non-healing radiation ulcer.

Cellular Substrates: Placental-Derived Wound Therapies

There has been a recent trend toward placental-derived materials such as EpiFix (MiMedx, Marietta, GA), Grafix (Osiris Therapeutics, Columbia, MD), AmnioBand (Musculoskeletal Transplant Foundation, Edison, NJ), and Neox (Amniox, Atlanta, GA). AmnioBand and EpiFix are examples of dehydrated human amnion/chorion allografts (dHACA). Though proprietary material processing can vary widely and significantly affect bioactivity, these products are thought to be rich in collagen types IV, V, and VII as well as bound and soluble platelet-derived growth factor-AA (PDGF-AA); PDGF-BB; transforming growth factor α (TGFα); TGFβ1; basic fibroblast growth factor (bFGF); epidermal growth factor (EGF); placental growth factor (PlGF); granulocyte colony-stimulating factor (GCSF); interleukin-4, interleukin-6, interleukin-8, and interleukin-10; and TIMP-1, TIMP-2, and TIMP-4 (Fig. 13.2) [25]. In vitro soluble extracts of dehydrated amnion/ chorion (reportedly similar to EpiFix) have been shown to increase cell proliferation and migration of mesenchymal stem cells, adipose-derived stem cells, and hematopoietic stem cells, though the clinical implications of these studies remain unknown [25, 26]. A recent multicenter, RCT compared AmnioBand, a dehydrated amnion/ chorion allograft, to standard-of-care off-loading, debridement, and moist wound dressings for the

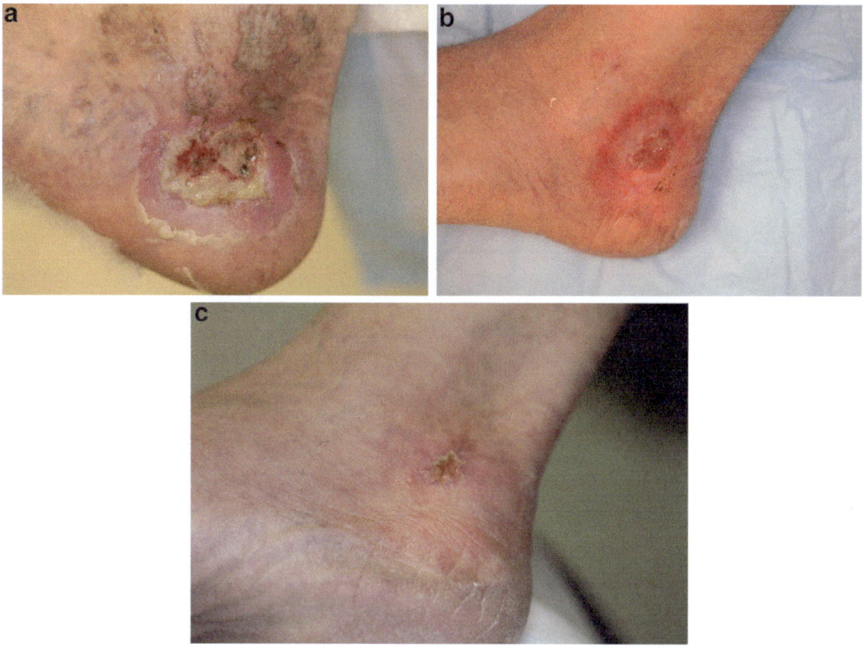

Fig. 13.1 Non-healing radiation ulcer treated with Apligraf. (**a**) Prior to debridement; (**b**) intermediate appearance following treatment with Apligraf; (**c**) healed ulcer at 6 weeks

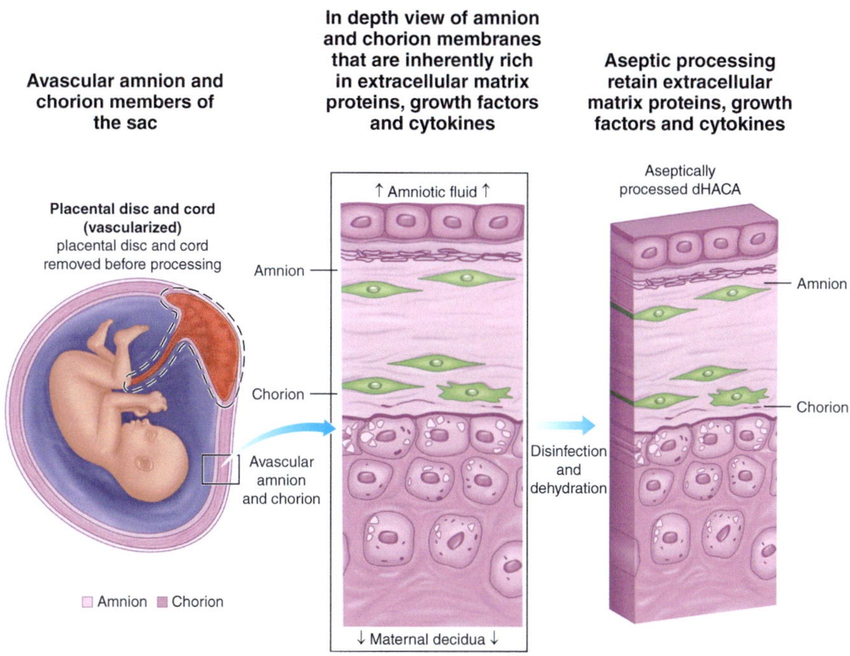

Fig. 13.2 Illustration of the structure of dehydrated human amnion/chorion allografts (Adapted from DiDomenico LA et al. Plastic and Reconstructive Surgery – Global Open. 4 (10):e1095, October 2016)

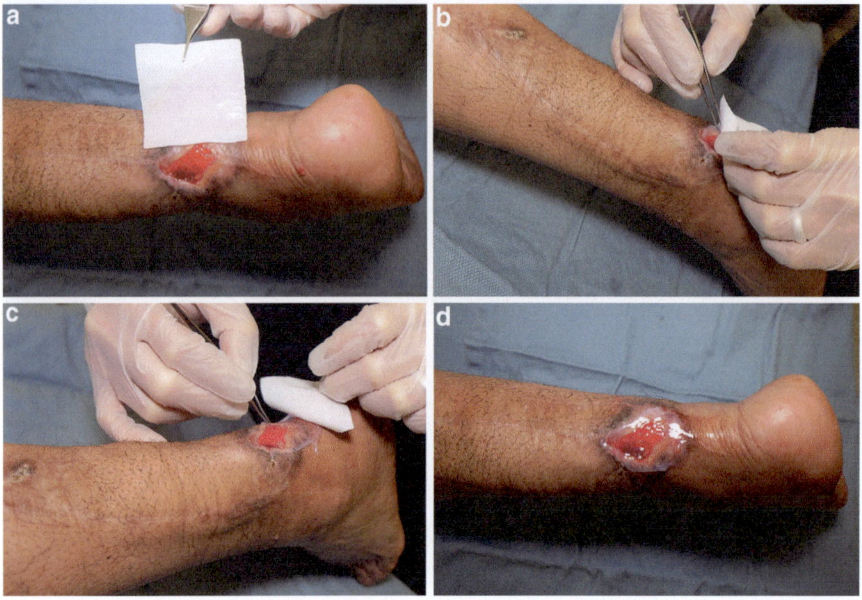

Fig. 13.3 Application of dehydrated amnion/chorion allograft (dHACA) to a diabetic lower-extremity wound. (**a**) AmnioBand membrane (Musculoskeletal Transplant Foundation, Edison, NJ) hydrated with sterile saline and placed on nonadherent gauze for handling. (**b, c**) Placement of dHACA onto wound with small overlap with wound edges. (**d**) Wound with dHACA applied. The wound was then dressed with a nonadherent dressing and left in place for 1 week

treatment of diabetic foot ulcers ($n = 20$ per group). At both 6 and 12 weeks, a significantly greater percentage of AmnioBand-treated diabetic wounds were healed compared to controls (70 versus 15% and 85 versus 25%, respectively) with shorter mean time to heal of 36 versus 70 days, respectively [27]. Application of the product and clinical photographs are shown in Figs. 13.3 and 13.4. In a separate comparative study of Apligraf, EpiFix (dehydrated human amnion/chorion allograft), and collagen-alginate dressings for diabetic foot ulcers, complete wound closure rates and mean time to heal within 12 weeks were 73% and 47.9 days ($n = 33$), 95% and 23.6 days ($n = 32$), and 51% and 57.4 days ($n = 35$), respectively [28].

Decellularized ECM-Based Wound Care Products

The next class of bioactive wound matrices sought to deliver growth factors to affect the wound healing milieu, without the sourcing or storage issues associated with cellular products. Led by Badylak and colleagues, the field of naturally derived, decellularized biomaterials grew through the 1990s. Acellular wound care devices were approved under the 510(k) process and were intended to be repopulated by host cells and absorbed into the wound bed. These substrates targeted impairments observed in diabetic foot ulcers, including TGF-beta controlled pathways, MMP-TIMP

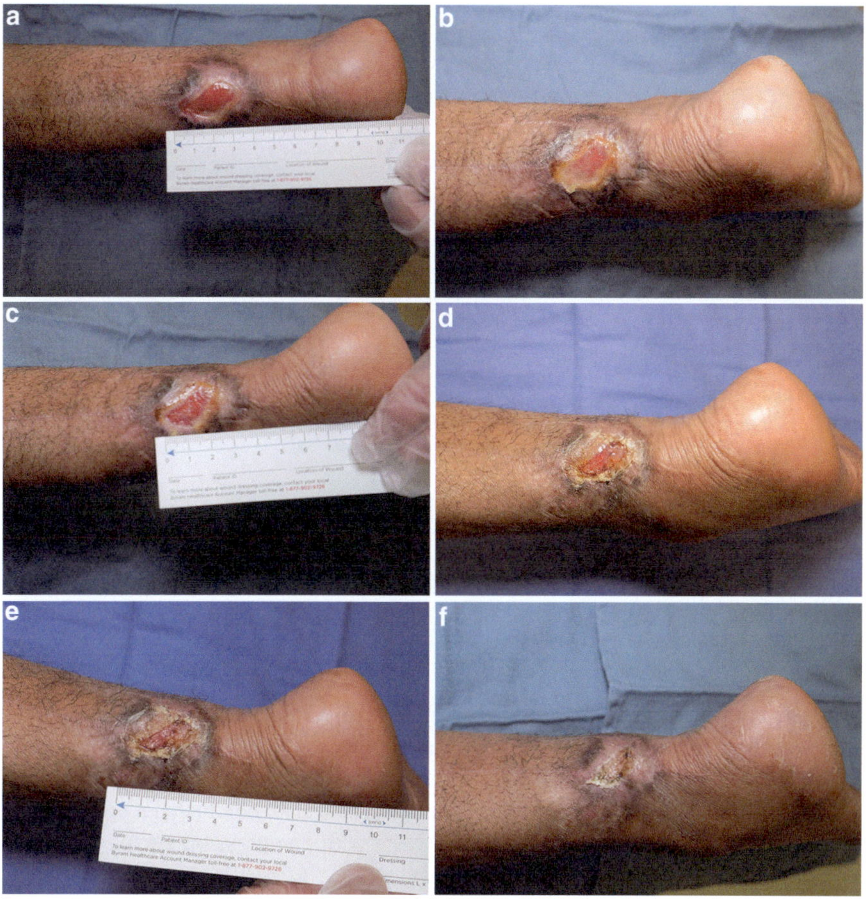

Fig. 13.4 Progression of wound healing after application of dehydrated amnion/chorion allograft (dHACA) to a diabetic lower-extremity wound from Fig. 13.3. (**a**) Clean wound prior to treatment; (**b**) 1-week follow-up; (**c**) 2-week follow-up; (**d**) 3-week follow-up; (**e**) 4-week follow-up; (**f**) 6-week follow-up

imbalance, and decreased responsiveness of HIF-1α and VEGF mediated angiogenesis [29–31] (Fig. 13.5). Decellularized products such as Oasis wound matrix (Smith & Nephew, Andover, MA) and ACell UBM (ACell, Inc., Columbia, MD) contain a "black box" of bioactive ECM molecules from various sources, including small intestinal submucosa (SIS), urinary bladder matrix (UBM), and foregut. Key mediators of cutaneous repair found within the ECM of most tissue types include structural proteins such as collagen and elastin, cell adhesion molecules such as fibronectin and laminin, and glycosaminoglycans and proteoglycans [32]. Growth factors including TGFβ, basic FGF, VEGF, and other tissue-specific cytokines have also been isolated from decellularized tissues [33–35]. A partial list of the many decellularized tissue-based wound dressings, focusing on those that claim to contain significant bioactive components beyond collagen, is listed in Table 13.6.

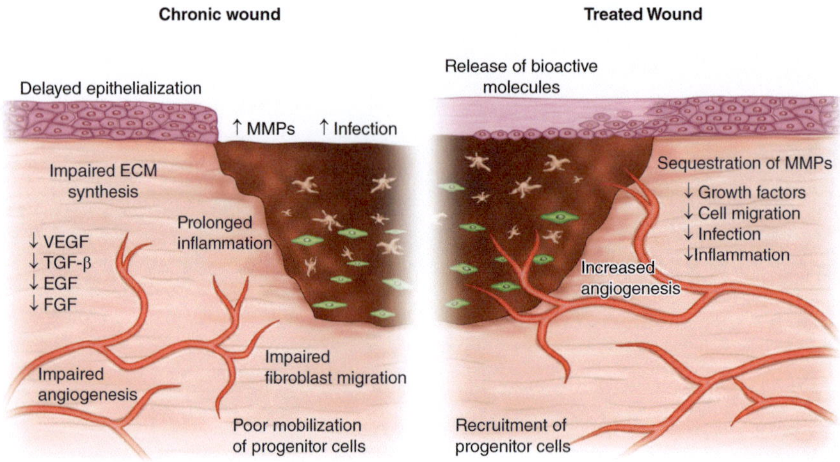

Fig. 13.5 Molecular derangements in impaired wound healing and the proposed mechanism of action of decellularized ECM-based matrices. Bioactive ECM fragments are released as the wound device is degraded. These ECM molecules promote cell migration and proliferation, sequester MMPs, and increase angiogenesis (Adapted from Turner NJ & Badylak SF. Adv Wound Care (New Rochelle). 2015 Aug 1; 4 (8): 490–500)

Oasis wound dressing (Smith & Nephew, Inc., Andover, MA) is manufactured from decellularized porcine small intestinal submucosa (SIS). As one of the earliest decellularized ECM-based materials for wound healing, several publications have studied its efficacy for various wound types. Mostow et al. conducted a prospective, randomized controlled trial (n = 120) of Oasis with compression versus compression alone for the treatment of chronic leg ulcers. At 12 weeks, modest but statistically significant differences in complete wound closure was observed (55% of Oasis group versus 34% of controls, p = 0.0196). At 6 months, no recurrences were reported from the Oasis group [36]. A similar RCT of Oasis versus moist wound dressings for chronic mixed vascular ulcers (n = 50) demonstrated complete healing in 80% with an average time to heal of 5.4 weeks in the Oasis group compared to a 65% rate of complete healing with an average time to heal of 8.3 weeks in the control group ($p < 0.05$) [37].

Management of Specific Wounds

General Wound Preparation and Substrate Selection

A problematic wound can be frustrating for both patient and practitioner. Despite weeks of serial debridements, mechanical off-loading, systemic optimization of comorbidities, and standard wound care, problematic, chronic wounds may fail to progress. In this frustrated state of mind, advanced wound matrices may be seen as either a potential magical solution or as an unlikely last effort to do something. The dizzying array of products contributes to the mystical nature of these wound care adjuncts. However, advanced wound care matrices are better thought of as biofunctional, targeted therapies for dysregulated, stalled, wound healing pathways. Designed to be placed on a properly prepared bed, biofunctional wound matrices are, in essence, avascular grafts – scaffolds that the host cells can populate and incorporate to reset and promote the healing environment. To the extent that a noninfected, not critically ischemic wound bed may be achieved, these substrates may accelerate wound healing in difficult wounds. The following represent general guidelines for selecting biofunctional matrices and dermal substitutes based on wound pathology. The reader is advised to consult specific insurance company guidelines for any required documentation for wound care adjunct use to be considered medically necessary.

Burns

Dermal substitute use in the burn patient differs from the majority of applications discussed in this publication, as acute burns may involve large areas with unavailable donor autograft sites, intense local and systemic inflammation, and different goals for time to healing to minimize scarring (ideally less than 2–3 weeks) [38, 39]. The burn wound bed contains high concentrations of reactive oxygen species and inflammatory mediators such as IL-1, TNF-α, PGE2, and hydrogen peroxide [40, 41]. Uncontrolled inflammation and edema may result in extension of the initial injury, while control of inflammation may limit tissue loss [42]. Primary goals in the management of the acute burn wound include temporary wound coverage to prevent evaporative fluid and heat losses, protection of the wound bed from infection, prevention of functional contracture, and minimization of pain [43].

Temporary wound coverage was initially accomplished with xenografts and allografts, which still remain widely used for this purpose. Xenografts and allografts will be rejected by the patient and will not incorporate, but may buy time while the patient's physiologic status is stabilized.

Synthetic dermal regenerative templates (Table 13.4) containing collagen are hypothesized to downregulate the local inflammatory response, while silicone layers serve to decrease heat and evaporative losses. For partial-thickness burns or split-thickness autograft donor sites, dermal regenerative templates such as Biobrane (no longer available in the USA) have been shown to prevent wound desiccation, reduce pain and dressing changes, and accelerate healing [44–46]. TransCyte, which is a fibroblast-seeded form of Biobrane, has been supported by multiple studies and RCT to decrease inpatient stay in children and adults [47, 48], stimulate epithelialization [49], and decrease hypertrophic scarring. For full-thickness burns, dermal regenerative templates such as Integra (Integra LifeSciences, Plainsboro, NJ) can protect exposed structures, such as tendon and bone, and prepare the wound bed prior to flap or autograft [12]. Briefly, Integra has also been successfully used to resurface chronic burn contractures.

A summary of dermal substitutes for burn care are listed in Table 13.7.

Table 13.7 Dermal substitutes and biologic matrices for acute burn care

Product	Indication
Integra	Full-thickness or severe burns with limited autograft options
Biobrane	Superficial partial-thickness burns and donor site after debridement, when autograft not available or not desirable due to patient's physiologic condition
TransCyte	Deep partial-thickness and full-thickness burns
Epicel	FDA approved for TBSA > 30% deep partial-thickness or full-thickness burns, in combination with split-thickness skin graft, or on its own
OrCel	Donor sites

Diabetic Foot Ulcers (DFUs)

Diabetic foot ulcers (DFUs) are prevalent, costly, and leading causes of hospitalizations and limb loss in the diabetic population [50, 51]. Diabetic neuropathy, repeated minor trauma, and foot deformity are implicated in pathogenesis of DFUs and can be found in 63% of all patients presenting with DFUs without concomitant arterial insufficiency [52]. Patients are likely to have associated comorbidities that further affect wound healing capacity, namely, renal insufficiency, immunosuppression, cardiac and vascular disease, and neuropathy. Biofunctional matrices for DFUs are indicated as an adjunct to comprehensive wound therapy (including but not limited to surgical debridement, complete off-loading, orthopedic correction, vascular intervention, and glucose control) in wounds that have not progressed toward healing after a period of 4–6 weeks, with no current evidence of infection in the wound bed, adequate perfusion of the limb, and adequate diabetes control (no current HbA1c reading above 12%).

Multiple derangements are recognized that contribute to poor wound healing in the diabetic patient on the molecular and cellular level. Reduced TGF-β signaling has been shown in a diabetic rat model to affect cell migration and decrease myofibroblast activity and wound contraction [53]. Derangements in the MMP-TIMP balance, with increased MMP and reduced TIMP levels beyond the early phases of wound healing, results in ECM degradation and an unstable foundation for cell migration [54]. High levels of matrix metalloproteinases and endopeptidases, which degrade extracellular matrix proteins and mediate apoptotic ligand release and cytokine inactivation, have been clinically observed in human diabetic foot wounds [31]. The responsiveness of hypoxia-inducible factor-1α (HIF-1α) in diabetic fibroblasts as well as in normal fibroblasts under high glucose conditions is diminished, resulting in poor hypoxic upregulation of VEGF and impaired angiogenesis [29, 30, 55]. As a result of the interplay of these processes, keratinocyte migration from the wound edge of diabetic patients is reduced by up to 60% [56]. Risk of infection is raised due to granulocyte dysfunction [57].

The role of biologic wound care matrices in DFUs is very different than in the burn setting. The normal wound healing pathways have been dysregulated, and the chronic wound is stalled in a state of excess inflammation, arrested epithelialization, extracellular matrix degradation, and impaired angiogenesis. The ideal cellular and decellularized ECM-based devices therefore function, in combination with debridement, to restore the wound to an acute wound state and to replace or stimulate the release of growth factors and appropriate cytokines. Restoring the regenerative state and providing a scaffold to stabilize the wound bed (as in the case of any device providing an ECM matrix) helps the MMP-TIMP balance that would allow for deposition of a healthy granulation tissue and neovascularization of the provisional matrix afforded by the device itself.

Clinical Trials

Tables 13.8 and 13.9 summarize the results of the landmark efficacy and comparative randomized controlled trials (RCTs) for biologically active matrices for the treatment of diabetic foot ulcers. Though many retrospective and prospective case series exist, they were not included in this review. Reported outcomes include higher rate of wound closure (defined as 100% epithelialization with no drainage) and shorter time to wound closure. These trials, while conducted as RCTs, are usually sponsored by the manufacturer, raising the possibility of bias toward findings in favor of the device. Study selection criteria often exclude patients with renal insufficiency, vascular compromise, taking immunosuppression or steroid medications, or ulcers with exposed deep structures. Many trials exclude patients whose wounds have shown progress over the preceding 30 days. They are designed to show non-inferiority of the device to the standard wound care (SWC) protocol in the ideal, optimized patient who has already demonstrated a low likelihood of wound closure with SWC. The outcomes of these studies have been consistently in favor of advanced wound care devices.

Comparative trials have evaluated multiple products within the same study while occasionally comparing to standard wound care as well. Attention must be given to study design since these can favor a particular product. The variability in patient cohorts owing to different sets of comorbidities, wound locations and size, and other patient variables can confound the results, leading to some conflicting data. Unfortunately, patient cohorts are often also small [68, 69], making it difficult to rely on the results for clinical guidance. At this time, adequate data exist to support the used of dermal substitute devices as indicated for DFUs failing standard wound care protocols, but more high-quality studies are needed to compare the devices in the clinical setting.

Venous Insufficiency Wounds

The pathogenesis of venous leg ulcers (VLUs) from incompetent valves in the veins of the lower extremities to the development of venous hypertension involves sluggish flow allowing leukocyte adhesion, chronic inflammation, destruction of endothelial cells, and ultimately degradation of the dermis with

Table 13.8 Summary of selected randomized controlled trials (RCT) for advanced wound care matrices in DFU care

Product	Author, year	Study design	Number of patients	Inclusion criteria	Exclusion criteria	Methods	Conclusions	LOE
Cellular substrates								
Apligraf	Veves et al. [24]	Prospective, RCT at 24 centers	208 total, 112 intervention, 96 control, 44 withdrew, but collected data was included in analysis	HbA1c between 6% and 12%, full-thickness neuropathic ulcers (excluding the dorsum of the foot and the calcaneus) 1 and 16 cm^2	Infection, clinically significant lower-extremity ischemia (ABI <0.65), active Charcot's disease, medical conditions that would impair wound healing	Serial debridement and application of Apligraf each week for 4 weeks compared to the control group of debridement and wet to dry dressings	Complete wound healing was higher by 12 weeks in the intervention group vs control group (56% vs 38%); median time to closure was shorter in the intervention group (65 vs 90 days)	I
Apligraf	Veves et al. [24]	Prospective, RCT at 24 centers	208 total, 112 intervention, 96 control, 44 withdrew but collected data was included in analysis	HbA1c between 6% and 12%, full-thickness neuropathic ulcers (excluding the dorsum of the foot and the calcaneus) 1 and 16 cm^2	Infection, clinically significant lower-extremity ischemia (ABI <0.65), active Charcot's disease, medical conditions that would impair wound healing	Serial debridement and application of Apligraf each week for 4 weeks compared to the control group of debridement and wet to dry dressings	Complete wound healing was higher by 12 weeks in the intervention group vs control group (56% vs 38%); median time to closure was shorter in the intervention group (65 vs 90 days)	I
Apligraf	Frykberg et al. [58]	Retrospective analysis of previously published data	314 total, 163 intervention, 151 control patients	Plantar foot ulcers on the heel or forefoot without exposure of tendon, muscle, joint capsule, or bone	Infection, ulcers due to Charcot deformity, ABI < 0.7, patients receiving immunosuppressant or cytotoxic agents	All patients received SWC for 12 weeks, intervention group received weekly applications of Apligraf up to eight times	Lower amputation rate in intervention group vs control group (5.5% vs 12.6%)	III

Dermagraft	Marston et al. [59]	Prospective, single-blind, RCT at 35 centers	245 total, 130 intervention, 115 control, 46 did not complete trial	Plantar foot ulcer 1.0 to 20 cm^2 present for a minimum of 2 weeks without exposure of muscle, tendon, bone, or joint capsule; ABI > 0.7	Gangrene, ulcer over Charcot deformity, albumin <2.0, infection, patients on corticosteroids, immunosuppressive or cytotoxic agents, Coumadin, or heparin	All patients received sharp debridement, saline-moistened gauze dressing, and off-loading. Intervention group received their first application at day 0 and up to seven additional weekly applications	Higher wound closure rate by 12 weeks in intervention group vs control group (30% vs 18.3%)	I
EpiFix	Zelen et al. [60]	Prospective single center RCT	25 total, 13 intervention, 12 control	Ulcer size between 1 and 25 cm^2 present for ≥4 weeks without clinical signs of infection; serum Cr <3.0 mg/dl, HbA1c < 12%. Dorsum transcutaneous oxygen test ≥30 mmHg, ankle-brachial index between 0.7 and 1.2 or triphasic or biphasic Doppler arterial waveforms at the ankle of affected leg	Charcot foot, ulcer probing to bone, currently receiving radiation or chemotherapy, known or suspected malignancy of current ulcer, diagnosis of autoimmune connective tissue disease, biomedical or topical growth factor within the preceding 30 days, taking medications considered to be immune system modulators	SWC was debridement, application of SilvaSorb gel and Aquacel AG and a compression dressing. Intervention received one application of EpiFix with nonadherent dressing, moisture-retentive dressing, and a compression dressing. EpiFix was reapplied at weeks 2, 4, 6, 8, and 10, if the ulcer was not healed. All wounds were off-loaded	Intervention group showed higher wound reduction rate by 1 week (80% vs 20%) and higher wound closure rate by 6 weeks (92% vs 8%) vs control group	II

(continued)

Table 13.8 (continued)

Product	Author, year	Study design	Number of patients	Inclusion criteria	Exclusion criteria	Methods	Conclusions	LOE
Grafix	Lavery et al. [61]	Prospective, multicenter, single-blinded RCT	97 total, 47 intervention, 47 control	DFU present between 4 and 52 weeks, DFU distal to malleolus on plantar or dorsal surface of the foot, size 1–15 cm^2	HbA1c > 12%, infection, inadequate circulation (ABI <0.7 or >1.3, toe-brachial index ≤0.5 or Doppler study with inadequate arterialpulsation), exposed muscle, tendon, bone, or joint capsule, reduction of wound area by ≥30% during the screening period	All wounds were debrided and received off-loading and nonadherent dressings. Control group received weekly SWC. Intervention group received Grafix weekly	Intervention group showed higher wound closure rate by 12 weeks (62% vs 21%), shorter median time to closure (42 vs 69.5 days), fewer adverse events (44% vs 66%), and infections (18% vs 26.2%) compared to the control group	I
Decellularized ECM substrates								
Oasis	Cazzell et al. [62]	Prospective, parallel-group, open-label RCT at 11 sites in the USA	82 total, 41 intervention, 41 control	Neuropathic foot ulcer on the plantar surface present between 6 and 52 weeks, between 0.5 and 10 cm^2 in size; albumin ≥2.0 g/dL, pre-albumin ≥10 mg/dL, HbA1c ≤12%	Clinical signs or symptoms of ulcer infection	SWC was sharp debridement and dressing changes, intervention was Oasis once each week to ulcers following cleansing with sterile saline and dressing	Higher wound closure rate by 12 weeks in intervention group vs control group (54% vs 32%), wound closure on average of 2 weeks earlier in intervention group	I
GraftJacket	Brigido [8]	Prospective, single-center RCT	28 total, 14 intervention, 14 control	Full-thickness wound for at least 6 weeks without epidermal coverage, palpable or Doppler audible pulses to the affected lower extremity	Evidence of active infection	Control group underwent weekly sharp debridement and Curasol (Healthpoint Ltd., Fort Worth, TX, USA) wound gel was applied. Intervention group underwent sharp debridement, application of GraftJacket, and a mineral oil-soaked fluff compressive dressing	Higher wound closure rate by 16 weeks in intervention group vs control group (86% vs 29%)	II

GraftJacket	Reyzelman et al. [63]	Prospective, RCT at 11 sites	93 total, 47 intervention, 39 control, 7 withdrew, and 6 of 7 were included in analysis	Ulcer size from 1 to 25 cm^2 without infection, adequate circulation defined by transcutaneous oxygen measurement at the dorsum of the foot greater or equal to 30 mmHg, ABI between 0.7 and 1.2, or at least biphasic Doppler arterial waveforms at the DP and PT arteries	HbA1c > 12%, serum Cr > 3.0 mg/dl, ulcers probing to bone, or ulcers treated with growth factors in the preceding 30 days	Intervention group received a single application of GraftJacket, dressed with a silver-based nonadherent dressing; additional applications were performed per the investigator. Control group SWC consisted of moist wound therapy with alginates, foams, hydrocolloids, or hydrogels at the discretion of the treating physician. Dressing changes occurred daily	Intervention group showed higher wound closure rate by 12 weeks (69.6% vs 46.2%) and shorter mean time to healing (5.7 +/− 3.5 weeks vs 6.8 +/−3.3 weeks) compared to the control group	II
Dermal regenerative scaffolds								
Integra	Driver et al. [20]	Prospective RCT at 32 sites	188 total, 106 intervention, 82 control	HbA1c <12%, full-thickness neuropathic ulcer distal to the malleolus present for >30 days, 1–12 cm^2 post debridement, ABI between 0.65 and 1.2 or toe pressure > 50 mmHg or TcPO2 > 40 mmHg or Doppler ultrasound consistent with adequate blood flow to the affected extremity	Infection, exposed capsule, tendon, or bone; reduction of wound 30% during the screening period	Control SWC was daily dressing changes. Intervention group received Integra +/− fenestration or meshing, and silicone layer was removed when the collagenlayer was replaced by new tissue (14–21 days after application). Reapplication of IDRT was performed at the discretion of the investigator	Intervention group showed higher wound closure rate by 16 weeks (51% vs 32%) and shorter median time to closure (43 vs 78 days) compared to the control group	I

Table 13.9 Summary of selected comparative trials for advanced wound care matrices in DFU care

Product	Author, year	Study design	Number of patients	Inclusion criteria	Exclusion criteria	Methods	Conclusions	LOE
EpiFix vs Apligraf vs standard wound care	Zelen et al. [64]	Prospective, parallel-group RCT at four centers	104 total, 34 EpiFix, 35 Apligraf, 35 control. 23 discontinued intervention, 18/23 in control group due to poor wound healing	DFU 1–25 cm^2 present ≥4 weeks and unresponsive to standard wound care, no infection, serum Cr <3.0 mg/dl, HbA1c <12%. Dorsum transcutaneous oxygen test ≥30 mmHg or ABI between 0.7 and 1.2 or triphasic or biphasic Doppler arterial waveforms at the ankle of affected leg	DFU present >52 weeks without intermittent healing; probing to tendon, muscle, capsule, or bone; receiving radiation or chemotherapy; autoimmune connective tissue disease; biomedical or topical growth factor within previous 30 days; immune system modulators or Cox2 inhibitors; wounds improving greater than 20% over the 2-week run-in period of the trial	Weekly graft applications and dressing change visits for 12 weeks; any wound improving by less than 50% within the first 6 weeks was excluded in the study. Standard wound care group received debridement weekly and changed their dressing daily using collagen-alginate and gauze dressing supplies. All wounds were off-loaded	Wound closure at 12 weeks was highest for EpiFix (97%), followed by Apligraf (73%), and lastly standard wound care (51%). Difference between Apligraf and SWC wound closure rates was not statistically significant; EpiFix was found to be more cost-effective than Apligraf ($1517 vs $8918 per wound closure)	II

EpiFix vs Apligraf	Kirsner et al. [65]	Retrospective study using deidentified data from the WoundExpert electronic medical record database (Net Health, Pittsburgh, PA)	226 total wounds, Apligraf 163 wounds, EpiFix 63 wounds	Patients received at least one treatment with Apligraf or EpiFix on a DFU with location coded as foot, toe, heel, metatarsal head, toe web space, toe amputation site, or transmetatarsal amputation site with an ulcer size ≥1 to ≤25 cm^2, ulcer duration ≤52 weeks, and ulcer area reduction ≤20% in the 14 days prior to the first treatment	Wounds receiving alternate skin substitute treatment or if follow-up wound area measurements were not available	All DFUs were followed from the first application of the product until wound closure. The proportion of wounds closed at 12 and 24 weeks, median time to wound closure, hazard ratio (HR) with 95% confidence interval (CI), and p-value were estimated	Patients treated with EpiFix required more applications of product Apligraf (3 versus 2). There was decreased median time to closure with Apligraf compared with EpiFix (13.3 weeks vs 26 weeks). The Apligraf group had a 97% better rate of complete wound healing compared to EpiFix (hazard ratio = 1.97; 95% CI 1.17, 3.33)	III

(continued)

Table 13.9 (continued)

Product	Author, year	Study design	Number of patients	Inclusion criteria	Exclusion criteria	Methods	Conclusions	LOE
Apligraf vs TheraSkin	DiDomenico et al. [66]	Prospective RCT with sequential enrollment into the two arms	39 total wounds, 17 treated with Apligraf and 12 with TheraSkin	DFU present >4 weeks size 0.5–4 cm^2, HbA1c < 12, ABI < 0.75, palpable pulses	Infection, exposed bone/tendon/joint, wound depth > 9 mm, no secondary etiology to ulcer	Both groups received a standard debridement; both groups received a single application of the chosen device, followed by daily or QOD dressing changes after a week of delay; with up to five reapplications	TheraSkin group showed higher closure rate by 12 weeks (66.7% vs 41.3%), shorter mean time to closure (5.00 weeks vs 6.86 weeks), and fewer average device applications (1.38 vs 1.53) compared to the Apligraf group	II

AlloPatch vs standard wound care	Zelen et al. [9]	Prospective multicenter RCT	40 total, 20 in each group	DFU present >4 weeks, >1cm^2, failure of prior therapy, no infection, adequate perfusion proven on objective testing	Wounds >25cm^2, wounds healing >20% in screening period, wounds probing to bone	All patients underwent debridement, AlloPatch group examined at 6 weeks and removed from study if >50% closure was not attained at that point; control dressing were hydrogel	Higher closure rate of DFUs with AlloPatch vs SWC at 6 weeks (65% vs 5%) and at 12 weeks (80% versus 20%); with 40 vs 77 days to complete wound closure for AlloPatch vs SWC, respectively	
Oasis vs Regranex	Niezgoda et al. [67]	Prospective multicenter RCT	73 total, 37 in Oasis group, 36 in Regranex group	DFU >1mo, non-healing, 1–49 cm^2, full thickness, granulation tissue in wound bed	Exposed bone/tendon/fascia, arterial insufficiency, HbA1c < 12%, Charcot disease, corticosteroids or immunosuppression, infection, hemodialysis	Patients were seen weekly for debridement and dressing changes as needed, Oasis and Regranex were reapplied at weekly visits as determined by practitioner	At 12 weeks, Oasis group showed 49% wound closure vs 28% in the Regranex arm ($p = 0.055$), no significant difference in time to healing was noted (67 vs 73 days, $p = 0.245$)	II

skin changes and ulcer formation. Once ulcers form, these wounds are inherently slow to heal due to derangements in blood flow and chronic changes in the tissue. Risk factors for VLUs include obesity, advanced age, prolonged standing, physical inactivity, greater height, and genetic predisposition. Compression and meticulous wound care is the gold standard treatment in treating venous stasis ulcers, but recurrence remains high. Compression therapy controls edema and reduces the effective distance between the capillary bed and the tissue, thus improving hypoxia [70].

While specifics may vary, advanced wound care substrates are indicated where conventional therapy (such as surgical debridement, elevation, standard dressing changes, and importantly compression) have been ineffective after a period of 3 weeks, with no current evidence of infection in the wound bed and adequate perfusion of the limb [2]. Treatment of VLUs using advanced skin substitutes relies on multiple factors. All devices provide the benefit of occlusion to provide a moist wound environment. Acellular products provide a scaffold for vascularization, integration, and eventual remodeling over time. Cell-containing substrates stimulate epithelialization and improve the local inflammatory milieu by acting as a temporary epithelial coverage, thereby downregulating the inflammatory response. Studies suggest that the recipient cells eventually replace the graft, likely due to stimulation by the graft cells, similar to the same mechanism by which autograft may stimulate wound closure [71]. Selected evidence of use of advanced wound care matrices for VLUs is included in Table 13.10. Many studies were excluded from review for low sample size or bias owing to inclusion/exclusion criteria. Further research is needed also comparing these products head to head in RCTs to help guide device choice.

Inflammatory Wounds

Biologic matrix use for inflammatory wounds has been limited to case reports (Level V) for treating pyoderma gangrenosum [74], sarcoid ulcer [74], and necrobiosis lipoidica [75]. These products can provide atraumatic coverage to restore a proper moisture balance and provide regeneration scaffolds and growth factors in much the same fashion as for DFUs and VLUs. As these wound care devices gain further acceptance, more data regarding outcomes will hopefully become available to support their use in treating these challenging wounds.

Practical Considerations

Biofunctional matrices are important adjuncts to standard wound care for chronic and difficult-to-heal wounds. New products are coming to market continuously, and the practitioner is cautioned to analyze the data critically. In a recent systematic review, Snyder et al. analyzed 15 studies comparing the effectiveness of skin substitutes in the care of DFUs and VLUs. Out of these 15 studies, the

Table 13.10 Summary of selected randomized controlled trials (RCT) for advanced wound care matrices in VLU care

Product	Author, year	Study design	Number of patients	Inclusion criteria	Exclusion criteria	Methods	Conclusions	LOE
Cellular substrates								
Apligraf	Falanga and Sabolinski [4]	Subgroup analysis of a previously published RCT	120 total, 72 Apligraf, 48 control	Ulcers present >1 year due venous insufficiency as determined by presence of clinical signs and symptoms, absence of arterial insufficiency, and evidence of venous insufficiency by air plethysmography or photoplethysmography	Infection, vasculitis, or collagen vascular diseases; pregnancy or lactation; uncontrolled diabetes mellitus or other clinically significant medical conditions or medications that would impair wound healing	Intervention group received Graftskin and compression with up to five reapplications within the first 3 weeks of the study, control group was compression only	Apligraf group showed 63% wound closure at 6 months vs 49% in control group; VLUs present >1 year, Apligraf group showed 47% wound closure vs 19% with compression alone	I

(continued)

Table 13.10 (continued)

Product	Author, year	Study design	Number of patients	Inclusion criteria	Exclusion criteria	Methods	Conclusions	LOE
Apligraf	Falanga et al. [3]	Prospective multicenter RCT	275 total, 146 in intervention group and 129 in control group	Clinical diagnosis of venous insufficiency, confirmation with air or photoplethysmography, ABI >0.65	Infection, vasculitis, uncontrolled DM, systemic disease impairing wound healing	Controls were treated with nonadherent dressing, Unna boot, and compression, with reapplication weekly; intervention group was treated with application of device, gauze, and compression, with up to five reapplications in the first 3 weeks of the study	Intervention group showed higher rate of healing (63% vs 49%, $p = 0.02$) at 6 months and shorter median time to wound closure (61 vs 181 days, $p = 0.003$)	I

EpiFix	Serena et al. [72]	Prospective multicenter RCT	84 total, 26 received one application of EpiFix, 27 received two applications of EpiFix, 31 multilayer compression therapy alone	ABI >0.75, VLU present >1mo, 2–20 cm^2, full thickness but not probing to muscle, tendon, or bone, failing compression therapy for at least 14 days	Clinical signs and symptoms of infection, HbA1c >10%, suspicion of malignancy, use of immunosuppressants, chemotherapy, or application of topical steroids within 1 month, history of radiation at ulcer site, or previously treated with tissue engineered materials or other scaffold materials within the last 30 days	EpiFix was applied once or twice 2 weeks apart depending on treatment group. The multilayer compression therapy bandage was used in all groups and applied at every visit. Endpoint was wound size reduction >40% by 4 weeks	EpiFix (single application) was similar to EpiFix (two applications) with 62% and 63% of patients achieving >40% wound size reduction at 4 weeks vs 32% in control group ($p < 0.05$)	I

(continued)

Table 13.10 (continued)

Product	Author, year	Study design	Number of patients	Inclusion criteria	Exclusion criteria	Methods	Conclusions	LOE
Decellularized ECM substrates								
Oasis	Mostow et al. [36]	Prospective multicenter RCT	120 total, 62 Oasis, 58 compression therapy	Ulcer size > = 1–64 cm^2 with no exposed bone or tendon. Duration >1 month with viable granulation tissue	Rheumatoid arthritis, radiotherapy to the ulcer site, uncontrolled congestive heart failure, corticosteroids or immune suppressives, collagen or vascular disease, malnutrition (albumin >2.5 g/dL), known allergy to porcine-derived products, infection, HgbA1c > 12%	Oasis group received weekly application of the graft and a four-layer compression bandaging system. The standard-care group received an identical nonadherent dressing and four-layer compression bandage. Dressing changes and evaluation occurred weekly	Oasis group showed higher wound closure rat by 12 weeks vs control group (55% vs 34%, $p = 0.02$)	I

Bio-active matrices for wound healing								
Talymed	Kelechi et al. [73]	Prospective, randomized, investigator-blinded, parallel-group, controlled study	82 total, 20 weekly application, 22 biweekly application, 20 triweekly application, 20 control	Partial-thickness VLU 2–20 cm^2 diagnosed within the past 4 weeks without recent skin grafts or use of growth factors; a viable and clean wound bed with granulation tissue and greater than or equal to 90% free of necrotic debris	Full-thickness ulcers, infection, insufficient blood supply to wound (ankle-brachial index <0.8 or >1.3); wound duration more than 6 months; collagen vascular disease, severe arterial disease, organ transplant, Charcot disease, or sickle cell disease	All patients received Unna boot and compression. Talymed group received one application immediately before administration of the primary nonadherent absorptive dressing. Reapplication of graft was performed according to randomization group	At 20 weeks, groups receiving Talymed every 2 or 3 weeks showed higher wound closure rates (86.4% and 65.0%) compared to the control group (45.0%) and the group receiving only one application of Talymed (45%), $p = 0.01$ for difference between biweekly application group and controls	II

conclusions of 6 studies were rated as low strength of evidence, and the other 9 studies were determined to be of inadequate quality to provide any recommendation whatsoever [13]. While these studies are RCTs, it is important to remember that inadequate sample size, overly restrictive inclusion and exclusion criteria, and bias due to sponsorship should all be factored into the final weighting of the study results.

These biologic products are significantly more costly than standard dressings, and this expense must be justified in today's value-driven environment. Cost-benefit analyses comparing advanced wound care products to SWC in caring for chronic wounds show superiority of the advanced wound care devices [76–78]. Langer and Rogowski conducted a systematic review of economic evaluations of human cell-derived wound care products for the treatment of venous leg and diabetic foot ulcers [79] and concluded that the current evidence supports the cost effectiveness of these devices compared to SWC. However, they aptly point out the multitude of methodological flaws present in the current cost-benefit analyses and draw the reader's attention to the lack of high-quality, prospective evidence to support these conclusions. Moreover, these cost-benefit analyses are predicted on critical assumptions inherent to such studies (i.e., cost to patient and society of a closed vs open wound, cost of amputation, standard wound care, etc.) [76].

Conclusions and Future Directions

Biofunctional matrices and dermal substitutes are a heterogenous and rapidly changing category of advanced wound care devices. The multitude of cellular and acellular options, as well as variations within each product, can be overwhelming at first glance. While these biologic substrates may not represent a holy grail for all wounds, there is ample evidence to conclude that advanced wound care matrices applied in the appropriate setting are beneficial in the treatment of problematic wounds. As we continue to identify molecular targets for aberrant wound healing and as our knowledge and experience with various bioactive and naturally derived materials grows, biofunctional matrices may become a routine part of a cost-effective, integrated wound care regimen. The future is bright as scientists and engineers pursue strategies that target specific wound healing pathways through small-molecule engineering [80] and develop emerging technologies such as three-dimensional bioprinting [81–83].

References

1. Sheehan P, Jones P, Giurini JM, Caselli A, Veves A. Percent change in wound area of diabetic foot ulcers over a 4-week period is a robust predictor of complete healing in a 12-week prospective trial. Plast Reconstr Surg. 2006;117(Suppl 7):239s–44s.

2. Phillips TJ, Machado F, Trout R, Porter J, Olin J, Falanga V. Prognostic indicators in venous ulcers. J Am Acad Dermatol. 2000;43(4):627–30.
3. Falanga V, Margolis D, Alvarez O, Auletta M, Maggiacomo F, Altman M, et al. Rapid healing of venous ulcers and lack of clinical rejection with an allogeneic cultured human skin equivalent. Human Skin Equivalent Investigators Group. Arch Dermatol. 1998;134(3):293–300.
4. Falanga V, Sabolinski M. A bilayered living skin construct (APLIGRAF) accelerates complete closure of hard-to-heal venous ulcers. Wound Repair Regen. 1999;7(4):201–7.
5. Sabolinski ML, Alvarez O, Auletta M, Mulder G, Parenteau NL. Cultured skin as a 'smart material' for healing wounds: experience in venous ulcers. Biomaterials. 1996;17(3):311.
6. Nyame TT, Chiang HA, Leavitt T, Ozambela M, Orgill DP. Tissue-engineered skin substitutes. Plast Reconstr Surg. 2015;136(6):1379–88.
7. Consensus I, editor. Acellular matrices for the treatment of wounds. An expert working group review. London: Wounds International; 2010.
8. Brigido SA. The use of an acellular dermal regenerative tissue matrix in the treatment of lower extremity wounds: a prospective 16-week pilot study. Int Wound J. 2006;3(3):181–7.
9. Zelen CM, Orgill DP, Serena T, Galiano R, Carter MJ, Didomenico LA, et al. A prospective, randomised, controlled, multicentre clinical trial examining healing rates, safety and cost to closure of an acellular reticular allogenic human dermis versus standard of care in the treatment of chronic diabetic foot ulcers. Int Wound J. 2017;14(2):307.
10. Raffetto JD, Mosti G, Santi M, Ligi D, Mannello F. Matrix metalloproteinase profiles in chronic venous ulcer wound fluid of inflammatory and granulating venous leg ulcers. J Vasc Surg Venous Lymphat Disord. 2015;3(1):119.
11. Yannas IV, Burke JF. Design of an artificial skin. I. Basic design principles. J Biomed Mater Res. 1980;14(1):65–81.
12. Yannas IV, Orgill DP, Burke JF. Template for skin regeneration. Plast Reconstr Surg. 2011;127(Suppl 1):60s–70s.
13. Snyder DL, Sullivan N, Schoelles KM. AHRQ technology assessments. Skin substitutes for treating chronic wounds. Rockville: Agency for Healthcare Research and Quality (US); 2012.
14. Moiemen NS, Staiano JJ, Ojeh NO, Thway Y, Frame JD. Reconstructive surgery with a dermal regeneration template: clinical and histologic study. Plast Reconstr Surg. 2001;108(1):93–103.
15. Komorowska-Timek E, Gabriel A, Bennett DC, Miles D, Garberoglio C, Cheng C, et al. Artificial dermis as an alternative for coverage of complex scalp defects following excision of malignant tumors. Plast Reconstr Surg. 2005;115(4):1010–7.
16. Taras JS, Sapienza A, Roach JB, Taras JP. Acellular dermal regeneration template for soft tissue reconstruction of the digits. J Hand Surg. 2010;35(3):415–21.
17. Weigert R, Choughri H, Casoli V. Management of severe hand wounds with Integra(R) dermal regeneration template. J Hand Surg Eur Vol. 2011;36(3):185–93.
18. Valerio IL, Masters Z, Seavey JG, Balazs GC, Ipsen D, Tintle SM. Use of a dermal regeneration template wound dressing in the treatment of combat-related upper extremity soft tissue injuries. J Hand Surg. 2016;41(12):e453–e60.
19. Helgeson MD, Potter BK, Evans KN, Shawen SB. Bioartificial dermal substitute: a preliminary report on its use for the management of complex combat-related soft tissue wounds. J Orthop Trauma. 2007;21(6):394–9.
20. Driver VR, Lavery LA, Reyzelman AM, Dutra TG, Dove CR, Kotsis SV, et al. A clinical trial of Integra template for diabetic foot ulcer treatment. Wound Repair Regen. 2015;23(6):891–900.
21. Dinh TL, Veves A. The efficacy of Apligraf in the treatment of diabetic foot ulcers. Plast Reconst Surg. 2006;117(7 Suppl):152S–7S. discussion 8S–9S
22. Griffiths M, Ojeh N, Livingstone R, Price R, Navsaria H. Survival of Apligraf in acute human wounds. Tissue Eng. 2004;10(7–8):1180–95.
23. Santema TBK, Poyck PPC, Ubbink DT. Systematic review and meta-analysis of skin substitutes in the treatment of diabetic foot ulcers: highlights of a Cochrane systematic review. Wound Repair Regen. 2016;24(4):737.
24. Veves A, Falanga V, Armstrong DG, Sabolinski ML. Graftskin, a human skin equivalent, is effective in the management of noninfected neuropathic diabetic foot ulcers: a prospective randomized multicenter clinical trial. Diabetes Care. 2001;24(2):290–5.

25. Koob TJ, Rennert R, Zabek N, Massee M, Lim JJ, Temenoff JS, et al. Biological properties of dehydrated human amnion/chorion composite graft: implications for chronic wound healing. Int Wound J. 2013;10(5):493–500.
26. Massee M, Chinn K, Lei J, Lim JJ, Young CS, Koob TJ. Dehydrated human amnion/chorion membrane regulates stem cell activity in vitro. J Biomed Mater Res B Appl Biomater. 2016;104(7):1495–503.
27. Didomenico LA, Orgill DP, Galiano RD, Serena TE, Carter MJ, Kaufman JP, et al. Aseptically processed placental membrane improves healing of diabetic foot ulcerations: prospective, randomized clinical trial. Plast Reconst Surg Glob Open. 2016;4(10):e1095.
28. Zelen CM, Gould L, Serena TE, Carter MJ, Keller J, Li WW. A prospective, randomised, controlled, multi-centre comparative effectiveness study of healing using dehydrated human amnion/chorion membrane allograft, bioengineered skin substitute or standard of care for treatment of chronic lower extremity diabetic ulcers. Int Wound J. 2015;12(6):724–32.
29. Lerman OZ, Galiano RD, Armour M, Levine JP, Gurtner GC. Cellular dysfunction in the diabetic fibroblast: impairment in migration, vascular endothelial growth factor production, and response to hypoxia. Am J Pathol. 2003;162(1):303–12.
30. Thangarajah H, Vial IN, Grogan RH, Yao D, Shi Y, Januszyk M, et al. HIF-1alpha dysfunction in diabetes. Cell Cycle. 2010;9(1):75–9.
31. Guo S, Dipietro LA. Factors affecting wound healing. J Dent Res. 2010;89(3):219–29.
32. Turner NJ, Badylak SF. The use of biologic scaffolds in the treatment of chronic nonhealing wounds. Adv Wound Care. 2015;4(8):490–500.
33. McDevitt CA, Wildey GM, Cutrone RM. Transforming growth factor-beta1 in a sterilized tissue derived from the pig small intestine submucosa. J Biomed Mater Res A. 2003;67(2):637–40.
34. Hodde JP, Ernst DM, Hiles MC. An investigation of the long-term bioactivity of endogenous growth factor in OASIS wound matrix. J Wound Care. 2005;14(1):23–5.
35. Hodde JP, Record RD, Liang HA, Badylak SF. Vascular endothelial growth factor in porcine-derived extracellular matrix. Endothelium. 2001;8(1):11–24.
36. Mostow EN, Haraway GD, Dalsing M, Hodde JP, King D. Effectiveness of an extracellular matrix graft (OASIS wound matrix) in the treatment of chronic leg ulcers: a randomized clinical trial. J Vasc Surg. 2005;41(5):837–43.
37. Romanelli M, Dini V, Bertone MS. Randomized comparison of OASIS wound matrix versus moist wound dressing in the treatment of difficult-to-heal wounds of mixed arterial/venous etiology. Adv Skin Wound Care. 2010;23(1):34–8.
38. Janzekovic Z. A new concept in the early excision and immediate grafting of burns. J Trauma. 1970;10(12):1103–8.
39. Cole JK, Engrav LH, Heimbach DM, Gibran NS, Costa BA, Nakamura DY, et al. Early excision and grafting of face and neck burns in patients over 20 years. Plast Reconstr Surg. 2002;109(4):1266–73.
40. Mileski W, Borgstrom D, Lightfoot E, Rothlein R, Faanes R, Lipsky P, et al. Inhibition of leukocyte-endothelial adherence following thermal injury. J Surg Res. 1992;52(4):334–9.
41. Youn YK, LaLonde C, Demling R. The role of mediators in the response to thermal injury. World J Surg. 1992;16(1):30–6.
42. Singer AJ, Taira BR, Lin F, Lim T, Anderson R, McClain SA, et al. Curcumin reduces injury progression in a rat comb burn model. J Burn Care Res. 2011;32(1):135–42.
43. Broughton G, Zbar RI. Burns and burn reconstruction. Sel Read Plast Surg. 2005;10(7):1–25.
44. Ehrenreich M, Ruszczak Z. Tissue-engineered temporary wound coverings. Important options for the clinician. Acta Dermatovenerol Alp Panonica Adriat. 2006;15(1):5.
45. Noordenbos J, Hansbrough JF, Gutmacher H, Dore C, Hansbrough WB. Enteral nutritional support and wound excision and closure do not prevent postburn hypermetabolism as measured by continuous metabolic monitoring. J Trauma. 2000;49(4):667–71. discussion 71-2
46. Kumar RJ, Kimble RM, Boots R, Pegg SP. Treatment of partial-thickness burns: a prospective, randomized trial using Transcyte. ANZ J Surg. 2004;74(8):622–6.
47. Lukish JR, Eichelberger MR, Newman KD, Pao M, Nobuhara K, Keating M, et al. The use of a bioactive skin substitute decreases length of stay for pediatric burn patients. J Pediatr Surg. 2001;36(8):1118–21.

48. Jones I, Currie L, Martin R. A guide to biological skin substitutes. Br J Plast Surg. 2002;55(3):185–93.
49. Hansbrough J. Dermagraft-TC for partial-thickness burns: a clinical evaluation. J Burn Care Rehabil. 1997;18(1 Pt 2):S25–8.
50. Yazdanpanah L, Nasiri M, Adarvishi S. Literature review on the management of diabetic foot ulcer. World J Diabetes. 2015;6(1):37–53.
51. Barshes NR, Sigireddi M, Wrobel JS, Mahankali A, Robbins JM, Kougias P, et al. The system of care for the diabetic foot: objectives, outcomes, and opportunities. Diabet Foot Ankle. 2013;4. https://doi.org/10.3402/dfa.v4i0.21847.
52. Reiber GE, Vileikyte L, Boyko EJ, del Aguila M, Smith DG, Lavery LA, et al. Causal pathways for incident lower-extremity ulcers in patients with diabetes from two settings. Diabetes Care. 1999;22(1):157–62.
53. Al-Mulla F, Leibovich SJ, Francis IM, Bitar MS. Impaired TGF-beta signaling and a defect in resolution of inflammation contribute to delayed wound healing in a female rat model of type 2 diabetes. Mol BioSyst. 2011;7(11):3006–20.
54. Martins VL, Caley M, O'Toole EA. Matrix metalloproteinases and epidermal wound repair. Cell Tissue Res. 2013;351(2):255–68.
55. Bento CF, Pereira P. Regulation of hypoxia-inducible factor 1 and the loss of the cellular response to hypoxia in diabetes. Diabetologia. 2011;54(8):1946–56.
56. Lan CC, Wu CS, Kuo HY, Huang SM, Chen GS. Hyperglycaemic conditions hamper keratinocyte locomotion via sequential inhibition of distinct pathways: new insights on poor wound closure in patients with diabetes. Br J Dermatol. 2009;160(6):1206–14.
57. Nolan CM, Beaty HN, Bagdade JD. Further characterization of the impaired bactericidal function of granulocytes in patients with poorly controlled diabetes. Diabetes. 1978;27(9):889–94.
58. Frykberg RG, Marston WA, Cardinal M. The incidence of lower-extremity amputation and bone resection in diabetic foot ulcer patients treated with a human fibroblast-derived dermal substitute. Adv Skin Wound Care. 2015;28(1):17–20.
59. Marston WA, Hanft J, Norwood P, Pollak R. The efficacy and safety of Dermagraft in improving the healing of chronic diabetic foot ulcers: results of a prospective randomized trial. Diabetes Care. 2003;26(6):1701–5.
60. Zelen CM, Serena TE, Denoziere G, Fetterolf DE. A prospective randomised comparative parallel study of amniotic membrane wound graft in the management of diabetic foot ulcers. Int Wound J. 2013;10(5):502–7.
61. Lavery LA, Fulmer J, Shebetka KA, Regulski M, Vayser D, Fried D, et al. The efficacy and safety of Grafix((R)) for the treatment of chronic diabetic foot ulcers: results of a multi-centre, controlled, randomised, blinded, clinical trial. Int Wound J. 2014;11(5):554–60.
62. Cazzell SM, Lange DL, Dickerson JE Jr, Slade HB. The management of diabetic foot ulcers with porcine small intestine submucosa tri-layer matrix: a randomized controlled trial. Adv Wound Care. 2015;4(12):711–8.
63. Reyzelman A, Crews RT, Moore JC, Moore L, Mukker JS, Offutt S, et al. Clinical effectiveness of an acellular dermal regenerative tissue matrix compared to standard wound management in healing diabetic foot ulcers: a prospective, randomised, multicentre study. Int Wound J. 2009;6(3):196–208.
64. Zelen CM, Serena TE, Gould L, Le L, Carter MJ, Keller J, et al. Treatment of chronic diabetic lower extremity ulcers with advanced therapies: a prospective, randomised, controlled, multicentre comparative study examining clinical efficacy and cost. Int Wound J. 2016;13(2):272–82.
65. Kirsner RS, Sabolinski ML, Parsons NB, Skornicki M, Marston WA. Comparative effectiveness of a bioengineered living cellular construct vs. a dehydrated human amniotic membrane allograft for the treatment of diabetic foot ulcers in a real world setting. Wound Repair and Regen. 2015;23(5):737–44.
66. Didomenico L, Landsman AR, Emch KJ, Landsman A. A prospective comparison of diabetic foot ulcers treated with either a cryopreserved skin allograft or a bioengineered skin substitute. Wounds. 2011;23(7):184.

67. Niezgoda JA, Van Gils CC, Frykberg RG, Hodde JP. Randomized clinical trial comparing OASIS wound matrix to Regranex Gel for diabetic ulcers. (Original investigation) (Author abstract). Adv Skin Wound Care. 2005;18(5):258.
68. Sanders L, Landsman AS, Landsman A, Keller N, Cook J, Cook E, et al. A prospective, multicenter, randomized, controlled clinical trial comparing a bioengineered skin substitute to a human skin allograft. Ostomy Wound Manage. 2014;60(9):26.
69. Landsman A, Roukis TS, Defronzo DJ, Agnew P, Petranto RD, Surprenant M. Living cells or collagen matrix: which is more beneficial in the treatment of diabetic foot ulcers? Wounds. 2008;20(5):111.
70. Gould LJ, Dosi G, Couch K, Gibbons GW, Howell RS, Brem H, et al. Modalities to treat venous ulcers: compression, surgery, and bioengineered tissue. Plast Reconstr Surg. 2016;138(Suppl 3):199s–208s.
71. Kirsner R, Falanga V, Eaglstein W. The biology of skin-grafts – skin-grafts as pharmacological agents. Arch Dermatol. 1993;129(4):481.
72. Serena TE, Carter MJ, Le LT, Sabo MJ, DiMarco DT. A multicenter, randomized, controlled clinical trial evaluating the use of dehydrated human amnion/chorion membrane allografts and multilayer compression therapy vs. multilayer compression therapy alone in the treatment of venous leg ulcers. Wound Repair Regen. 2014;22(6):688–93.
73. Kelechi TJ, Mueller M, Hankin CS, Bronstone A, Samies J, Bonham PA. A randomized, investigator-blinded, controlled pilot study to evaluate the safety and efficacy of a poly-N-acetyl glucosamine-derived membrane material in patients with venous leg ulcers. J Am Acad Dermatol. 2012;66(6):e209–15.
74. Climov M, Bayer LR, Moscoso AV, Matsumine H, Orgill DP. The role of dermal matrices in treating inflammatory and diabetic wounds. Plast Reconstr Surg. 2016;138(Suppl 3):148s–57s.
75. Gilmour A, Shah A, Telfer JR. Use of Integra ® dermal regeneration template in excision and reconstruction of pre-tibial necrobiosis lipoidica: a case report. Br J Diabetes Vasc Dis. 2012;12(5):261.
76. Steinberg J, Beusterien K, Plante K, Nordin J, Chaikoff E, Arcona S, et al. A cost analysis of a living skin equivalent in the treatment of diabetic foot ulcers. Wounds. 2002;14(4):142.
77. Redekop WK, McDonnell J, Verboom P, Lovas K, Kalo Z. The cost effectiveness of Apligraf treatment of diabetic foot ulcers. PharmacoEconomics. 2003;21(16):1171–83.
78. Sibbald RG, Torrance GW, Walker V, Attard C, MacNeil P. Cost-effectiveness of Apligraf in the treatment of venous leg ulcers. Ostomy Wound Manage. 2001;47(8):36–46.
79. Langer A, Rogowski W. Systematic review of economic evaluations of human cell-derived wound care products for the treatment of venous leg and diabetic foot ulcers. BMC Health Serv Res. 2009;9:115.
80. Webber MJ, Tongers J, Newcomb CJ, Marquardt KT, Bauersachs J, Losordo DW, et al. Supramolecular nanostructures that mimic VEGF as a strategy for ischemic tissue repair. Proc Natl Acad Sci U S A. 2011;108(33):13438–43.
81. Lee W, Debasitis JC, Lee VK, Lee JH, Fischer K, Edminster K, et al. Multi-layered culture of human skin fibroblasts and keratinocytes through three-dimensional freeform fabrication. Biomaterials. 2009;30(8):1587–95.
82. Murphy SV, Atala A. 3D bioprinting of tissues and organs. Nat Biotechnol. 2014;32(8):773–85.
83. Valerio IL, Hammer DA, Rendon JL, Latham KP, Fleming ME. A case report of the first nonburn-related military trauma victim treated with spray skin regenerative therapy in combination with a dermal regenerate template. Plast Reconstr Surg Glob Open. 2016;4(12):e1174.

Part II
Interventional Techniques

Chapter 14
Arterial Diagnostics

Kaspar Trocha and Samir K. Shah

Peripheral Arterial Disease

Peripheral arterial disease, interchangeably referred to as peripheral vascular disease, is the pathologic spectrum of chronic and progressive diseases involving stenotic or occluded non-cardiac, extracranial arteries resulting in compromised perfusion. Hemodynamically it is defined as a resting ABI of <0.90, reflecting significant arterial disease, and can be subclassified based on anatomy into proximal aortoiliac disease or more distal, infra-inguinal disease. It is estimated that PAD globally affects 200 million people, with 8.5 million in the United States alone. Moreover its prevalence is rapidly increasing with an increase of 23.5% from 2001 to 2010 [1]. Progressive atherosclerotic disease is the principal culprit of PAD, accounting for 90% of the disease. For this reason the clinician must also be aware that PAD is a comorbidity associated with systemic atherosclerosis and is a predictor of coronary artery disease and cerebrovascular disease [2–6].

Uncommon in those younger than 50 years of age (<3%), PAD increases to a prevalence of 14.5% in patients over the age of 70 [7]. The strongest modifiable risk factors ranked in order for both low-income and high-income countries for the development of PAD are cigarette smoking, diabetes mellitus, hypertension, and hypercholesterolemia [8]. Patients who smoke cigarettes are often diagnosed earlier than non-smokers and have more severe consequences of the disease [7]. It is therefore vital to educate the patient that smoking is the most important modifiable risk factor. Diabetics are also another high-risk group with a fourfold increased

---

Electronic Supplementary Material: The online version of this chapter (https://doi.org/10.1007/978-3-319-66990-8_14) contains supplementary material, which is available to authorized users.

K. Trocha, MD • S.K. Shah, MD (✉)
Division of Vascular and Endovascular Surgery, Brigham and Women's Hospital, 75 Francis Street, Boston, MA, USA, 02115
e-mail: ktrocha@partners.org; skshah@bwh.harvard.edu

D.P. Orgill (ed.), *Interventional Treatment of Wounds*,
https://doi.org/10.1007/978-3-319-66990-8_14

likelihood of progression to critical limb ischemia (CLI) [7]. Other important risk factors include black race, elevated levels of C-reactive protein, and hyperhomocysteinemia [7].

Critical limb ischemia is the most severe form of PAD, represented by a state of chronic inadequate perfusion and is defined clinically by the presence of rest pain or tissue loss (ischemic ulcer or gangrene). Disease can be further suggested in patients with tissue loss together with an ankle pressure of <70 mmHg; however, there continues to be a discussion regarding the hemodynamic parameters required for a diagnosis of CLI. The natural history of CLI is dismal: at 1 year there is a 25% mortality rate with only 45% being alive with both limbs at 1 year [7]. As such, if technically possible and medically appropriate, patients with CLI should be offered revascularization to prevent limb loss and improve quality of life [9].

Clinical Evaluation

Intermittent claudication (IC) is the most common complaint of the vasculopathic patient. It is characterized by reproducible pain, discomfort, or fatigue in muscles of the lower extremity following exertion that is relieved by short rest. However, it is estimated that the prevalence of asymptomatic patients exceeds symptomatic patients with PAD [10]; thus relying on symptomatology will underdiagnose the disease. The presence or absence of peripheral pulses provides subjective information yet cannot confirm or disprove the diagnosis. Clinical suspicion of PAD therefore necessitates further objective evaluation. The indications for screening patients with the use of ABI measurements include all patients over the ages of 70, patients between 50 and 69 with cardiovascular risk factors (especially smokers and diabetics), those with lower extremity claudication, and, finally, any patient with a 10-year 10–20% risk for a cardiovascular event [7]. It is important to note, however, that according to the current US Preventive Services Task Force guidelines, there is insufficient data to support PAD screening using ABI measurements [11].

A physical exam of the circulatory system should focus on the palpation of peripheral pulses and observe for signs of ischemia. Palpation of upper and lower extremity pulses should be included as well as the evaluation of exaggerated pulses or bruits. Specific attention should be paid to the femoral, popliteal, dorsalis pedis, and posterior tibial pulses. The absence of palpable distal pulses can be quickly confirmed at bedside with a handheld audible Doppler, and noting the phasicity or absence of signals can help assess the severity of disease. The skin and its integrity may often be compromised resulting in changes such as dry, smooth, or shinny skin; ulcerations; and hair loss. Other changes may include cool extremities, color changes, hypertrophied skin, or slow-growing nails.

Ankle Brachial Index

The ankle-brachial systolic pressure index or ABI is recommended as the first-line noninvasive study to establish a diagnosis of PAD in individuals with signs or symptoms suggestive of disease [7](Fig. 14.1). Recent pooled data from a Cochrane meta-analysis reported a 95% sensitivity and 89% specificity using oscillometric ABI [12]. Despite its accuracy in the diagnosis of PAD, some dispute that its prognostic value in predicting wound healing is significantly lower compared to other modalities [13]. Nevertheless the ABI continues to serve as an invaluable diagnostic assessment. It is performed by obtaining brachial pressures and ankle pressures at the dorsalis pedis and posterior tibial arteries using a Doppler ultrasound probe, cuff, and sphygmomanometer. The highest ankle pressure is then divided by the highest brachial pressure for each limb.

A resting ABI of ≤0.90 has been shown to have a higher sensitivity than invasive angiography [7] in the diagnosis of PAD and is a strong correlate for future cardiovascular events [14]. An ABI from 1.00 to 1.30 is considered normal, mild to moderate diminished values are from 0.41 to 0.90, and severely diminished values are equal to or less than 0.40 [15]. However, a subset of patients will present with exertional leg symptoms and a normal or borderline ABI. To distinguish vasculogenic symptoms from neurogenic and other causes, an exercise ABI is recommended. Using a treadmill protocol, symptoms of claudication are reproduced, and the ABI is collected immediately following the exercise. A drop in baseline ABI by 20% or a 30 mm Hg decrement in ankle pressures is generally considered diagnostic.

While this diagnostic modality has a high sensitivity and specificity, it is limited in the presence of non-compliant, stiff, and calcified vessels frequently seen in diabetics, the elderly, and patients with end-stage renal disease. These patients can have falsely elevated ABI values >1.30. In these patients toe brachial index (TBI) pressures are indicated. TBIs can be reliable even in the face of more proximal arterial calcification, and values less than 0.70 are suggestive of PAD, and a toe systolic pressure less than 30 mmHg may represent CLI. Finally, it is important to recognize that the ABI serves not only as a diagnostic test but also correlates with mortality, with low and high values associated with increased cardiovascular mortality [16–18].

Plethysmography: PVR and Segmental Pressure

Plethysmography in the vascular context refers to measurements of arterial inflow volumes during the cardiac cycle. Indirect arterial pressure measurements are recorded using an air plethysmograph to provide data using pressure variances as a

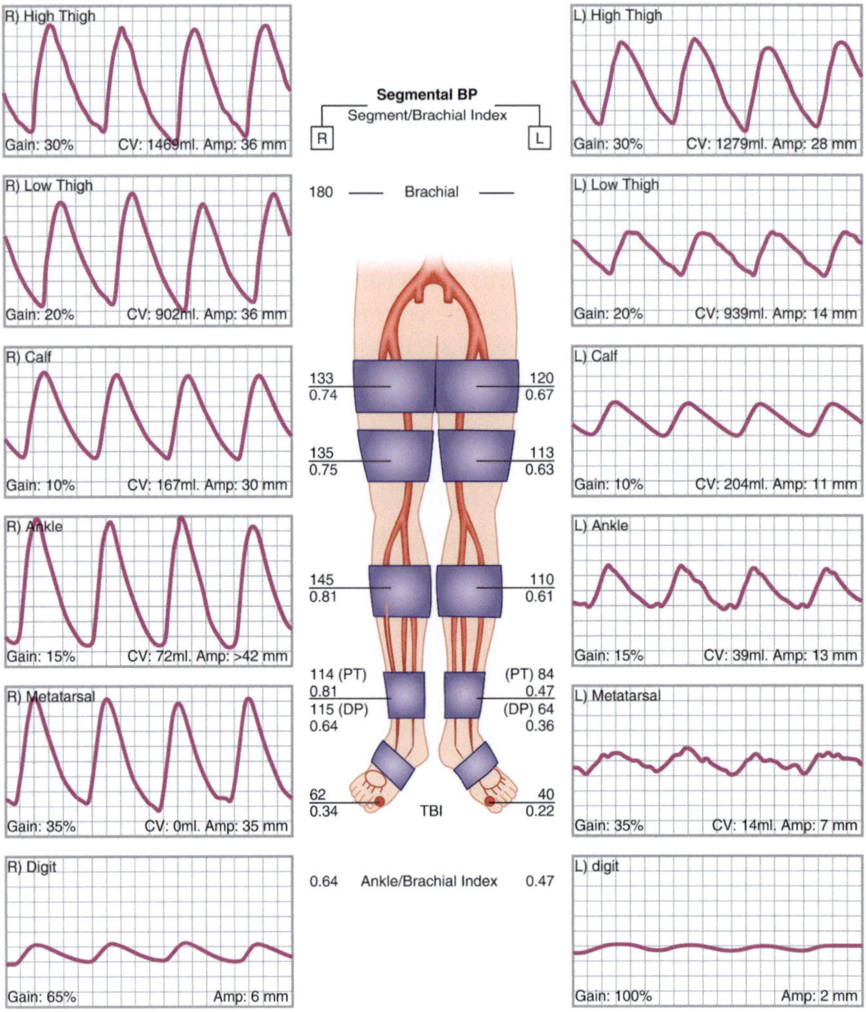

Fig. 14.1 ABI with segmental limb pressures and pulse volume recordings. This patient had bilateral multilevel disease that is worse on the *left*. This is confirmed by lower segmental pressures, diminished amplitudes of the pulse volume recording, and lower ABI and toe brachial index on the *left*

correlate of flow. PVR is a technique that employs multiple pneumatic cuffs and pressure sensors at different levels on each leg. Waveforms are then analyzed for amplitude and contour. The normal arterial waveform will include a rapid upstroke followed by a sharp peak, a dicrotic notch, and a downslope bowed toward the baseline. Abnormal waveform patterns such as slow upstroke or flattened waveforms can indicate disease. Especially in the diabetic population and other groups affected by medial calcification where segmental pressures and ABIs may be nondiagnostic, PVRs, which are unaffected by noncompressibility artifact, are helpful in diagnosing and localizing disease [19]. Limitations include patients with cardiac valvular disease, hypotension, or tachycardia. Moreover, a lack of standardized, reproducible quantification methods has limited the use of PVRs in many centers.

Another use of plethysmography is segmental limb pressures, which are obtained by using a cuff to measure pressures at different levels of the lower extremity. A decrease in the systolic arterial pressure of 20 mm Hg or more at any one level in relation to the proximal segment may represent significant disease. Location of disease can then be comparatively assessed between different levels of the limb. Considerable diagnostic information can be obtained from this modality; however, this is not recommended as a stand-alone diagnostic test and should be coupled with DUS or with ABI, which increases sensitivity and specificity [20]. Incompressible vessels, multilevel disease, and isolated iliac lesions are limitations of its accuracy [7].

Transcutaneous Oxygen Pressures ($TcPO_2$)

Recently $TcPO_2$ has been described as a more reliable predictor of wound healing in diabetic foot ulcers when compared to ABI in a systematic review comparing ABI, TBI, $TcPO_2$, and toe systolic blood pressure (TBP) [13]. $TcPO_2$ is a reflection of the metabolic function of tissue obtained by measuring oxygen (pO_2) and carbon dioxide (pCO_2) tension on the surface of the skin. Normal values are approximately >60 mm Hg, and critical values less than 30 mm Hg are suggestive of inadequate perfusion [7]. However, this method is highly variable and influenced by various factors such as limb temperature, edema, age, obesity, thickness of the skin, and cellulitis. Therefore, caution should be taken when obtaining and interpreting $TcPO_2$ values.

Imaging

Duplex Ultrasound

Arterial duplex ultrasound (DUS) is the most versatile modality in the vascular lab, and once severity of disease is characterized by ABI, TBI, or treadmill testing, the next step is to determine the disease location, often with DUS. DUS is an inexpensive, noninvasive method that uses real-time 2D B-mode gray scale

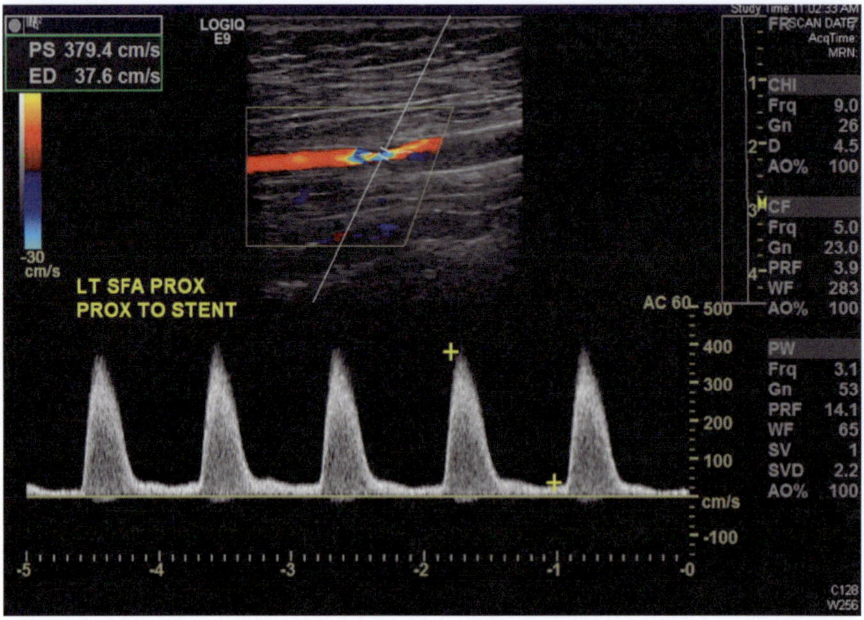

Fig. 14.2 Ultrasound demonstrating narrowing of a segment of the superficial femoral artery. Note the elevated peak systolic velocity on the spectral Doppler with turbulent flow also noted on the color Doppler picture above

images and color Doppler. This is commonly combined with spectral Doppler to provide anatomic and hemodynamic assessments of arterial flow (Fig. 14.2). Evaluation of PAD using DUS is highly operator dependent and should be ideally performed by an accredited vascular lab. In trained hands arterial DUS has proven to be an accurate diagnostic modality comparable to CTA, MRA, and DSA [21, 22]. At reliable centers, it may also be used as a sole imaging modality to plan revascularization [23–25], but this is uncommon due to lack of clinician confidence in DUS alone [26].

Grading stenoses using duplex entails measuring peak systolic velocities (PSV), end diastolic velocities (EDV) and velocity ratios (V_r) of adjacent segments of vessels. For example, a lesion with a PSV > 300 cm/s, EDV < 90 cm/s, and a Vr > 4.0 generally correlates with a > 75% stenosis. When an occlusion is present, no color flow will be visualized, distal waveforms will be significantly dampened, and collateralization may be present. Limitations of DUS arise with the visualization of iliac vessel presence of multi-segmental disease [27] and lower extremity wounds that could hinder the ability to perform a detailed exam. As technology continues to evolve and the need for noninvasive testing increases, DUS will continue to serve as a fundamental tool for diagnosing, localizing, and monitoring disease.

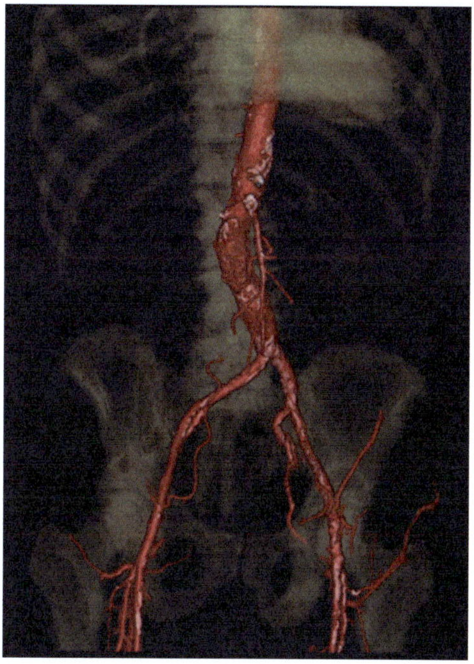

Fig. 14.3 3D CTA reconstruction demonstrating diffuse calcific disease of the aorta and iliac arteries

Computed Tomography Angiography and Magnetic Resonance Angiography

Digital subtraction angiography has long been considered the gold standard diagnostic modality for the evaluation of location and extent of luminal stenosis in patients with vascular disease [28]. However, its sole use for diagnostic purposes is decreasing. This is in part due to improving technology and accuracy of CTA and MRA [29–33].

Despite requiring both iodinated contrast and ionizing, CTA is emerging as a more convenient modality for diagnosis of PAD compared to MRA (Fig. 14.3). Generally, the choice of imaging modality will depend on availability, cost, and experience. The advantages of CTA compared to MRA include but not limited to quicker scan times and the ability to image patients with pacemakers, defibrillators, and other metal implants. Technological improvements in spatial resolution, slice thickness, and the ability to scan the entire vascular tree with decreased radiation dose using multi-detector CT will continue to improve.

The use of CTA is not without limitations, however. Two of these – ionizing radiation and contrast – have been mentioned; however, the average dose of 7.47 mSv [34] may have limited impact on an older patient with extensive comorbid conditions, while effects of radiation on a younger patient should be considered. Contrast-induced nephropathy continues to be a potential side effect of contrast agents associated with high morbidity and mortality. It is worth noting that this association is currently being questioned, with a recent meta-analysis from the Mayo Clinic showing no independent correlation between contrast administration and acute kidney injury, death, or dialysis [35].

MRA is an imaging technique that does not use ionizing radiation (Fig. 14.4). The most common methods are time-of-flight (TOF) non-contrast modalities and gadolinium-based angiography. TOF relies on flow-related enhancement in which circulating blood results in a high signal compared to adjacent tissues but may take up to 90 minutes. Three-dimensional contrast-enhanced MRA is generally considered to have superior diagnostic performance when compared to 2D TOF-MRA [36]. MRA has several disadvantages. First, gadolinium-based MRA is associated with nephrogenic systemic fibrosis in patients with pre-existing renal dysfunction (glomerular filtration rate [GFR], less than 30 mL/min/1.73 m^2) or acute kidney injury [37] with an approximate incidence of 2–5% in patients with severe renal insufficiency [38]. Conversely, a recent prospective cohort study revealed no cases of nephrogenic systemic fibrosis in patients at an increased risk of its development over a 2-year time period [39]. Nevertheless, nephrogenic systemic fibrosis is an incurable chronic condition carrying significant morbidity marked by skin thickening, hyperpigmentation, flexion contractures of joints, and extracutaneous fibrosis. However, patients with a GFR of 30–59 mL/min together with a dose of 0.2 mL/kg or less of gadolinium-based agents are considered at low or no risk for the development of NSF [38]. Also, MRA may be contraindicated or limited by the presence of metal stents and devices, such as pacemakers. Last, vascular calcification, which may be critical to surgical planning, is underappreciated by MR.

In any event, both CTA and MRA have accuracies comparable to that of conventional angiography [32, 33]. CTA is a modality with fast acquisition times that is widely available and highly reliable with the ability to obtain 3D images (Video 14.1). MRA on the other hand obviates the need for ionizing radiation and has established itself as a highly accurate diagnostic modality [40] with newer MR machines utilizing less contrast, requiring shorter scan times, and less susceptibility to arterial calcifications that can obscure the accurate interpretation of a stenosis. Finally, despite powerful imaging techniques, physiologic testing should precede anatomic evaluations, followed by carefully selected imaging studies to more precisely identify sites of disease and plan for revascularization.

Angiography

Digital subtraction angiography (DSA) (Video 14.2) has been considered the gold standard for diagnosis of PAD; however, it is now being challenged by evolving noninvasive approaches (Figure 14.5a, b). The use of DSA as a first-line imaging modality for patients with PAD is no longer typical [41]. Its principal advantage lies in the ability to view flow in real time and ability to intervene via catheter-based techniques. Major risks, classified as requiring hospitalization, having permanent adverse sequelae or death following catheter angiography are low: 0.7% [7].

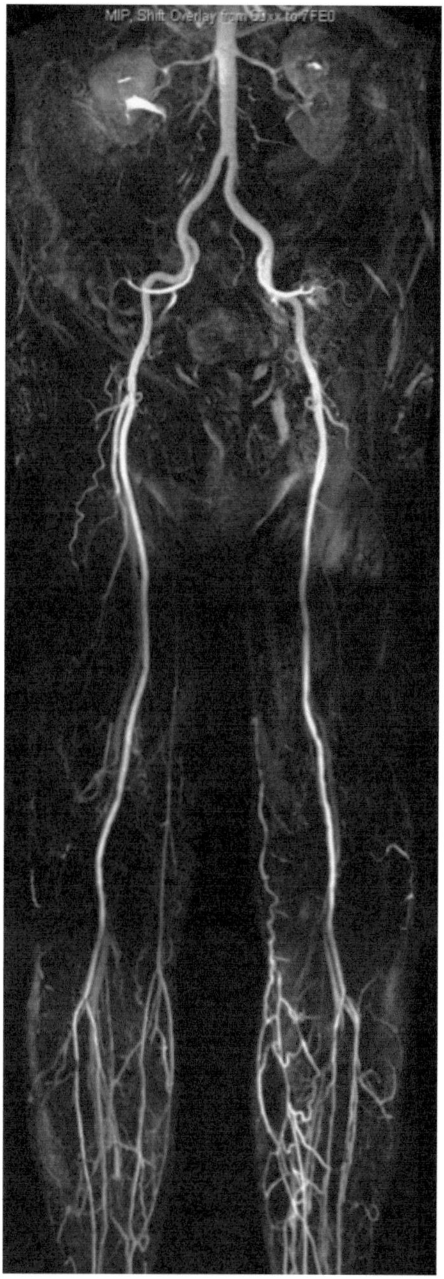

Fig. 14.4 Three-dimensional reconstruction of a gadolinium-based MRA demonstrating the arterial vasculature from the abdominal aorta to the ankles. Note the bilateral tibial arterial disease

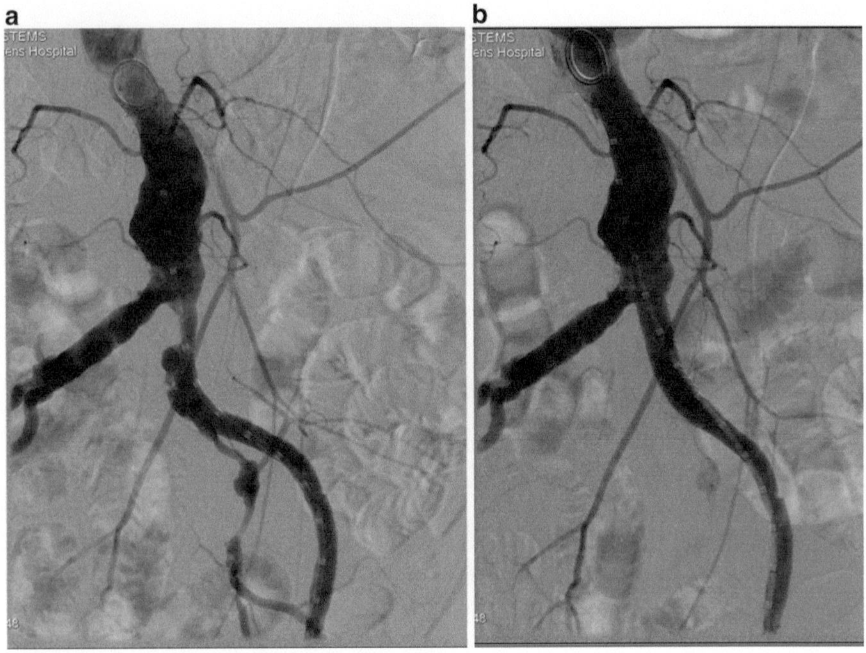

Fig. 14.5 (**a**) Angiography demonstrating a proximal *left* common iliac artery stenosis prior to intervention. (**b**) Angiography demonstrating resolution of a proximal *left* common iliac artery stenosis after stent placement and balloon angioplasty

Catheter-related complications such as hematoma are reported to be as high as 10% [42]. Contrast agents have the potential to produce nephropathy, cardiac toxicity, and allergic reactions secondary to histamine release such as bronchospasm or laryngeal edema. Limitations are its underestimation of stenosis [43], inability to provide 3D images, and crural vessel visualization. For these reasons, and with the advancement of CTA, MRA, and DUS, the use of catheter angiography is often reserved as a final diagnostic modality or treatment adjunct (Fig. 14.6).

Emerging as an exciting addition to angiography is the use of intravascular ultrasound (IVUS) , which provides real-time 360-degree cross-sectional intra-arterial images with the ability to assess luminal morphology and plaque distribution (Fig. 14.7). IVUS is particularly useful as an adjunct to endovascular interventions, with the ability to provide a more precise location for deployment of stent grafts as well as limiting the use of radiation and contrast agents [44]. Nevertheless, IVUS requires additional resources and skills, but its use as an adjunct to angiography has proven to be instrumental.

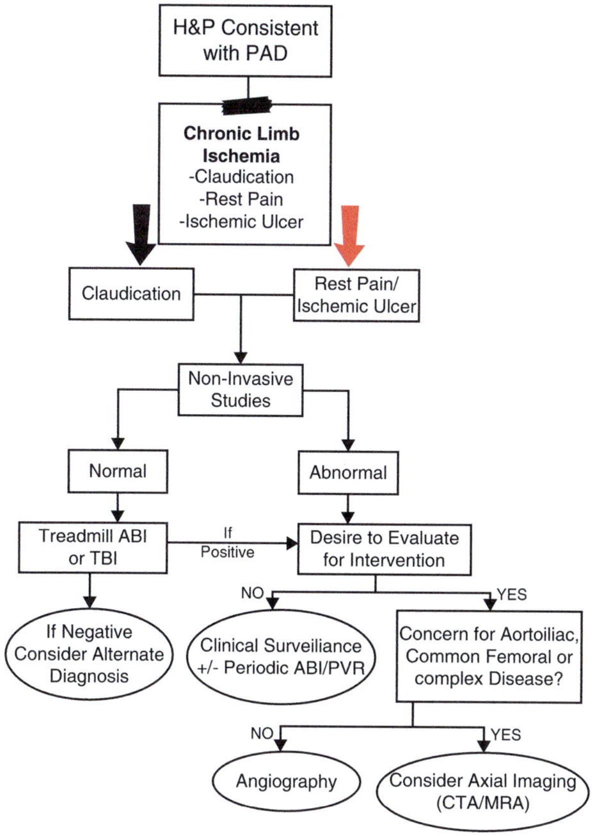

Fig. 14.6 Choice of diagnostic modality flowchart

Wound Healing and Emerging Techniques

Assessment of wound healing potential involves measures directly related to vascular supply such as flow, oxygen saturation, and hemoglobin content. Similar factors have also been described in the angiosome concept, in which the three runoff vessels in the limb supply six areas of the foot. Revascularization is thus targeted to the relevant angiosome to improve limb salvage rate. This concept remains controversial but there is some evidence supporting its use in patients with CLI and below the knee lesions, showing that angiosome-directed endovascular treatment resulted in improvements in amputation free survival and freedom from major amputation [40].

There are a number of instruments to assess morphology of a wound and evaluate tissue perfusion. For the purposes of this chapter, only a few of these technologies will be mentioned. Hyperspectral imaging (HSI) relies on spectroscopy to quantify chromophores of interest such as oxyhemoglobin and deoxyhemoglobin. These values are then reported, with lower mean values predicting poorer wound

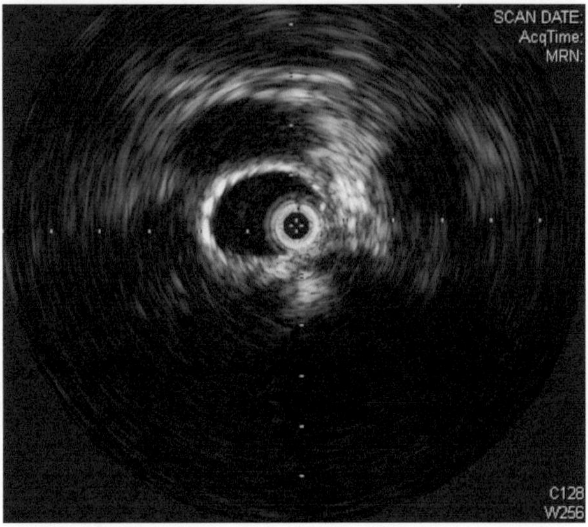

Fig. 14.7 Intravascular ultrasound image of a patent common iliac vein stent. Note the lucency at 12 o'clock consistent with an overlying common iliac artery

healing in a small study of 54 patients comparing healing of diabetic foot ulcers [45]. Other measures of tissue perfusion include microvascular oxygen saturation and skin perfusion pressure, which rely on spectrophotometry and laser Doppler in attempts to predict treatment outcomes on wound healing. However, with limited availability and few studies [46, 47], evaluating the accuracy of these methods as measures and predictors of wound healing requires additional research.

Optical coherence tomography (OCT) can be applied as an intraluminal diagnostic modality similar to IVUS albeit with higher definition to characterize intravascular morphology or to evaluate properties of the surface of wounds. It employs near-infrared light to produce a cross-sectional image in which the reflected near-infrared light measures the thickness of various tissue sections [48]. As an intra-arterial device it has become increasingly promising for the evaluation of vulnerable plaques in carotid and coronary vessels, as well as to monitor the progression of peripheral arterial atherosclerosis with the unique advantage of being able to evaluate the intimal layer of a vessel [49, 50]. Additionally, it can be used to evaluate the structural integrity of the skin such as the epidermal layer of the skin, allowing noninvasive tracking of wound reepithelialization.

Conclusion

PAD is a multifactorial disease that requires deliberate workup and treatment. PAD has many consequences including the disruption of the cellular and molecular mechanisms involved in wound healing. As the US population ages and the prevalence of risk factors such as diabetes increases, accurate and efficient diagnosis of PAD is essential. Noninvasive vascular studies, such as the ABI, and cross-sectional imaging remain crucial tools alongside conventional angiography.

References

1. Fowkes FG, Rudan D, Rudan I, Aboyans V, Denenberg JO, McDermott MM, et al. Comparison of global estimates of prevalence and risk factors for peripheral artery disease in 2000 and 2010: a systematic review and analysis. Lancet. 2013;382(9901):1329–40.
2. Cordero A, Morillas P, Bertomeu-Gonzalez V, Quiles J, Soria F, Guindo J, et al. Pathological ankle-brachial index is equivalent of advanced age in acute coronary syndromes. Eur J Clin Investig. 2011;41(12):1268–74.
3. Zheng ZJ, Sharrett AR, Chambless LE, Rosamond WD, Nieto FJ, Sheps DS, et al. Associations of ankle-brachial index with clinical coronary heart disease, stroke and preclinical carotid and popliteal atherosclerosis: the Atherosclerosis Risk In Communities (ARIC) Study. Atherosclerosis. 1997;131(1):115–25.
4. Diehm C, Allenberg JR, Pittrow D, Mahn M, Tepohl G, Haberl RL, et al. Mortality and vascular morbidity in older adults with asymptomatic versus symptomatic peripheral artery disease. Circulation. 2009;120(21):2053–61.
5. Gronewold J, Hermann DM, Lehmann N, Kroger K, Lauterbach K, Berger K, et al. Ankle-brachial index predicts stroke in the general population in addition to classical risk factors. Atherosclerosis. 2014;233(2):545–50.
6. Hajibandeh S, Hajibandeh S, Shah S, Child E, Antoniou GA, Torella F. Prognostic significance of ankle brachial pressure index: a systematic review and meta-analysis. Vascular. 2016;25(2):208–24.
7. Norgren L, Hiatt WR, Dormandy JA, Nehler MR, Harris KA, Fowkes FG, et al. Inter-society consensus for the management of peripheral arterial disease (TASC II). J Vasc Surg. 2007;33(45 Suppl S):S5–67.
8. Writing Group M, Mozaffarian D, Benjamin EJ, Go AS, Arnett DK, Blaha MJ, et al. Heart disease and stroke statistics-2016 update: a report from the American Heart Association. Circulation. 2016;133(4):e38–360.
9. Shahab H, Shahin H, Sohan S, Emma C, George AA, Francesco T, et al. Prognostic significance of ankle brachial pressure index: A systematic review and meta-analysis. Vascular. 2016; 25(2):208–24
10. Society for Vascular Surgery Lower Extremity Guidelines, Writing G, Conte MS, Pomposelli FB, Clair DG, Geraghty PJ, JF MK, et al. Society for vascular surgery practice guidelines for atherosclerotic occlusive disease of the lower extremities: management of asymptomatic disease and claudication. J Vasc Surg. 2015;61(3 Suppl):2S–41S.
11. Moyer VA. Force USPST. Screening for peripheral artery disease and cardiovascular disease risk assessment with the ankle-brachial index in adults: U.S. Preventive Services Task Force recommendation statement. Ann Intern Med. 2013;159(5):342–8.
12. Crawford F, Welch K, Andras A, Chappell FM. Ankle brachial index for the diagnosis of lower limb peripheral arterial disease. Cochrane Database Syst Rev. 2016;9:CD010680.
13. Wang Z, Hasan R, Firwana B, Elraiyah T, Tsapas A, Prokop L, et al. A systematic review and meta-analysis of tests to predict wound healing in diabetic foot. J Vasc Surg. 2016;63 2 Suppl:29S–36S. e1–2.
14. Aboyans V, Criqui MH, Abraham P, Allison MA, Creager MA, Diehm C, et al. Measurement and interpretation of the ankle-brachial index: a scientific statement from the American Heart Association. Circulation. 2012;126(24):2890–909.

15. Hirsch AT, Haskal ZJ, Hertzer NR, Bakal CW, Creager MA, Halperin JL, et al. ACC/AHA 2005 practice guidelines for the management of patients with peripheral arterial disease (lower extremity, renal, mesenteric, and abdominal aortic): a collaborative report from the American Association for Vascular Surgery/Society for Vascular Surgery, Society for Cardiovascular Angiography and Interventions, Society for Vascular Medicine and Biology, Society of Interventional Radiology, and the ACC/AHA Task Force on Practice Guidelines (Writing Committee to Develop Guidelines for the Management of Patients With Peripheral Arterial Disease): endorsed by the American Association of Cardiovascular and Pulmonary Rehabilitation; National Heart, Lung, and Blood Institute; Society for Vascular Nursing; TransAtlantic Inter-Society Consensus; and Vascular Disease Foundation. Circulation. 2006;113 11:e463–654.
16. Dormandy JA, Murray GD. The fate of the claudicant – a prospective study of 1969 claudicants. Eur J Vasc Surg. 1991;5(2):131–3.
17. Suominen V, Uurto I, Saarinen J, Venermo M, Salenius J. PAD as a risk factor for mortality among patients with elevated ABI – a clinical study. Eur J Vasc Endovasc Surg. 2010;39(3):316–22.
18. Hyun S, Forbang NI, Allison MA, Denenberg JO, Criqui MH, Ix JH. Ankle-brachial index, toe-brachial index, and cardiovascular mortality in persons with and without diabetes mellitus. J Vasc Surg. 2014;60(2):390–5.
19. Carter SA, Tate RB. The value of toe pulse waves in determination of risks for limb amputation and death in patients with peripheral arterial disease and skin ulcers or gangrene. J Vasc Surg. 2001;33(4):708–14.
20. Hashimoto T, Ichihashi S, Iwakoshi S, Kichikawa K. Combination of pulse volume recording (PVR) parameters and ankle-brachial index (ABI) improves diagnostic accuracy for peripheral arterial disease compared with ABI alone. Hypertens Res. 2016;39(6):430–4.
21. Collins R, Burch J, Cranny G, Aguiar-Ibanez R, Craig D, Wright K, et al. Duplex ultrasonography, magnetic resonance angiography, and computed tomography angiography for diagnosis and assessment of symptomatic, lower limb peripheral arterial disease: systematic review. BMJ. 2007;334(7606):1257.
22. Collins R, Cranny G, Burch J, Aguiar-Ibanez R, Craig D, Wright K, et al. A systematic review of duplex ultrasound, magnetic resonance angiography and computed tomography angiography for the diagnosis and assessment of symptomatic, lower limb peripheral arterial disease. Health Technol Assess. 2007;11 20:iii–iv, xi–xiii, 1–184.
23. Mandolfino T, Canciglia A, D'Alfonso M, Carmignani A. Infrainguinal revascularization based on duplex ultrasound arterial mapping. Int Angiol. 2006;25(3):256–60.
24. Canciglia A, Mandolfino T. Infrainguinal endovascular procedures based upon the results of duplex scanning. Int Angiol. 2008;27(4):291–5.
25. Sultan S, Tawfick W, Hynes N. Ten-year technical and clinical outcomes in TransAtlantic inter-society consensus II infrainguinal C/D lesions using duplex ultrasound arterial mapping as the sole imaging modality for critical lower limb ischemia. J Vasc Surg. 2013;57(4):1038–45.
26. de Vos MS, Bol BJ, Gravereaux EC, Hamming JF, Nguyen LL. Treatment planning for peripheral arterial disease based on duplex ultrasonography and computed tomography angiography: consistency, confidence and the value of additional imaging. Surgery. 2014;156(2):492–502.
27. Allard L, Cloutier G, Durand LG, Roederer GO, Langlois YE. Limitations of ultrasonic duplex scanning for diagnosing lower limb arterial stenoses in the presence of adjacent segment disease. J Vasc Surg. 1994;19(4):650–7.
28. Oser RF, Picus D, Hicks ME, Darcy MD, Hovsepian DM. Accuracy of DSA in the evaluation of patency of infrapopliteal vessels. J Vasc Interv Radiol. 1995;6(4):589–94.
29. Jens S, Koelemay MJ, Reekers JA, Bipat S. Diagnostic performance of computed tomography angiography and contrast-enhanced magnetic resonance angiography in patients with critical limb ischaemia and intermittent claudication: systematic review and meta-analysis. Eur Radiol. 2013;23(11):3104–14.

30. Met R, Bipat S, Legemate DA, Reekers JA, Koelemay MJ. Diagnostic performance of computed tomography angiography in peripheral arterial disease: a systematic review and meta-analysis. JAMA. 2009;301(4):415–24.
31. Menke J, Larsen J. Meta-analysis: accuracy of contrast-enhanced magnetic resonance angiography for assessing steno-occlusions in peripheral arterial disease. Ann Intern Med. 2010;153(5):325–34.
32. Kock MC, Adriaensen ME, Pattynama PM, van Sambeek MR, van Urk H, Stijnen T, et al. DSA versus multi-detector row CT angiography in peripheral arterial disease: randomized controlled trial. Radiology. 2005;237(2):727–37.
33. Huegli RW, Aschwanden M, Bongartz G, Jaeger K, Heidecker HG, Thalhammer C, et al. Intraarterial MR angiography and DSA in patients with peripheral arterial occlusive disease: prospective comparison. Radiology. 2006;239(3):901–8.
34. Kock MC, Dijkshoorn ML, Pattynama PM, Myriam Hunink MG. Multi-detector row computed tomography angiography of peripheral arterial disease. Eur Radiol. 2007;17(12):3208–22.
35. McDonald JS, McDonald RJ, Comin J, Williamson EE, Katzberg RW, Murad MH, et al. Frequency of acute kidney injury following intravenous contrast medium administration: a systematic review and meta-analysis. Radiology. 2013;267(1):119–28.
36. Koelemay MJ, Lijmer JG, Stoker J, Legemate DA, Bossuyt PM. Magnetic resonance angiography for the evaluation of lower extremity arterial disease: a meta-analysis. JAMA. 2001;285(10):1338–45.
37. Kitajima K, Maeda T, Watanabe S, Ueno Y, Sugimura K. Recent topics related to nephrogenic systemic fibrosis associated with gadolinium-based contrast agents. Int J Urol. 2012;19(9):806–11.
38. Sadowski EA, Bennett LK, Chan MR, Wentland AL, Garrett AL, Garrett RW, et al. Nephrogenic systemic fibrosis: risk factors and incidence estimation. Radiology. 2007;243(1):148–57.
39. Soulez G, Bloomgarden DC, Rofsky NM, Smith MP, Abujudeh HH, Morgan DE, et al. Prospective cohort study of nephrogenic systemic fibrosis in patients with stage 3-5 chronic kidney disease undergoing MRI with injected Gadobenate Dimeglumine or Gadoteridol. AJR Am J Roentgenol. 2015;205(3):469–78.
40. Iida O, Soga Y, Hirano K, Kawasaki D, Suzuki K, Miyashita Y, et al. Long-term results of direct and indirect endovascular revascularization based on the angiosome concept in patients with critical limb ischemia presenting with isolated below-the-knee lesions. J Vasc Surg. 2012;55(2):363–70. e5
41. Hessel SJ, Adams DF, Abrams HL. Complications of angiography. Radiology. 1981;138(2):273–81.
42. Dariushnia SR, Gill AE, Martin LG, Saad WE, Baskin KM, Caplin DM, et al. Quality improvement guidelines for diagnostic arteriography. J Vasc Interv Radiol. 2014;25(12):1873–81.
43. Kashyap VS, Pavkov ML, Bishop PD, Nassoiy SP, Eagleton MJ, Clair DG, et al. Angiography underestimates peripheral atherosclerosis: lumenography revisited. J Endovasc Ther. 2008;15(1):117–25.
44. Nishanian G, Kopchok GE, Donayre CE, White RA. The impact of intravascular ultrasound (IVUS) on endovascular interventions. Semin Vasc Surg. 1999;12(4):285–99.
45. Nouvong A, Hoogwerf B, Mohler E, Davis B, Tajaddini A, Medenilla E. Evaluation of diabetic foot ulcer healing with hyperspectral imaging of oxyhemoglobin and deoxyhemoglobin. Diabetes Care. 2009;32(11):2056–61.
46. Rajbhandari SM, Harris ND, Tesfaye S, Ward JD. Early identification of diabetic foot ulcers that may require intervention using the micro lightguide spectrophotometer. Diabetes Care. 1999;22(8):1292–5.
47. Castronuovo JJ Jr, Adera HM, Smiell JM, Price RM. Skin perfusion pressure measurement is valuable in the diagnosis of critical limb ischemia. J Vasc Surg. 1997;26(4):629–37.

48. Rieber J, Meissner O, Babaryka G, Reim S, Oswald M, Koenig A, et al. Diagnostic accuracy of optical coherence tomography and intravascular ultrasound for the detection and characterization of atherosclerotic plaque composition in ex-vivo coronary specimens: a comparison with histology. Coron Artery Dis. 2006;17(5):425–30.
49. Meissner OA, Rieber J, Babaryka G, Oswald M, Reim S, Siebert U, et al. Intravascular optical coherence tomography: comparison with histopathology in atherosclerotic peripheral artery specimens. J Vasc Interv Radiol. 2006;17(2 Pt 1):343–9.
50. Jang IK, Bouma BE, Kang DH, Park SJ, Park SW, Seung KB, et al. Visualization of coronary atherosclerotic plaques in patients using optical coherence tomography: comparison with intravascular ultrasound. J Am Coll Cardiol. 2002;39(4):604–9.

Chapter 15
Minimally Invasive Arterial Interventions for Wounds

Dean J. Arnaoutakis and Edwin C. Gravereaux

Introduction

Atherosclerosis of the lower extremities can affect multiple segments of the arterial tree resulting in symptoms ranging from mild claudication to limb-threatening tissue loss. Critical limb ischemia (CLI) encompasses rest pain and ischemic ulceration or gangrene of the forefoot and/or toes (Table 15.1). Fortunately, CLI represents a minority of patients with peripheral arterial disease; however, its incidence is seven times higher in diabetics, and it carries a very poor prognosis reflected by nearly 60% mortality rate at 5 years [1]. Ischemic ulceration develops after repetitive soft tissue trauma resulting in skin erosion, wound formation, and moderate to severe pain (Fig. 15.1). Wound healing usually does not occur because resting limb blood flow is inadequate to meet metabolic demands. Without intervention, further tissue death ensues which can ultimately lead to limb loss.

Endovascular interventions of the lower extremity are distinctly different than traditional open bypass surgery in that the native, diseased vessel is relied upon to provide adequate blood flow distally. As such, minimally invasive treatments must sufficiently improve the culprit arterial stenosis or occlusion in order to restore distal perfusion thereby resolving claudication or tissue loss. Naturally, endovascular therapies have advantages and disadvantages that must be balanced when selecting the best treatment option for each patient.

D.J. Arnaoutakis, MD, MBA (✉) • E.C. Gravereaux, MD
Division of Vascular and Endovascular Surgery, Brigham and Women's Hospital, Boston, MA, USA
e-mail: dean.arnaoutakis@surgery.ufl.edu

D.P. Orgill (ed.), *Interventional Treatment of Wounds*,
https://doi.org/10.1007/978-3-319-66990-8_15

Table 15.1 Rutherford classification system of chronic peripheral arterial disease

Rutherford classification		
Grade	Category	Clinical description
0	0	Asymptomatic
I	1	Mild claudication
I	2	Moderate claudication
I	3	Severe claudication
II	4	Ischemic rest pain
III	5	Minor tissue loss
III	6	Major tissue loss

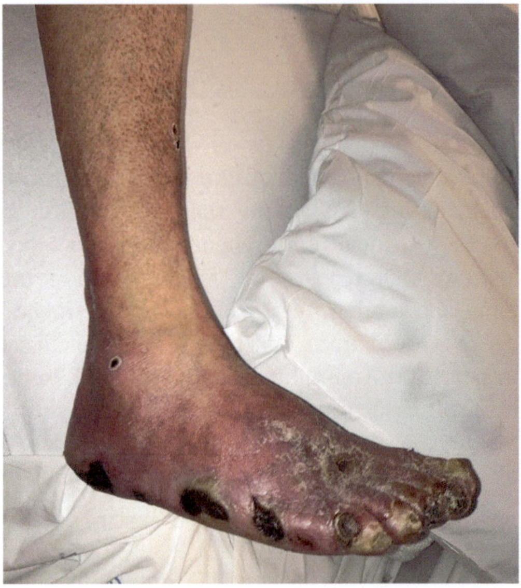

Fig. 15.1 Critical limb ischemia of right lower extremity. Chronic ischemic ulceration of the toes, forefoot, and heel in a patient with severe, multilevel peripheral arterial disease

Historical Background

Infrainguinal bypass surgery was the gold standard treatment for revascularization of lower extremity arterial disease for decades due to its durable and reproducible results [2]. However, this procedure can be morbid, especially in the cardiovascular patient population, one that is full of frail, elderly patients who suffer from multiple comorbid conditions. For example, wound complications have been reported in up to 40% of patients postoperatively after infrainguinal bypass [3]. Many have underlying coronary artery disease, and thus the 5% incidence of postoperative myocardial infarction is not trivial [4]. As such, a need arose to provide arterial treatment in a minimally invasive manner – the endovascular revolution was born.

The first intravascular intervention can be traced back to 1964 when Charles Dotter, an interventional radiologist in Oregon, dilated an iliac artery by serial insertion of coaxial catheters of increasing diameter [5]. Ten years later, Grüntzig performed the first balloon angioplasty using a "distensible" catheter [6]. However, elastic recoil following balloon angioplasty of atherosclerotic plaques was quickly identified as a limitation to these procedures. Metal stents were consequently developed to address elastic recoil, first with balloon expandable devices as described by Palmaz, and subsequently self-expanding technologies gave rise [7]. Since these initial techniques and devices, endovascular therapies have evolved tremendously over the past 20 years to include thrombolytic catheters, drug-eluting balloons and stents, and atherectomy devices. The current day armamentarium is endless thereby providing the interventionalist with multiple treatment options; however, the surplus of devices makes it incredibly difficult to discern which intervention is the most clinically and economically effective.

Role of Endovascular Surgery

Given some of the aforementioned disadvantages of open surgical bypass, endovascular treatment options have flourished over the past 20 years. In fact, the number of peripheral interventions has more than tripled during that period of time [8]. Percutaneous lower extremity interventions are typically performed using conscious sedation in an outpatient interventional suite. The avoidance of general anesthesia along with the lack of a surgical incision is a major benefit that reduces overall complications and enables patients a quick recovery. Complications from percutaneous arterial access do occur (hematoma, pseudoaneurysm, bleeding, thrombosis, and infection) in up to 8% of cases, but their incidence is much less compared to the complications after surgical bypass procedures [9]. Finally, conduit type and quality is irrelevant with endovascular surgery, which can be of critical importance in select patients.

Limitations to endovascular treatment involve attempts at intervention in heavily calcified vessels. In these situations, crossing the culprit lesion with a wire and catheter may not be feasible. Even if the lesion can be crossed, the durability of interventions in these scenarios is questionable. Additionally, many of these patients have had prior arterial interventions (i.e., aortic endograft) which can alter the anatomy of the aortic bifurcation thereby limiting arterial access for the procedure.

Patients with CLI (Rutherford categories 4–6) typically have multilevel arterial disease that can make percutaneous intervention more complicated and less durable. The goal should be to restore in-line blood flow to the foot in an expeditious manner. Ulceration and gangrene should be evaluated using the WIfI classification system as it has been shown to reliably predict amputation, reintervention, and wound healing [10, 11]. Oftentimes, pre-procedure imaging with a computed tomography or magnetic resonance angiography scan can help plan the procedure most effectively. Standard noninvasive studies, such as pressure volume recordings and ankle-brachial indexes, should be obtained as they can aid in localizing disease and provide a quantitative measure of flow.

Technique

Access

All interventions require intra-arterial access. Fluoroscopy and ultrasound can be very useful to safely achieve this goal. The most common manner to achieve this is via the contralateral common femoral artery (CFA). A 4F micropuncture kit or an 18-gauge needle is passed into the CFA, and then using Seldinger technique an access sheath is inserted over a guide wire. The target lesion can then be addressed in a retrograde fashion. An alternative point of entry is the ipsilateral CFA, which can be useful in those patients who have had prior aortic reconstruction as there is no need to navigate the aortic bifurcation. Gaining this access can be difficult, especially in obese patients as the abdominal wall pannus can limit the amount of working length proximal to the profunda femoris artery. Additional access points include the brachial artery as well as the ipsilateral tibial vessels. Limitation to using the brachial artery, besides its relatively small size, is its distance to the target lesion(s) as the working lengths of necessary devices may not reach.

Diagnostic Imaging

Typically, after inserting a 5F sheath in the contralateral CFA, a flush catheter is advanced in a retrograde fashion to the abdominal aorta to obtain angiographic images of the aortoiliac segment. Doing so not only provides information regarding the need for intervention in the inflow vessels but also provides a roadmap for sending a wire and catheter over the bifurcation toward the iliac artery of the affected leg. Once the catheter is positioned at the inguinal ligament, images are obtained of the CFA, superficial femoral artery (SFA), and profunda femoris artery using digital subtraction angiography (DSA) (Fig. 15.2a). In order to best visualize the femoral bifurcation, the image intensifier should be rotated 30–45 degrees in the ipsilateral direction. The remainder of the leg (popliteal and tibial segments) can be imaged in stations after adjusting the contrast rate and volume (Fig. 15.2b–d). Next, the images are reviewed to identify the lesion(s) of interest so as to best devise an interventional plan.

Lesion Crossing

Crossing the target lesion with a wire and catheter is required for percutaneous intervention. A plethora of wires, catheters, and devices in different diameters and lengths, which are beyond the scope of this chapter, are available to assist in this regard. In order to maximize the chance of successful lesion crossing and

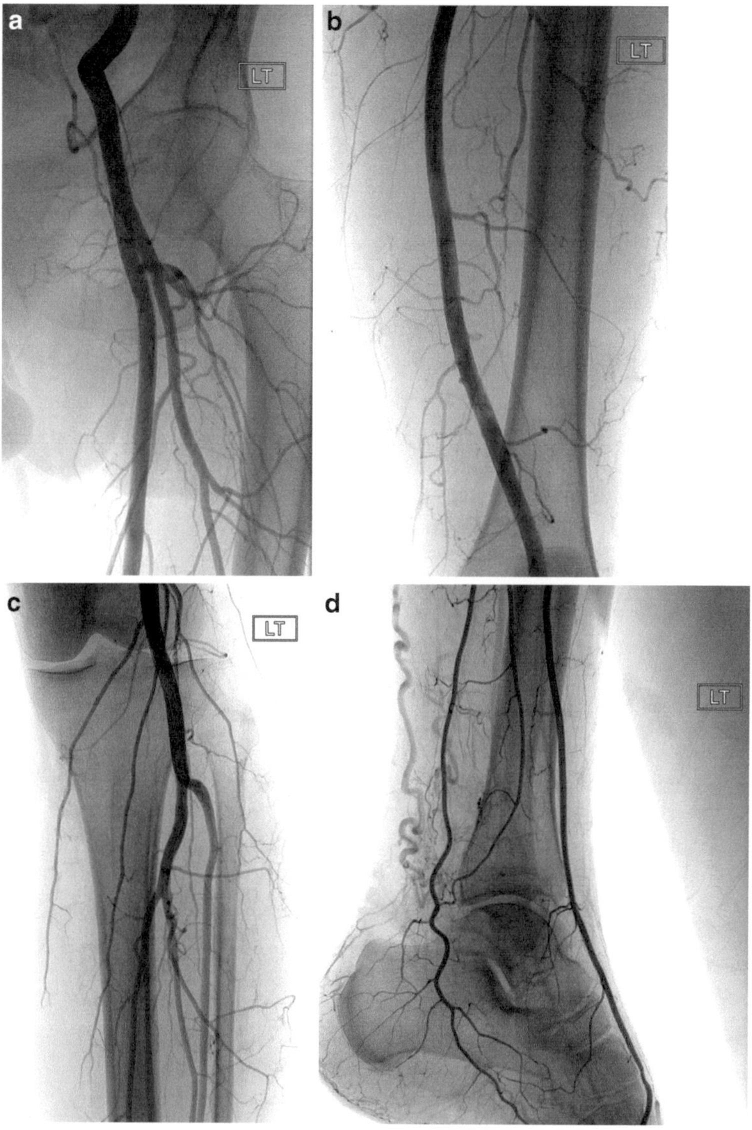

Fig. 15.2 Diagnostic angiogram of the left lower extremity. Series of diagnostic images using digital subtraction imaging of the left lower extremity showing normal anatomy. (**a**) Depicts the common femoral artery and its bifurcation into the superficial femoral and profunda femoris arteries. (**b**) Depicts the superficial femoral artery as it crosses the adductor canal becoming the above-knee popliteal artery. (**c**) Shows the popliteal artery and the three tibial vessels. (**d**) Lateral view of the foot showing the dorsalis pedis and posterior tibial arteries

subsequent intervention, a long, flexible 6F sheath should be inserted to the CFA of the affected leg in order to provide additional support to the coaxial system. Systemic heparin sulfate (100 units/kg) should then be administered.

Staying within the true lumen of the vessel while crossing an area of stenosis is critical so as to not create a dissection plane. A hydrophilic wire with a floppy tip is usually used with the help of a torque device to slowly navigate through the narrow lumen. A support catheter can be employed to provide directionality to the wire tip. Chronic total occlusions can prove more difficult to traverse. In these situations, the wire can create a subintimal plane as it passes the chronic occlusion. Once the wire and catheter are beyond the lesion and positioned in the area of presumed target lesion reconstitution, the wire should be withdrawn to check for back bleeding from the catheter as this suggests successful reentry into the true lumen. Small volume of contrast can also be injected into the catheter under fluoroscopy to confirm that the catheter is within the true lumen. If not, the catheter and wire should be withdrawn back to the area of occlusion; then, subsequent attempts to direct the system across the lesion and naturally into the true lumen should ensue. If this fails despite multiple attempts, a reentry device can be used to facilitate this process; however, these devices are expensive and can be cumbersome to use. These principles are applicable in whether crossing a lesion in the femoral, popliteal, or tibial segment.

Intervention Options

Once the target lesion has been crossed with a wire, multiple different treatment options exist that rely on either lumen distention (angioplasty, stenting) or plaque reduction (atherectomy). Oftentimes, these modalities are combined.

Balloon Angioplasty

Angioplasty balloons have evolved and improved over the past decade such that they are smaller profile and more "trackable" across tight lesions. The balloon is placed at the distal-most extent of the disease and then slowly inflated to its profile diameter (Fig. 15.3a–b). The balloon is deflated, moved more proximally, and then reinflated; this process is repeated until the entire length of disease vessel has been treated. A completion angiogram is then performed to assess the result (Fig. 15.3c). Balloons come in a variety of diameters and lengths and are used over three main guidewire platforms (0.014″, 0.018″, or 0.035″ wires). Typical diameters utilized for the femoropopliteal segment range from 4 to 7 mm and 1.5 to 3 mm for the tibials. More recently, angioplasty balloons can be coated with drug-eluting medications (i.e., paclitaxel) with the intent of decreasing rates of intimal hyperplasia. The cost-effectiveness of these new balloons has yet to be determined.

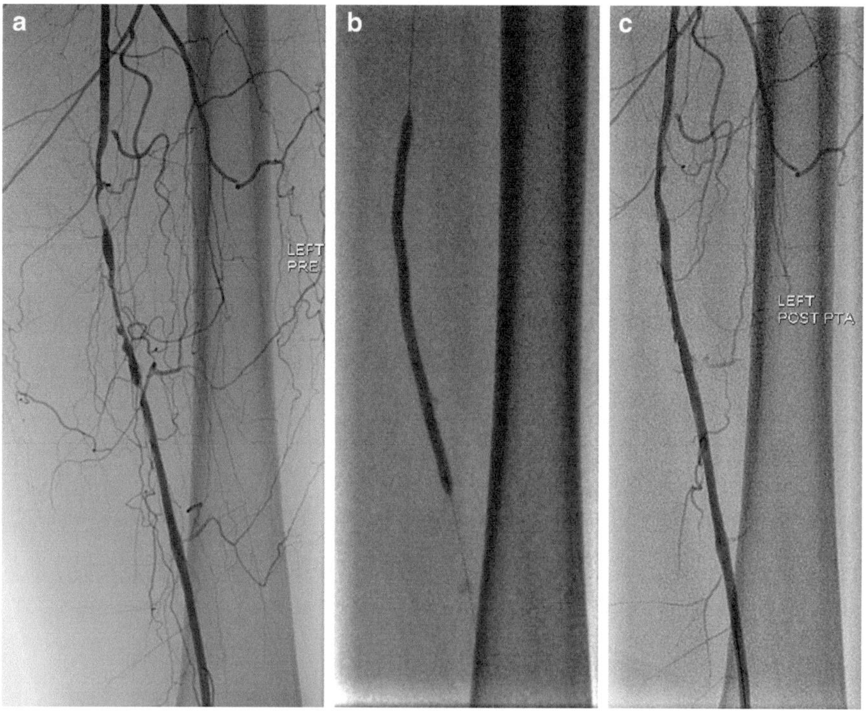

Fig. 15.3 Balloon angioplasty of the left lower extremity. Balloon angioplasty of a diseased distal superficial artery in a patient tissue loss of the toes. (**a**) Depicts the area of stenosis pretreatment. (**b**) A 4 × 150 mm balloon catheter is positioned and inflated to its nominal size. (**c**) Completion angiogram showing improved flow

An advantage of using balloon angioplasty alone is that no foreign substrate (i.e., metal stent) remains within the vessel arguably decreasing a nidus for intimal hyperplasia. However, inflation of the balloon inherently traumatizes the arterial wall which may not only instigate the inflammatory process underlying intimal hyperplasia but also can cause an arterial dissection (Fig. 15.4) or even rupture. If a dissection occurs, stenting is selectively utilized in a "bailout" fashion. In addition, a heavily calcified lesion may have a poor response to balloon angioplasty alone (> 30% residual stenosis) in which case stenting is needed.

Stenting

The purpose of stenting is to provide support for the expansion of a heavily calcified arterial lumen that did not respond well to angioplasty or to treat an iatrogenic flow-limiting dissection that occurred after angioplasty, as previously mentioned. Most stents used currently in the femoropopliteal level are self-expanding nitinol stents as

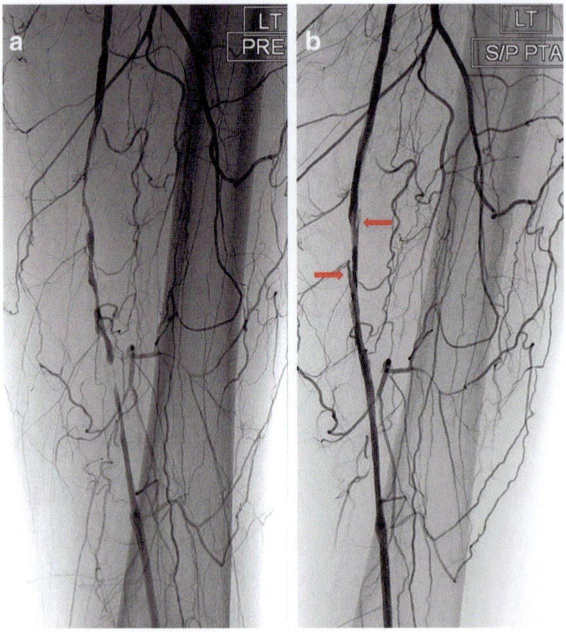

Fig. 15.4 Iatrogenic dissection from balloon angioplasty. Angiogram of heavily diseased superficial femoral artery pre-balloon angioplasty. Completion angiogram post-balloon angioplasty showing areas of iatrogenic focal dissection (*red arrows*) of the treated vessel. Such a result requires "bailout" stenting

opposed to stainless steel. Nitinol offers improved flexibility, excellent radial force, and decreased kinking or fracturing. Notably, self-expanding stents cease to exert an outward radial force once their nominal diameter is reached. As such, these stents are oversized by 1 mm–2 mm to the true arterial lumen diameter so that the stent continually applies radial force on the arterial lumen. Once deployed, self-expanding stents may require a brief balloon angioplasty to facilitate their expansion (Fig. 15.5).

Covered stents (Viabahn, W. L. Gore & Associates, Flagstaff, AZ), which have been approved for use in the SFA, are another stenting option. Some believe this stent design decreases intimal hyperplasia since the fabric prevents tissue ingrowth [12]. Covered stents can also be very useful in emergency settings when there is an arterial injury resulting in extravasation.

Finally, based on the experience and data from the coronary circulation, some peripheral self-expanding stents are now designed with drug-eluting capabilities with the goal of minimizing intimal hyperplasia and increasing patency rates. Local delivery of antiproliferative agents to the vessel wall via an eluting polymer inhibits endothelial cell migration and proliferation, which form the basis for restenosis. Similar to the drug-eluting balloons, there have been some encouraging early results, but more data is needed to verify their clinical and economic utility [13].

Options for stenting in the tibial vessels are much more limited than the femoropopliteal segment. Stenting is often avoided in these vessels, but if needed there are small diameter, balloon-expandable coronary stents that can be used off-label.

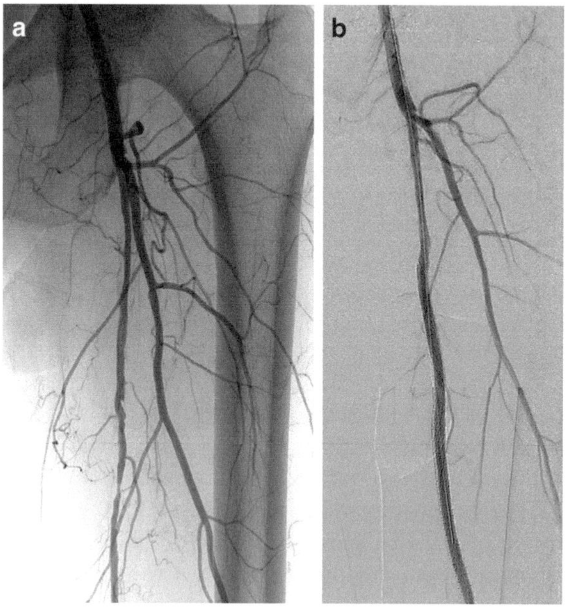

Fig. 15.5 Stenting of the left superficial femoral artery. (**a**) Pretreatment angiogram showing moderate proximal-mid superficial femoral artery atherosclerotic disease. (**b**) Completion angiogram after the deployment of a 7 × 200 mm self-expanding stent

As alluded to multiple times, the main complication with stenting is the development of restenosis invariably due to intimal hyperplasia. Additionally, stents are placed in very dynamic parts of the leg, and thus they can fracture after repeated flexion, extension, and twisting. Stent fracture can be a benign event, or it can lead to thrombus formation with subsequent ischemia.

Atherectomy

Atherectomy devices shave away calcified plaque thereby increasing luminal diameter. Some devices use a rotational design which sand the plaque whereas others use laser energy. The devices come in different sizes making them useable in both femoral and tibial vessels. This technique, much like the others previously mentioned, emanated from the coronary circulation experience. The theoretical advantage of atherectomy is that reducing the plaque burden eliminates the need for stenting and subsequent restenosis. However, inevitably debris is produced during this process which can embolize distally leading to ischemia. Embolic protection devices can be used concomitantly, but these add substantial expense to an already expensive device and have not been shown to clinically improve results. In general, there has been no substantial evidence that atherectomy in the lower extremities is superior to plain old balloon angioplasty and/or stenting. Its utility may be in select situations where stenting is known to have very poor results – when treating a focal plaque directly behind the knee.

Outcomes

Multiple outcome measures have been created for assessing the success of an endovascular intervention. Technical success, patency rates (primary, primary assisted, and secondary), and restenosis rates are frequently reported, but these measures do not provide any commentary on the patient's clinical status. Accordingly, many studies capture clinical response to treatment – namely, whether there has been resolution of claudication or rest pain (improved Rutherford category), healing of ulcers, or freedom from either minor or major amputation.

Outcomes mostly depend upon several important items including the lesion length and character, pattern of disease, clinical indication, comorbid conditions, and intraprocedural findings. Not surprisingly, patients with CLI and multiple comorbidities who have long segment lesions at multiple levels have the worst outcomes. In a meta-analysis of over 900 angioplasty procedures of the femoropopliteal vessels, the 3-year primary patency rate was 61% in claudicants with stenosis, 48% in claudicants with occlusions, 43% in those with CLI and stenosis, and 30% in those with CLI and occlusions [14]. Generally, these rates drop off when performing balloon angioplasty below the popliteal artery as demonstrated by a meta-analysis showing a 3-year primary patency of 48% [15].

The benefit of stenting over angioplasty alone in the femoropopliteal segment is not entirely clear. In the Femoral Artery Stenting Trial (FAST), no difference was found in the 1-year restenosis rates between angioplasty (39%) versus angioplasty and stenting (31%) [16]. In contrast, another randomized controlled trial comparing angioplasty with selective stenting versus primary stenting found a benefit toward stenting with regard to 1-year restenosis rates (63% vs 37%) [17]. With regard to infrapopliteal disease, randomized trials comparing these two modalities have yet to be performed. Several prospective series describe similar short-term results between angioplasty and stenting with 1-year patency rates in the 70–80% range [18].

Translating these patency and restenosis rates into clinically meaningful metrics of ulcer healing, limb salvage, and amputation-free survival is essential. The 3-year limb salvage rate was 82% in a meta-analysis of infrapopliteal balloon angioplasty for CLI, an outcome that is comparable to rates seen after infrapopliteal bypass surgery [15]. In the Bypass versus Angioplasty in Severe Ischemia of the Leg (BASIL) trial, which compared angioplasty alone to open bypass in patients with severe leg ischemia, the 5-year amputation-free survival in the angioplasty group was nearly 50%. So, even though the long-term patency rates after endoluminal treatment of patients with CLI are average at best (and certainly worse than bypass surgery), the limb salvage rates are acceptable (and on par to surgical bypass). This finding suggests that many patients with CLI require a relatively brief period of revascularization to heal their ischemic wound (Fig. 15.6). However, these encouraging results should not translate into the broad application of endovascular therapy first in all CLI patients (a practice that is common in many centers). Patients in the BASIL trial who had a failed initial angioplasty had significantly worse limb salvage rates, even if they underwent a subsequent bypass, suggesting that an endovascular first approach should not be employed routinely [19].

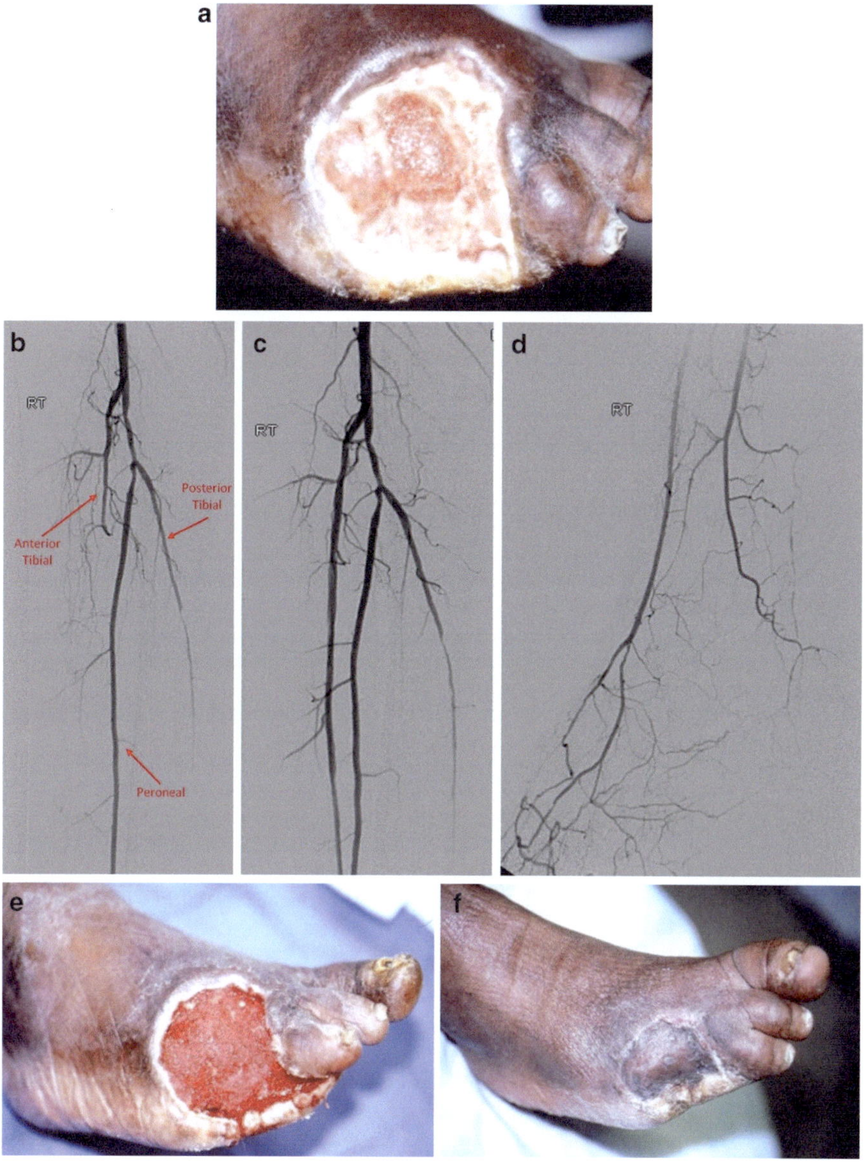

Fig. 15.6 Healing of chronic ischemic ulcer following tibial angioplasty. (**a**) Chronic ischemic right foot ulcer in diabetic patient with severe tibial disease. (**b**) Diagnostic angiogram showing single-vessel runoff (severely disease posterior tibial artery, occluded anterior tibial artery, and patent peroneal artery). (**c–d**) Post-angioplasty angiogram showing two-vessel flow to the foot. (**e**) Healthy granulation tissue at base of wound following 4 weeks of negative pressure dressing treatment. (**f**) Skin grafting of wound with ultimate limb salvage

Conclusion

The introduction and evolution of minimally invasive therapies have changed the landscape of managing ischemic wounds of the extremities. Balloon angioplasty, stenting, and atherectomy can attain limb salvage rates that are equitable to those after open bypass surgery but without the prolonged and morbid recovery periods seen after bypass surgery. Much more organized data, preferably from randomized trials, is needed to discern which technique and device are clinically superior yet financially palatable.

References

1. Abu Dabrh AM, Steffen MW, Undavalli C, Asi N, Wang Z, Elamin MB, Conte MS, Murad MH. The natural history of untreated severe or critical limb ischemia. J Vasc Surg. 2015;62:1642–51.
2. Veith FJ, et al. Six-year prospective multicenter randomized comparison of autologous saphenous vein and expanded polytetrafluoroethylene grafts in infrainguinal arterial reconstructions. J Vasc Surg. 1986;3:104–14.
3. Arnaoutakis DJ, Scully RE, Sharma G, Shah SK, Ozaki CK, Belkin M, Nguyen LL. Impact of body mass index and gender on wound complications after lower extremity arterial surgery. J Vasc Surg. 2017;65(6):1713–8. pii: S0741–5214(17)30107–6
4. Soden PA, Zettervall SL, Shean KE, et al. Effect of femoral endarterectomy in lower extremity bypass on perioperative and 1-year outcomes. J Vasc Surg. 2017;65(3):711–9.
5. Dotter CT, Judkins MP. Transluminal treatment of arteriosclerotic obstruction: description of a new technique and preliminary report of its application. Circulation. 1964;30:645–70.
6. Grüntzig A, Hopff H. Perkutane rekanalisation chronischer arterieller Verschlüsse mit einen neuen Dilatationskatheter: Modifikation der Dotter-technik. Dtsch Med Wochenschr. 1974;99:2502–51.
7. Palmaz JC, Siggitt RR, Reuter SR, et al. Expandable intraluminal graft: preliminary study. Radiology. 1985;156:73–7.
8. Goodney PP, Beck AW, Nagle J, Welch HG, Zwolak RM. National trends in lower extremity bypass surgery, endovascular interventions, and major amputations. J Vasc Surg. 2009;50(1):54–60.
9. Schultz-Schupke S, Heide S. Comparison of vascular closure device vs manual compression after femoral artery puncture: the ISAR-CLOSURE randomized controlled trial. JAMA. 2014;312(18):1981–7.
10. Darling JD, McCallum JC, Soden PA, Meng Y, Wyers MC, Hamdan AD, Verhagen HJ, Schermerhorn ML. Predictive ability of the Society for Vascular Surgery Wound, ischemia, and foot infection (WIfI) classification system following infrapopliteal endovascular interventions for critical limb ischemia. J Vasc Surg. 2016;64(3):616–22.
11. Mills JL Sr, Conte MS, Armstrong DG, Pomposelli FB, Schanzer A, Sidawy AN, Andros G; Society for Vascular Surgery Lower Extremity Guidelines Committee. The Society for Vascular Surgery Lower Extremity Threatened Limb Classification System: risk stratification based on wound, ischemia, and foot infection (WIfI). J Vasc Surg. 2014;59(1):220–234.e1–2.
12. McQuade K, Gable D, Hohman S, Pearl G, Theune B. Randomized comparison of ePTFE/nitinol self-expanding graft vs prosthetic femoral-popliteal bypass in the treatment of superficial femoral artery occlusive disease. J Vasc Surg. 2009;49(1):109–15.

13. Dake MD, Ansel GM, Jaff MR, Ohki T, Saxon RR, Smouse HB, Machan LS, Snyder SA, O'Leary EE, Ragheb AO, Zeller T, Zilver PTX Investigators. Durable clinical effectiveness with paclitaxel-eluting stents in the femoropopliteal artery: 5-year results of the zilver ptx randomized trial. Circulation. 2016 Apr 12;133(15):1472–83.
14. Muradin GS, Bosch JL, Stijnen T, Hunink MG. Balloon dilation and stent implantation for treatment of femoropopliteal arterial disease: meta-analysis. Radiology. 2001;221(1):137–45.
15. Romiti M, Albers M, Brochado-Neto FC, et al. Meta-analysis of infrapopliteal angioplasty for chronic critical limb ischemia. J Vasc Surg. 2008;47:975–81.
16. Krankenberg H, Schlüter M, Steinkamp HJ, et al. Nitinol stent implantation versus percutaneous transluminal angioplasty in superficial femoral artery lesions up to 10 cm in length: the femoral artery stenting trial (FAST). Circulation. 2007;116:285–92.
17. Schillinger M, Sabeti S, Loewe C, Dick P, et al. Balloon angioplasty versus implantation of nitinol stents in the superficial femoral artery. N Engl J Med. 2006;354:1879–88.
18. Peregrin JH, Smirova S, Koznar B, et al. Self-expandable stent placement in infrapopliteal arteries after unsuccessful angioplasty failure: one-year follow-up. Cardiovasc Intervent Radiol. 2008;31:860–4.
19. Bradbury AW, Adam DJ, Bell J, Forbes JF, Fowkes FG, Gillespie I, Ruckley CV, Raab GM, BASIL Trial Participants. Bypass versus angioplasty in severe ischaemia of the leg (BASIL) trial: analysis of amputation free and overall survival by treatment received. J Vasc Surg. 2010;51(5 Suppl):18S–31S.

Chapter 16
Endovascular Venous Interventions

Chieh-Min Fan

Introduction

Effective treatment of venous ulcers requires a coordinated approach between meticulous local wound care, infection control, patient education and lifestyle modification, and mechanical reversal of underlying treatable venous insufficiency and obstruction. While conventional surgical vein stripping and ligation may be indicated in select situations, open surgical procedures have largely been superseded by imaging-guided minimally invasive endovenous techniques. Endovenous thermal or chemical vein ablation can selectively close incompetent veins, while venous thrombolysis and stenting can restore flow in segments with post-thrombotic obstruction. These modern vein treatments, performable through needles or small catheters through micro-incisions, facilitate treatment of venous disease without requiring surgical incisions in a tissue bed compromised by chronic inflammation and poor wound healing. Endovenous procedures can also often be done in an outpatient setting without general anesthesia or sedation, thus promoting post-procedural mobility with decreased thrombotic complications and recovery time. This chapter will provide an overview of the role of endovenous therapies in the treatment of venostasis ulcers.

Background

Venous Anatomy and Physiology The venous system of the lower extremity is comprised of three components: a deep venous system, a superficial venous system, and a system of connecting perforator veins linking the deep and superficial veins.

C.-M. Fan, MD (✉)
Interventional Radiology, Beverly Hospital, Beverly, MA 01915, USA
e-mail: chieh-min.fan@lahey.org

D.P. Orgill (ed.), *Interventional Treatment of Wounds*,
https://doi.org/10.1007/978-3-319-66990-8_16

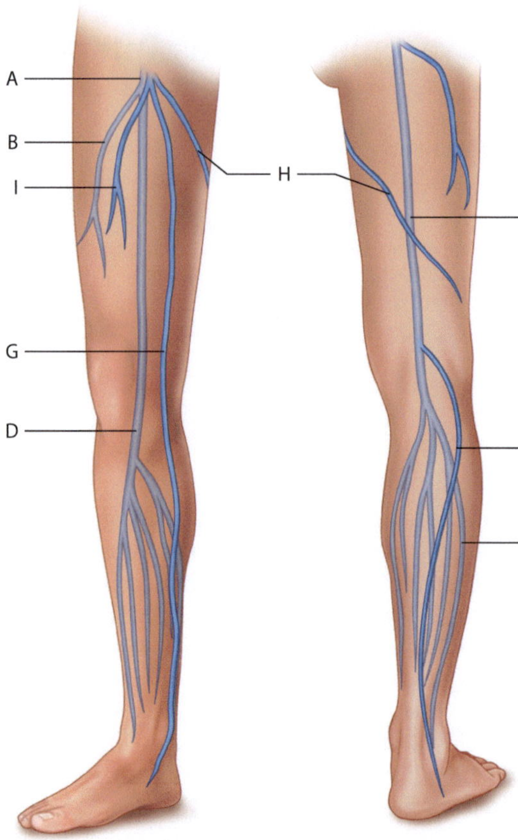

Fig. 16.1 Venous anatomy of the lower extremity: (**A**) common femoral vein; (**B**) deep femoral vein; (**C**) femoral vein; (**D**) popliteal vein; (**E**) paired calf veins (anterior tibial, peroneal, posterior tibial); (**F**) small saphenous vein; (**G**) great saphenous vein; (**H**) posterior accessory saphenous vein; (**I**) anterior accessory saphenous vein

The deep venous system is a series of large capacitance veins running in the core of the limb deep to the deep fascia and large muscle groups. From peripheral to central location, the named deep veins include the paired calf veins (peroneal, posterior tibial, and anterior tibial), major calf muscular tributaries (gastrocnemius and soleal veins and their sinuses), and the popliteal, femoral, deep femoral, and common femoral veins (Fig. 16.1). Above the inguinal ligament, the deep system continues in the pelvis as the external iliac and internal iliac veins that converge into the common iliac veins that terminated at the inferior vena cava. The deep veins provide the dominant venous drainage for the lower extremity, carrying approximately 90% of the venous return. Extending from central to peripheral, the superficial venous system consists of the saphenous veins (great, small, and accessory saphenous) which receive inflow from tributary and reticular branches. These in turn receive venous return from the small veins of the skin. The saphenous veins reside in the saphenous space between the superficial and deep fascial layers, while the other components of the superficial venous system reside outside the superficial fascia in the subdermal tissues and skin. Retrograde flow is prevented by a series of bicuspid one-way valves spaced along the course of the veins. The deep and superficial venous systems connect at the saphenofemoral and saphenopopliteal junctions and through approximately 60 valved perforator veins that connect the superficial and deep venous structures and promote predominantly unidirectional flow of venous blood from the superficial to deep veins [1–3].

Unlike circulation in the pressurized arterial system, flow in the veins is a passive process, driven by external compression of venous structures by surrounding muscular contraction and cyclical variation in abdominal pressure during the respiratory cycle. During contraction of the thigh and calf muscles, the deep veins compress and empty in the cephalad direction resulting in a sudden drop in deep venous pressure. Lubrook demonstrated that with rhythmic exercise, the venous blood volume is reduced by 65% in the calf and 15% in the thigh. During muscular relaxation, the lower pressure in the empty veins promotes passive flow of blood from the higher pressure superficial veins via perforator veins. As deep veins refill and pressure increases, the perforator valves close and the cycle repeats [1, 4–6].

Pathophysiology of Venous Ulcers Venous ulceration represents the damaging end-organ effects of advanced chronic venous hypertension resulting from the presence of valvular insufficiency (reflux), venous obstruction, or both. Valvular reflux can involve the deep, superficial, and perforator systems and is characterized as primary in the absence of prior thrombotic event, or secondary as the result of post-thrombotic damage. There is a strong causal relationship between deep vein thrombosis and the development of axial venous reflux. Yamaki et al. performed serial duplex US on 67 limbs with DVT and noted that while at 1 year 76% of thrombose segments had recanalized, deep venous reflux developed in 43% of limbs with multisegment DVT and in 20% in limbs with single segment thrombosis [7]. Venous reflux is not limited to sites of thrombosis-related valve damage only, and can develop in vein segments remote from the site of thrombosis likely from downstream effects of regional obstruction-related venous hypertension [8]. Post-thrombotic venous insufficiency may develop into a clinical *post-thrombotic syndrome (PTS)*, characterized by chronic limb swelling, pain, venous claudication, inflammatory skin changes, and ulceration. Approximately 20–50% of patients with symptomatic DVT will develop PTS within 2 years despite adequate DVT treatment, and 25–30% of these cases will be severe with risk of ulceration [9]. Risk factors for developing PTS include multilevel DVT, proximal iliofemoral DVT, recurrent ipsilateral DVT, and inadequate anticoagulation treatment [10–12].

The pathogenesis of primary venous insufficiency is not fully known but is believed to be a multifactorial process with age, gender, parity, body habitus, lifestyle, and genetics all playing a role. The Tampere study of 3284 men and 3590 women ranging from 40–60 years in age demonstrated that the prevalence of venous insufficiency was greater in women than men (48% versus 18%) and increased with age and increasing parity [13]. Obesity may be a minor risk factor for primary venous insufficiency as shown by the Edinburgh vein study and Callum's review of 21 epidemiological studies on varicose veins [14, 15]. A hereditary component to primary venous insufficiency has long been postulated, with Cornu-Thenard et al.

showing the risk of varicose in subjects with unaffected parents was 20%, 25–62% with one affected parent, and 90% with two affected parents [16]. The recent advances in human genome analysis have stimulated increasing interest in the genetic basis of venous disease. Markovic et al. showed through DNA microarray analysis that compared with normal controls, patients with chronic venous insufficiency exhibit downregulation of regulatory genes of collagen synthesis and overexpression of hydroxyprostaglandin dehydrogenase-15 enzyme (HPGD), a molecule that decreases prostaglandin activity and downregulates inflammation in vivo [17].

The role of perforator veins in ulcer formation deserves special discussion. Isolated perforator incompetence is present in only 3.2% of venous ulcer patients [18] indicating that it is unlikely to play a primary role in the pathogenesis of venous ulcers. However, perforators are intermediary conduits that once recruited into the disease process play a key role in the extension of disease between the superficial and deep zones. Labropoulos et al. demonstrated an incompetent perforator vein (IPV) prevalence of 28% in the setting of chronic venous disease versus none in normal controls. Both Delis and Labropoulos found that perforator diameter and flow increased in patients with advanced CEAP C3–6 disease compared with CEAP C1–2 disease [19, 20]. There are two mechanisms by which perforator dysfunction can develop: antegrade overload of the perforator valve due to excess inflow from superficial venous reflux or retrograde blowout of the perforator valve from chronic deep venous hypertension. It is common to find pathological perforators in proximity to the ulcer bed, and the SVS/AVF clinical practice guidelines for care of patients with venous disease define three criteria for a pathologic perforator: diameter $\geq$ 3.5 mm, $\geq$ 500 ms of retrograde flow, and anatomic location of the IPV beneath a healed or active ulcer. These guidelines recommend treatment of pathological perforators occurring in the setting of healed or open venous ulcers [21].

The presence of chronic ambulatory venous hypertension incites ulcer formation through a complex inflammatory cascade. High venous pressure transmits to the capillary bed resulting in leakage of macromolecules such as fibrin, fibrinogen, and α-macroglobulin into the pericapillary tissues and subdermal space. The fibrin and fibrinogen may form a barrier to oxygen and nutrient transfer as well as causing downregulation of collagen synthesis, while α-macroglobulin may act as a scavenger of growth factors. These processes act collectively to slow tissue repair. Venous hypertension also incites leukocyte trapping in the microcirculation of the wound with subsequent release of cytotoxins, proteolytic enzymes, and free radicals resulting in tissue injury [22].

Mitigation of ambulatory venous hypertension by eliminating treatable reflux and restoring flow through obstructed segments abates the inflammatory cascade and promotes stable wound healing. As such, venous ulcer management should include a systematic evaluation and treatment of correctable components of venous insufficiency in conjunction with use of local wound therapies. Endovenous treatments for chronic venous disease can be divided into two general categories: (a) techniques for closing or removing incompetent components of the superficial venous system and (b) techniques to relieve deep venous obstruction through clot dissolution and stenting of fixed stenoses.

Patient Evaluation

Clinical Evaluation The Society for Vascular Surgery and American Venous Forum (SVS/AVF) clinical practice guidelines for care of patients with chronic venous disease outline best practice recommendations for evaluation of the chronic venous insufficiency patient. This includes obtaining a complete patient history with targeted review of prior vein treatments including compression therapy, thrombotic events, disorders of coagulation, family history of venous disease, and a survey of vein-related symptoms (leg heaviness, pain, itching, swelling, restless legs, and nocturnal cramps.) The physical exam is done with the patient in standing position to facilitate accurate documentation varicose veins and inspection for stigmata of CVI (corona phlebectatica, varicose veins, edema, pigmentation, lipodermatosclerosis, and ulcers). Examples of physical findings of chronic venous insufficiency are shown in Fig. 16.2. Certain findings such as prominent cross-pelvic venous collateral veins and total limb swelling may suggest the presence of central pelvic venous outflow obstruction and direct further imaging evaluation. Selected use of laboratory testing for thrombophilias, infection, or coagulation status may be helpful. The use of validated venous disease clinical assessment instruments at baseline and after treatment is recommended to promote objective outcomes assessment. Such metrics include the CEAP classification, venous severity scoring (VSS) system, Villalta scoring system for post-thrombotic syndrome, and venous disease-specific quality of life questionnaires among others. The SVS/AVF guidelines specifically recommend CEAP clinical classification and venous clinical severity scoring (VCSS) for all patients at baseline and ongoing during treatment [21, 23–26].

Imaging Evaluation Venous mapping with a standing duplex US reflux study is essential for accurate diagnosis and treatment planning of endovenous therapies. This exam assesses for site and severity of valvular incompetence in both deep and superficial veins, depth and diameter of target vessels, source of reflux for all major varicosities, presence of acute or chronic thrombosis, and should include a targeted search for perforators in ulcer patients. The Union Internationale de Phlebologie (UIP) consensus document on the topic [27] summarizes the technique for duplex US reflux scanning for evaluation of chronic venous disease. Patients with history of DVT or severe venous disease suggesting deep venous involvement warrant additional evaluation of deep vein status by selective use of duplex US exam for DVT, CT or MR venography, catheter-based venography, and intravascular US. Functional assessment studies by plethysmography and ambulatory venous pressure monitoring can provide quantitative assessment of global venous function in the limb [28–30]. Figure. 16.3 provides a suggested algorithm for venous testing in the evaluation of patients with chronic venous disease.

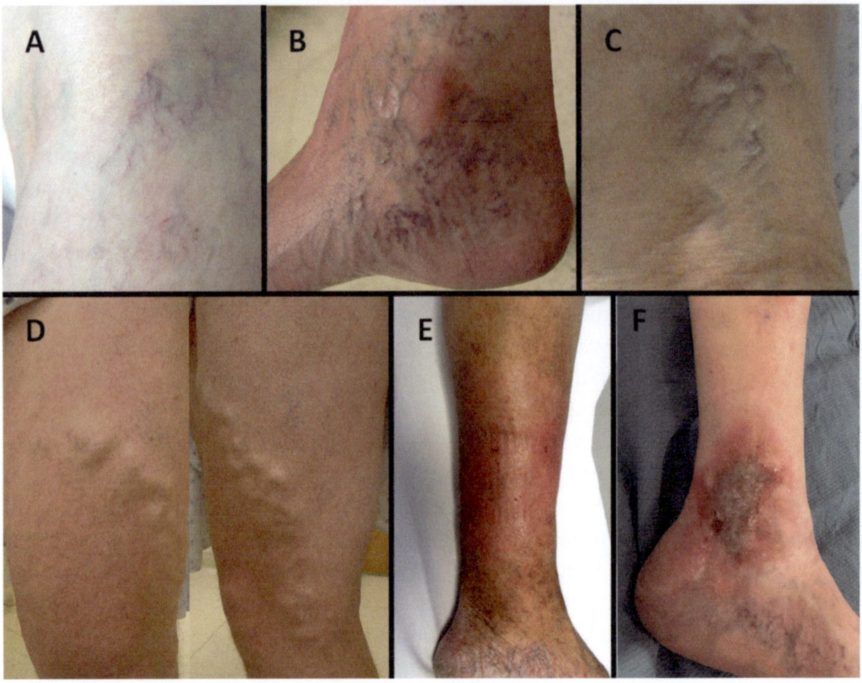

Fig. 16.2 The spectrum of chronic venous insufficiency: (**A**) telangiectasia (spider veins). (**B**) Venulectasia: "corona phlebectatica," pattern indicative of significant deep or superficial reflux. (**C**) Reticular varicose veins. (**D**) Tributary varicose veins from saphenous reflux. (**E**) Lipodermatosclerosis: reactive inflammation, often a precursor to ulceration. (**F**) Venostasis ulcer

Endovenous Treatments for Superficial Venous Disease

Potentially correctable isolated superficial venous reflux contributes to venous hypertension in approximately 40% of patients with CEAP clinical class 4–6 disease, and an additional 40% of ulcer patients have a combined pattern of superficial and deep reflux [18, 31]. Elimination of the superficial reflux component is an important step in improving the venous hemodynamics in these patients. Endovenous saphenous vein ablation has largely replaced surgical vein stripping as the first-line treatment for incompetent great and small saphenous veins, while thermal and chemical ablation methods have largely replaced open surgical and subfascial endoscopic ligation of perforators. Endovenous ablation methods include endovenous thermal ablation (ETA), chemical ablation (sclerotherapy), mechanochemical ablation (MOCA), and adhesive closure with cyanoacrylate (CAE). Figure 16.4 illustrates some of currently available devices for endovenous saphenous vein ablation.

Endovenous Thermal Ablation (ETA) Endovenous thermal ablation involves using a heating element (either radiofrequency probe or laser fiber) to heat the vessel wall from the endoluminal side. The thermal injury results in contraction of the

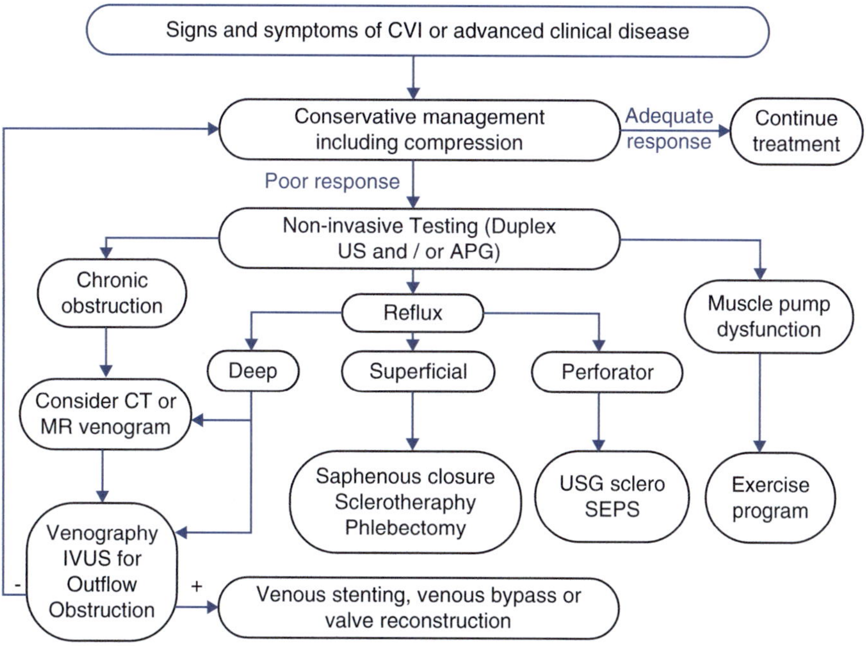

Fig. 16.3 Algorithm for evaluation and management of CVI patient (Modified from Eberhardt and Raffetto [30])

vein wall collagen, shrinkage of the vein, and ultimately a permanent fibrotic closure. The technique initially targeted the great and small saphenous veins but is also applicable to accessory saphenous veins, perforators, and tributary branches provided the target vessel is relatively straight and not superficially subdermal in location.

Radiofrequency Ablation (RFA) RFA was the first method of endovenous thermal ablation introduced in the USA in 1999, specifically for closure of incompetent great saphenous veins. The original device has passed through many modifications to its current form consisting of a 3 or 7 cm heating element mounted on a catheter (ClosureFast™; Medtronic, Inc. Fridley, MN). The device is inserted into the target vein under sonographic guidance through a 7 French introducer sheath and positioned within 1–2 cm of the saphenofemoral or saphenopopliteal junction. Under US guidance, tumescent anesthesia (typically 0.1 or 0.2% lidocaine solution) is injected circumferentially around the target vein in the saphenous space to form a 10 mm thick halo of fluid (see Fig. 16.5c). The tumescent fluid isolates the vein from surrounding tissues and prevents nontarget thermal injury, anesthetizes the vein, and compresses the vein wall onto the heating unit. Catheter position is reconfirmed sonographically, and then overlapping vein segments are sequentially heated in 20 s bursts, with peak temperature of 120°C achieved [32].

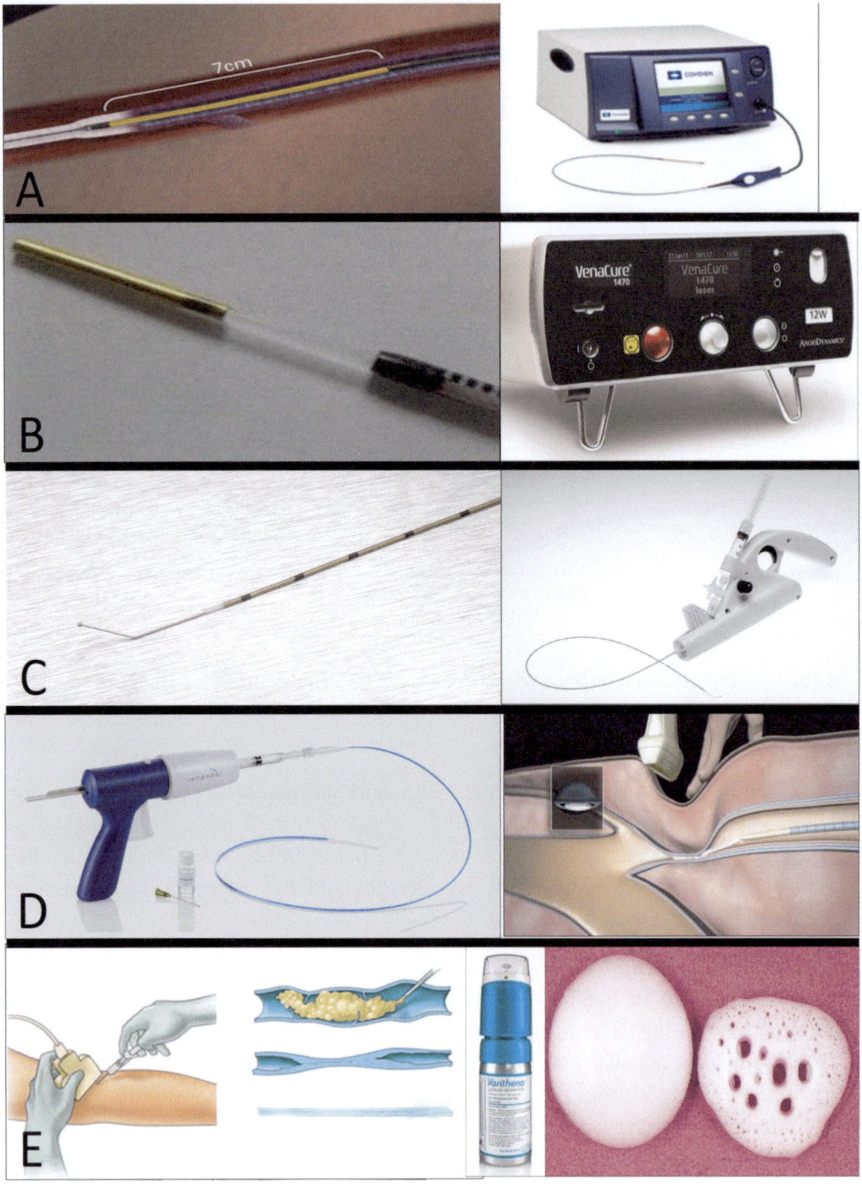

Fig. 16.4 Devices for saphenous vein ablation: (**A**) ClosureFast™ radiofrequency ablation system. (**B**) VenaCure™ (AngioDynamics, Latham NY) endovenous laser. (**C**) Clarivein™ mechanochemical ablation device. (**D**) VenaSeal™ cyanoacrylate embolization system. (**E**) Varithena™ polidocanol foam

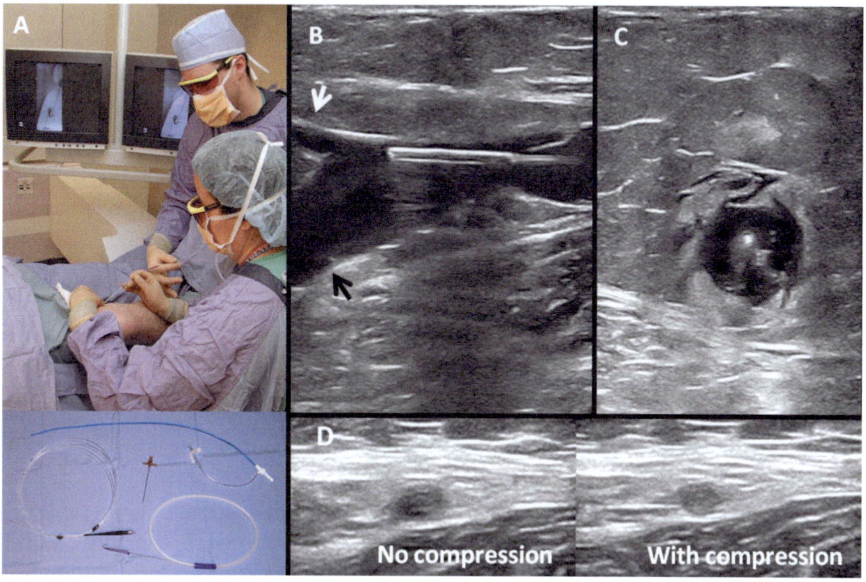

Fig. 16.5 Endovenous laser ablation procedure: (**A**) procedure and laser kit components. (**B**) Laser positioning below the saphenous femoral junction (*black arrow*) and terminus of the inferior epigastric vein (*white arrow*). (**C**) Injection of 0.1% lidocaine tumescent anesthesia around the target. (**D**) Posttreatment appearance of occluded and noncompressible GSV

Endovenous Laser Ablation (EVLA) In 2001, endovenous laser ablation was introduced as another method for thermal ablation of saphenous veins [33]. The procedure for endovenous laser ablation is very similar to that of RFA with a few technical differences related to laser devices. Laser safety training and strict adherence to laser safety procedure are mandatory prerequisites. Many wavelengths of light ranging from 810 to 1500 nm have been approved and used for EVLA application. The actual heating element is typically a 400–600 micron fiber optic that is introduced through a vascular sheath into the target vein. Various fiber tip configurations have been marketed (bare flat tip, metal jacketed tip, round tip) without clear evidence to support differences in clinical efficacy. Positioning of the laser fiber tip and application of tumescent anesthesia are procedurally the same as for RFA. Once the tumescent anesthesia is administered, the laser is activated and withdrawn slowly while firing continuously [34]. Figure 16.5 illustrates some salient aspects of the EVLA procedure.

The mechanism by which heat transfer occurs from the laser tip to the vein wall continues to be debated. Proposed mechanisms include light absorption directly into the vein wall, light absorption by residual blood in the lumen, heat transfer via steam bubbles, carbonization at the fiber tip resulting in a light absorbing black layer that can become superheated, and the effects of thermally induced coagula within the lumen. Energy delivered in EVLA is expressed as the linear endovenous energy density (LEED, joules/cm) which is the product of the laser power (joules/

sec) times duration of treatment (sec) divided by length of treated vein (cm). At light wavelengths less than 1000 nm, the dominant chromophore for light absorption is hemoglobin which is confined to the vessel lumen, while at longer wavelengths water becomes the dominant chromophore. Since blood and tissue have a 75–80% water content, longer wavelength light is postulated to be more penetrating and therefore equally efficacious for EVLA at lower LEED. However, the optimal LEED for EVLA has not been scientifically determined, and in clinical practice, target LEED of 80–100 J/cm for shorter wavelength lasers and 40–50 J/cm for longer wavelength lasers has been accepted as standardizing parameters. In actuality, success of EVLA vein closure is likely impacted by many factors other than LEED including laser power, pullback rate, vein diameter, and inflow from tributary branches [34, 35].

Post-ETA Management Following ETA, the patient is placed into multilayer compression wrap or 30–40 mm HG full-length compression stocking for 1–2 weeks. Patients typically can ambulate and return to work and resume normal daily activities immediately. Minor ecchymoses and soreness often described as a "pulling" sensation can occur along the treated vein. These symptoms respond readily to oral nonsteroidal anti-inflammatory medication. Clinical post-procedural follow-up with duplex US within 1–2 weeks is recommended to confirm successful vein closure and assess for thrombotic complications. Long-term follow-up at 3, 6, and 12 months with symptom assessment using proven metrics enables outcomes evaluation [33, 34].

Complications of ETA Endovenous thermal ablation is associated with a low rate of complications, most of which are minor. Potential adverse effects include DVT, paresthesias, pulmonary embolus, thrombophlebitis, hyperpigmentation, infection, and skin burns. Post-ETA extension of thrombus across the saphenofemoral junction is a well-described phenomenon termed endothermal heat-induced thrombosis (EHIT). Lawrence et al. described a six-tier EHIT classification system for EHIT lesions: EHIT-1,2 lesions stop below the SFJ, EHIT-3 terminates at the SFJ, EHIT-4,5 show nonocclusive extension into the common femoral vein, and EHIT-6 represents occlusion of the common femoral vein. EHIT1-3 lesions do not require treatment, whereas anticoagulation is recommended for EHIT4–6 lesions [36]. Figure 16.6 illustrates an EHIT-3 lesion with progression to EHIT-5. In randomized clinical trial of 500 subjects comparing EVLA, RFA, USG foam sclerotherapy, and surgical stripping, Rasmussen noted 6.4% phlebitis, 4.4% hyperpigmentation, 3.6% paresthesias, 0.4% infection and bleeding, and no DVT or PE [37]. In a meta-analysis of 17 RCT comparing RFA or EVLA to ligation/stripping, Dermody found EVLA associated with complication rates of 0.5% wound infection, 5.6% superficial phlebitis, 3.8% paresthesias, 0.85 DVT/EHIT, and 0.3% skin burn. With the exception of higher paresthesia rate, RFA demonstrated comparable complication profile: 1.5% wound infection, 4–8% superficial phlebitis, 12% paresthesia, 0% DVT/EHIT, and 0.7% skin burn [38].

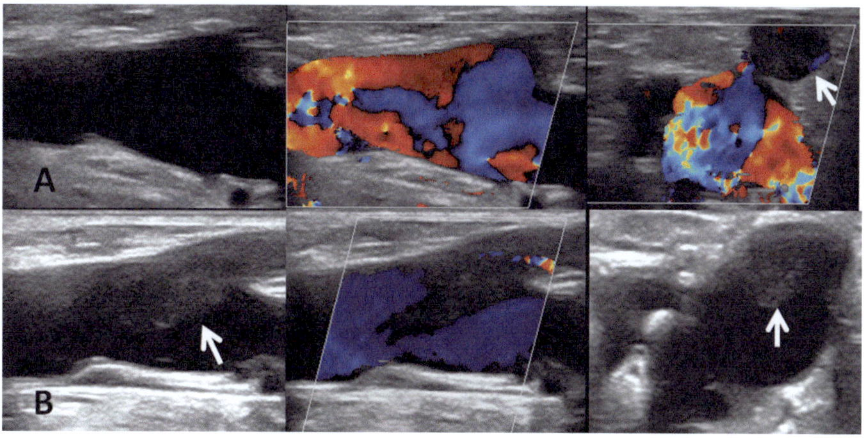

Fig. 16.6 Endothermal heat-induced thrombosis (EHIT) complication of EVLA: (**A**) EHIT-3 terminating at the saphenofemoral junction, which subsequently progressed to (**B**) EHIT-5 (> 50% lumenal occlusion)

Tumescentless Methods of Saphenous Vein Closure Injection of tumescent anesthesia is often a procedural rate-limiting step for the practitioner and the most uncomfortable step for the patient undergoing thermal vein ablation. This has led to the emergence of several tumescentless and nonthermal methods of saphenous vein ablation which eliminate risk of nontarget thermal injury to the nerves and skin, require no tumescent anesthesia, and obviate the need for laser safety precautions. Early and midterm results from these newer methods of GSV closure appear comparable to thermal ablation and surgery, but long-term outcomes data on some of these newer treatments is limited.

Chemical Ablation (Sclerotherapy) Sclerotherapy is a well-established technique of injecting a vein with a chemical agent that causes endothelial damage, fibrosis, and vascular occlusion. Sclerotherapy is most commonly used to treat telangiectasias and small 3–7 mm superficial varicosities, but with ultrasound and/or flouroscopic guidance, the technique readily translates to larger and deeper venous structures including saphenous and perforator veins. FDA-approved sclerosants include detergents (sodium tetradecyl sulfate (STS), polidocanol, sodium morrhuate, and ethanolamine), hypertonic saline, and chemical irritants (glycerin, absolute ethanol). At the present time, the most commonly used agents for lower extremity venous applications are polidocanol, STS, and hypertonic saline. Agent selection is determined by location and size of the target vessel, degree of desired inflammatory effect, and operator preference. Optimal results require appropriate matching of sclerosant type and strength to size of target vein since an overly powerful agent can itself incite excessive inflammation, while too low concentration of agent results in recanalizable thrombus rather than permanent fibrotic closure or failure of closure altogether [39].

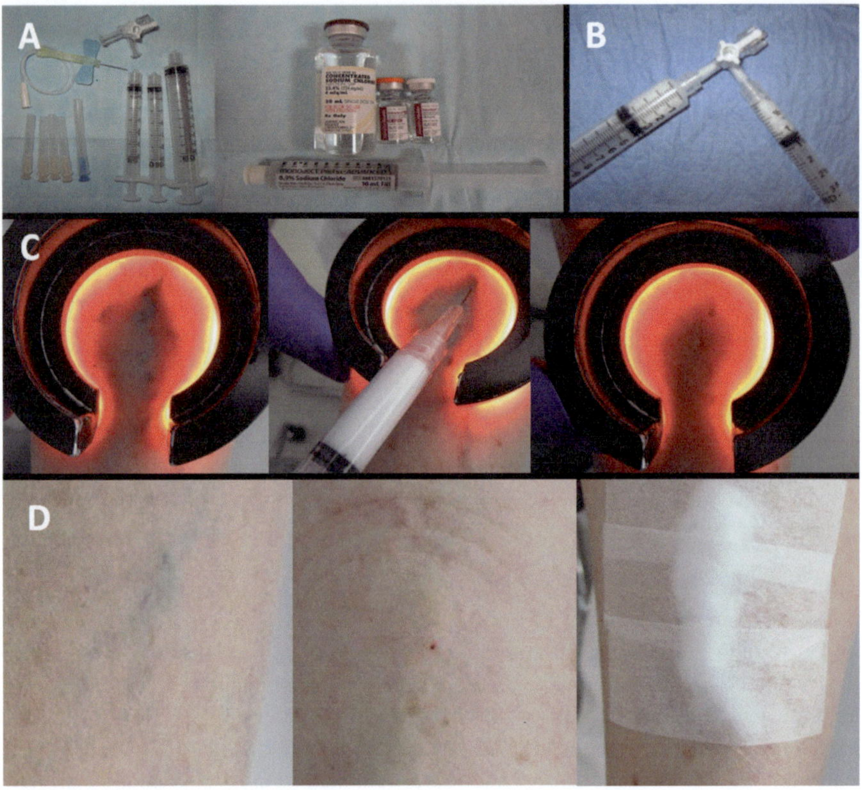

Fig. 16.7 Sclerotherapy: (**A**) sclerotherapy equipment and agents. (**B**) Tessari method of making foamed sclerosant. (**C**) Injection of foam into a varicose vein under transillumination with disappearance of the vein. (**D**) Pre- and post-injection appearance, with post-injection dressing

Detergent sclerosants such as polidocanol and STS can be administered in liquid form or converted to an injectable foam by agitation with 2–4 parts gas such as room air or carbon dioxide (CO_2) using the Tessari method described by Cabrera [40] (see Fig. 16.7b). Foaming enhances sclerosant effect by resisting dilutional mixing with blood and prolonging wall contact time. Foam is highly visible on ultrasound which is technically advantageous for targeted treatments such as perforator sclerotherapy and enables effective sclerotherapy with lesser amounts of sclerosant. However, foam sclerotherapy has been associated with well-documented neurological side effects including visual scotomata, migraine-like aura, chest tightness, and very rarely ischemic stroke which was reported in three patients worldwide [41, 42]. Transcranial Doppler studies have demonstrated intracranial gas bubbles in up to 42% of subjects undergoing foam sclerotherapy [43]. Multiple clinical studies have shown that the vast majority of these neurological sequelae are transient and resolve rapidly and spontaneously, but the potential for permanent neurological deficit remains a concern for practitioners [44–46]. An example of foam sclerotherapy of a reticular varicose vein is shown in Fig. 16.7.

Ultrasound-guided foam sclerotherapy (UGFS) has gained international acceptance as a method for saphenous vein ablation due to the advantages of being easy to perform, tumescentless, low cost, and without thermal injury risk. The first commercially available proprietary polidocanol-based foam (Varithena™, BTG International LTD, West Conshohocken, PA) recently received FDA approval for great saphenous vein closure [47, 48]. Prior to that, the only foam available for clinical use in the US was physician compounded foam (PCF), a non-FDA-approved usage of detergent sclerosants. For UGFS, access is obtained into the vein under ultrasound guidance with a butterfly needle or catheter. The saphenous vein is occluded cephalad to the injection site at the SFJ or SPJ by manual compression or balloon occlusion to prevent nontarget delivery of the sclerosant to the deep veins during injection. Another technique is to use a long vascular sheath with a coaxially placed balloon occlusion catheter. The balloon is inflated proximally, while the sclerosant is injected from the sheath distal to point of balloon occlusion. The system is then repositioned to the next untreated segment, and the process is repeated. Leg elevation is another maneuver used to prolong retention of the sclerosant in the target vein, particularly with foamed agents. Following treatment, the limb is placed into 30–40 mm HG compression similarly to thermal ablation.

Compared to ETA and surgical stripping, foam sclerotherapy for saphenous vein closure has comparable early closure rates but higher rates of recanalization (16–20% at 1 year versus 5% for thermal ablation) [37, 46]. Van den Bos et al. conducted a meta-analysis of 12,320 limbs undergoing saphenous vein treatment by surgical stripping, EVLT, RFA, or UGFS. This study showed success rates of 78%, 77%, 84%, and 94% for surgery, UGFS, RFA, and EVLA, respectively [49].

Mechanochemical Ablation (MOCA) The Clarivein™ occlusion catheter (Vascular Insights, Madison CT, USA) is a saphenous vein closure device that combines mechanical disruption of the endothelium by means of a rotating catheter tip with simultaneous deliver of sclerosant from the catheter tip. The combined effects of endothelial mechanical excoriation and chemical injury result in vein closure. The device is inserted into the target vein through a 5 French sheath and positioned with the tip 10 cm below the saphenopopliteal or saphenofemoral junction. The rotating catheter, which is driven by a 9 volt battery-operated handle mounted with a syringe of sclerosant (1.5–2.0 STS), is withdrawn slowly at a rate of 1 cm/7–10 s while activated and with simultaneous injection of the sclerosant at 0.1–0.2 ml/cm of pullback. Following ablation the patient is placed into compression as with ETA.

Two prospective series of MOCA of the GSV or SSV with phlebectomy demonstrated 100% technical saphenous vein closure rate, with 97% and 94% closure at 2 and 6 months, respectively [50, 51]. In a randomized controlled trial comparing MOCA to RFA in 170 subjects, technical closure rates at 6 months were 93% and 87% for RFA and MOCA, respectively. Clinical outcomes by VCSS and QOL measurements were not significantly different between the two modalities, but MOCA was associated with less procedural pain by visual analog scale assessment [52].

Cyanoacrylate Embolization (CAE) Cyanoacrylate (CA) is a fast-acting adhesive with established medical applications in wound closure and intravascular embolization procedure. Recently, the VenaSeal™ (Sapheon, Inc., Morrisville, NC) device received FDA approval for saphenous vein closure by intravenous application of CA. This system consists of an introducer sheath, a delivery catheter, and a delivery gun for injection of 0.09 ml aliquots of a proprietary preparation of CA at 3 cm intervals. Thirty seconds of external compression is applied to each injection site before proceeding to the next. CAE requires no tumescent anesthesia and also does not require posttreatment compression.

The VeClose trial, a multicenter RCT of 220 subjects comparing CAE to RFA for GSV closure, noted 3 months closure rates of 99% and 96%, respectively, for CAE and RFA. Both groups demonstrated significant and similar reductions in VCSS, CEAP, and AVVQ QOL scores. The prevalence and severity of complications were also similar between the two treatments aside from slightly higher rate of phlebitis in the CAE group which did not reach statistical significance [53]. In a prospective multicenter study (eSCOPE) of CAE for GSV closure in 70 subjects, Proebstle et al. reported 93% freedom from recanalization at 12 months and statistically significant improvement of VCSS and AVVQ scores compared to baseline with few complications, predominantly phlebitis in 11.4% [54]. In a retrospective comparison of EVLA with CAE with 1-year follow-up, Koramaz et al. found no significant difference in total occlusion rates or clinical VCSS response but less adverse effects in the CAE group with decrease in hyperpigmentation and phlebitis [55]. CAE has been shown to be effective treatment for veins up to 20 mm in diameter [56].

Endovenous Treatment of Incompetent Perforator Veins Current practice guidelines support treatment of pathologic perforators in advanced CEAP 4–6 venous disease, preferentially using percutaneous ablation methods. Percutaneous ablation of perforators (PAPs) techniques has increasingly replaced SEPS as primary therapy for IPVs. These techniques include RFA, EVLA, and UGFS. The SVS/AVF clinical practice guidelines for management of leg ulcers recommend PAPs as primary treatment over surgical techniques for perforator ablation to minimize incisions in the diseased peri-ulcer tissues [21, 57].

Endovenous Thermal Ablation Closure of perforators by RF or laser ablation is very analogous to saphenous vein closure, although perforator closure remains a non-FDA-approved application of these devices. The target perforator is localized by US, cannulated with a wire over which an introducer sheath with the RF or laser system is coaxially positioned. Tumescent anesthesia is injected and the thermal ablation performed. This approach is best suited to relatively large and straight perforator veins and is of limited applicability to tortuous perforators. Following thermal ablation, standard compression therapy is applied for 2 weeks with clinical and duplex US follow-up [58–60].

Ultrasound-Guided Foam Sclerotherapy (UGFS) UGFS is a simple and minimally invasive method of perforator closure. Under US guidance, needle access into

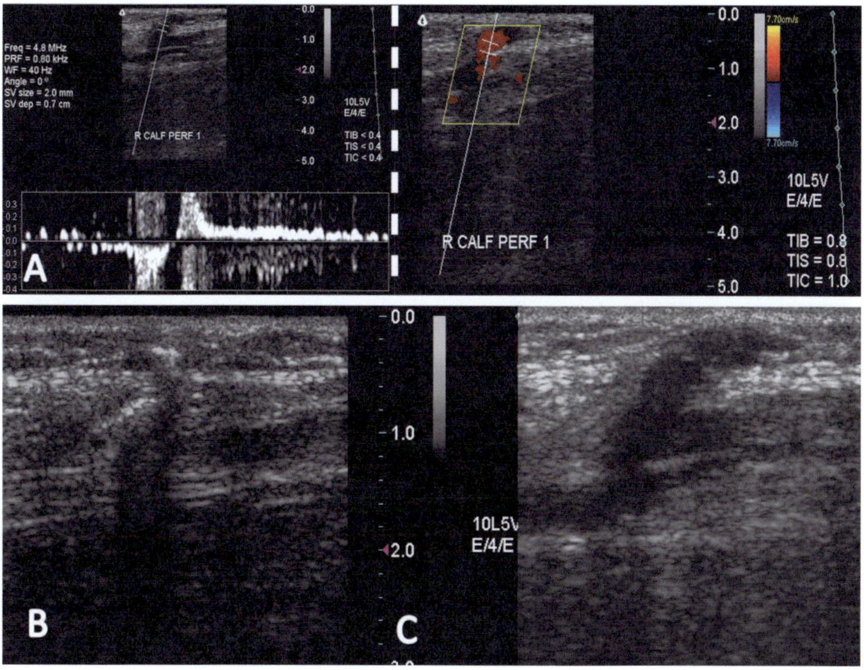

Fig. 16.8 Ultrasound-guided foam sclerotherapy of an incompetent. (**A**) Spectral and color Doppler demonstrating severe reflux in the perforator. (**B**) Injection of hyperechoic foam sclerosant into the perforator. (**C**) Occluded perforator 2-week posttreatment

a varicosity feeding into the perforator is established and venous blood return confirmed. Direct access into the perforator itself within the perforator canal is avoided to prevent inadvertent injection of the perforator artery which can result in nontarget damage to the skin. Under US observation, foamed sclerosant is injected until the column of foam reaches the perforator and then allowed to flow passively into the perforator without additional active injecting. While a small amount of sclerosant entry into the deep vein is unavoidable, care is also taken to avoid over-injection of the perforator and infusion of excessive amount of sclerosant into the deep venous system. Post-sclerotherapy management includes 2 weeks of compression therapy with US follow-up [61, 62]. An example of UGFS of a perforator is provided in Fig. 16.8.

Masuda et al. reported 98% initial perforator occlusion and 75% persistent occlusion at 20 months with liquid sodium morrhuate USG sclerotherapy [61]. Lawrence et al. reported a 58% initial perforator closure rate with RFA, with 71% closure success after retreatment [62]. A recent retrospective comparison of RFA, EVLT, and UGFS in 296 perforators in 112 subjects demonstrated better closure rate with RFA (73%) compared to EVLA (61%) or UGFS (57%). Vein size, anticoagulation,

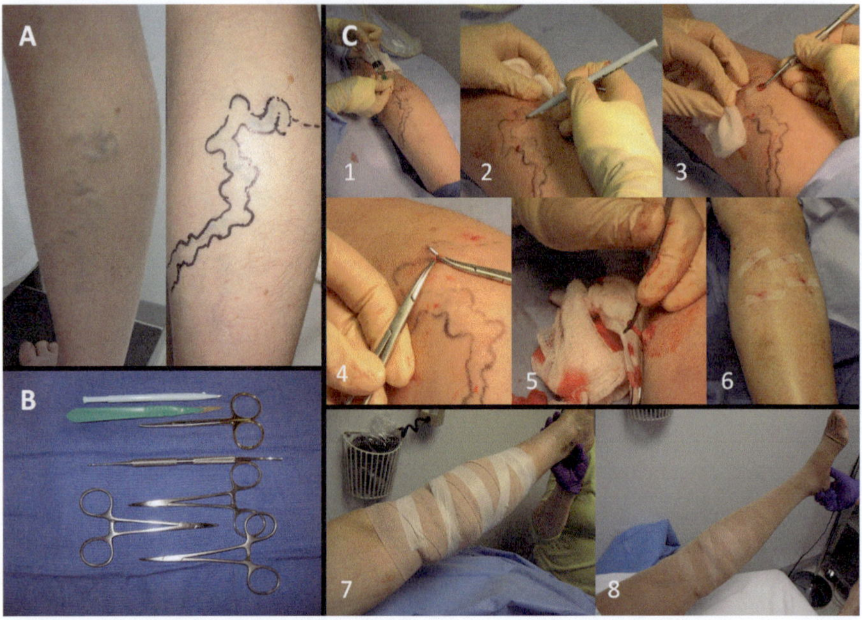

Fig. 16.9 Microphlebectomy: (**A**) identification and marking of target vein. (**B**) Surgical instruments for phlebectomy. (**C1**) Injection of 0.1% lidocaine tumescent anesthesia around the vein. (**C2**) Incising skin. (**C3–5**) Extracting the vein with gentle traction. (**C6**) Steri-strips applied to incisions. (**C7–8**) Applying pressure dressing and compression stocking to the leg

and deep vein reflux did not affect closure rates, while body mass index > 50 was associated with decreased closure rate (37%) with all modalities [63].

Microphlebectomy Microphlebectomy is a surgical technique for removal of reticular and tributary varicosities through small 2–3 mm incisions. This technique, also referred to as stab phlebectomy or ambulatory phlebectomy, is an important and useful adjunct for large branch varicosities that are more difficult to successfully treat with sclerotherapy. The vein targeted for removal is mapped visually and marked on the skin indelibly prior to surgical prepping and draping. The vein is anesthetized by infiltration of the perivenous tissues with 0.1% lidocaine tumescent anesthesia. A small incision is made with an ophthalmologic blade, and the vein is extracted with a phlebectomy hook. The vein is pulled out and removed in segments through additional incisions placed sequentially along its course. The incisions are closed with adhesive strips, and the leg is dressed with a pressure bandage and compression wrap or stocking. To minimize bleeding, coagulopathies should be corrected, and higher sources of reflux into the vein, e.g., saphenous reflux, should be treated prior to performing a phlebectomy [64]. The steps for performing phlebectomy are illustrated in Fig. 16.9.

Endovenous Treatment for Deep Venous Disease

Deep venous obstruction is an important but often under-detected contributor to chronic venous insufficiency. The clinical signs and symptoms of venous disease are often nonspecific to the level of obstruction, making it challenging to identify by clinical evaluation and history alone the subset of ulcer patients with central venous lesions. Such lesions can be characterized as primary nonthrombotic iliac vein lesions (NIVL) or post-thrombotic chronic total occlusions (CTO). Clinical findings that increase suspicion for central venous outflow obstruction include total limb swelling, venous claudication, prominent patterns of groin or cross-pelvic venous collaterals, and the presence of axial deep venous reflux. Labropoulos et al. showed that at 1 year out, multisegment DVT was associated with more severe post-thrombotic symptoms, higher rate of rethrombosis, and higher prevalence of skin changes and ulceration compared to limited single segment DVT. Venous claudication developed only in subjects with iliac vein involvement [65]. CEAP clinical class 4–6 disease should raise suspicion for the presence of deep venous pathology, even without history of prior thrombotic event. Marsten et al. evaluated 78 limbs in ulcer patients with no history of DVT by duplex US and CT or MR venography and found a high incidence of iliocaval venous obstruction: 37% with >50% stenosis and 28% with >80% stenosis [66]. The combination of obstruction with reflux appears to be more detrimental than either obstruction or reflux alone, according to Neglen et al. who examined outcomes of iliac stenting in 447 limbs with chronic nonmalignant obstruction, comparing those with obstruction alone to those with both obstruction and reflux. He found the rate of advanced C4-C6 disease to be 54% in the group with reflux and obstruction versus 24% with obstruction only, and venous ulcer prevalence was 24% versus 3% in these two groups, respectively [67].

While there are surgical methods such as valve transposition or valve reconstruction to restore venous competency, endovenous methods for rebuilding an incompetent valve have not yet been developed. In current practice, endovenous treatment of chronic deep venous disease aims to ameliorate reflux and venous hypertension by restoring iliocaval patency via stenting in conjunction with thrombolysis when clinically appropriate. Infrainguinal venoplasty and stenting of chronic venous occlusions are not routinely performed due to high rates of rethrombosis due to inadequate restoration of inflow and the tendency for stents in the popliteal region to fracture and occlude [68]. For severe CVI due to infrainguinal deep venous obstruction refractory to conservative management, surgical revascularization through endophlebectomy, venous bypass, or valve reconstruction may be beneficial.

Technique for Iliac Vein Thrombolysis and Stenting The strategy for deep vein recanalization entails accessing and traversing the length of the occluded segment, removal of acute thrombus if present, followed by evaluation and stenting of the underlying culprit lesion. Access to the thrombosed segment can be achieved from an antegrade femoral or calf vein approach or retrograde from a jugular approach. The target vein is localized and accessed under US guidance using standard Seldinger technique, and the access site coaxially dilated to admit a vascular sheath. A selective catheter and wire combination is used to negotiate through the thrombus to a patent segment of vein. If acute thrombus is present, thrombolysis is performed prior to stent placement. Mechanical disruption of the clot burden increases surface area exposed to the thrombolytic agent, and this can be done through balloon angioplasty, the use of pulse spray rheolytic thrombolysis (Angiojet™, Boston Scientific, Marlborough MA), or sonicating infusion systems (EKOS®,EKOS Corp, Bothwell, WA). Once a flow channel is restored, further removal of clot is achieved with a continuous infusion of the thrombolytic agent over several hours, in conjunction with anticoagulation to prevent rethrombosis. Once the acute thrombus is removed, the underlying vessel is assessed by venography and intravascular ultrasound if indicated. Residual stenoses are stented and brisk antegrade flow reestablished. Optimal stent outcomes in the venous system require use of large diameter stents (14–20 mm diameter) in the iliocaval zones and establishment of brisk inflow and outflow through the stented segment. To prevent early stent rethrombosis, temporary or lifelong anticoagulation may be indicated, particularly in patients with post-thrombotic damage or impaired inflow [69]. Fig. 16.10 illustrates the process of thrombolysis and stenting of an occluded iliac vein.

Wound Healing Outcomes with Endovenous Therapies

Saphenous Vein Closure In terms of the secondary endpoint of vein closure, endovenous methods of saphenous ablation compare favorably to conventional vein stripping. Van den Blos et al. conducted a meta-analysis of 64 studies including 12,320 limbs comparing saphenous vein closure rates 5 years after surgical stripping, ultrasound-guided foam sclerotherapy, EVLA, or RFA. He found the highest closure rate associated with EVLA (94.5%), with comparable closure rates of 75.7%, 73.5%, and 79.9% for surgery, UGFS, and RFA, respectively [49]. Rasmussen et al. conducted an RCT of 580 limbs in 500 consecutive patients comparing RFA, UGFS, EVLA, and surgical vein stripping for treatment of CEAP clinical class 2–4 disease. The study revealed similar 5–6% closure failure rates at 1 year for EVLA, RFA, and surgery and a significantly higher closure failure rate of 16% for UGFS. All four treatment modalities had comparable improvement in QOL scores and similar varicose vein recurrence rates [36].

Vein closure success notwithstanding, current evidence indicates that correction of saphenous reflux by surgery or endovenous methods may reduce ulcer recurrence but does not necessarily improve primary ulcer healing rates. The ESCHAR study which randomized 500 patients to compression therapy versus saphenous surgery and compression therapy with 3-year follow-up showed no statistical difference in the rate of ulcer healing between the two groups (89% healing with compression, 93% with surgery and compression, $p = 0.73$) but did show significant reduction of ulcer recurrence in the surgery group (31% versus 56%, $p < 0.01$) and prolongation of time to recurrence [70]. These findings were corroborated by Mauck et al. in a

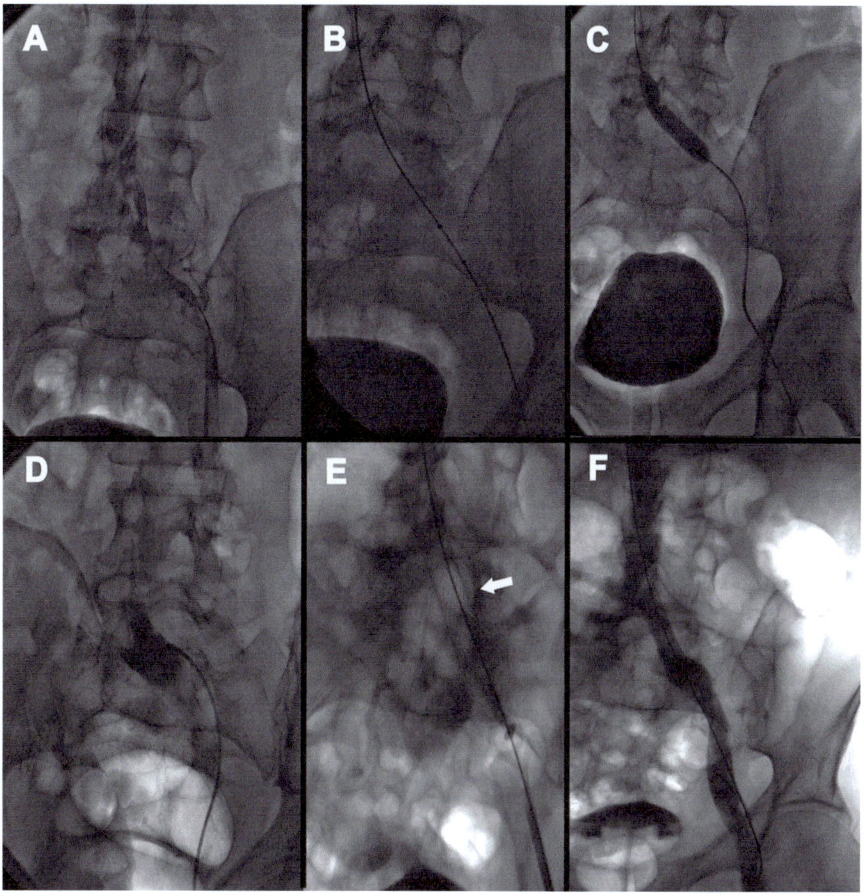

Fig. 16.10 Thrombolysis and stenting of *left* common iliac stenosis with acute thrombosis. (**A**) Venogram depicting thrombosed *left* iliac outflow. (**B**) Angiojet™ pharmacomechanical thrombolysis of the clot. (**C**) Balloon disruption of the clot, also demonstrating a likely stenosis in the proximal common iliac vein. (**D**) Residual common iliac vein obstruction after 24 h more thrombolysis. (**E**) Deployment of an endovenous stent across the obstructed segment. (**F**) Venogram showing restoration of brisk antegrade flow

meta-analysis of seven RCT and four observational studies comparing surgical interventions (including endovascular) to conservative management for venous ulcer treatment. This study showed minimal improvement in ulcer healing with surgery (rendered insignificant when RCT were analyzed separately), a significant reduction in ulcer recurrence, and no change in time to ulcer healing [71]. Kheirelseid et al. reviewed the evidence for varicose vein interventions for ulcer treatment in a meta-analysis of 15 studies [72] and also concluded that overall saphenous intervention improved ulcer healing rates slightly, but this difference was not sustained when only RCT were analyzed. Stratification of open surgery versus endovenous therapy showed improved ulcer healing compared to compression with open surgery but not by endovenous methods. The authors concluded this difference likely reflected limited and poorer quality data in the endovenous group.

Perforator Vein Closure It is difficult to quantify the contribution of IPV treatment toward venous ulcer healing from the existing published data because the majority of studies involving IPV treatment are confounded by concurrent treatment of other veins, e.g., saphenous reflux. Prior to the advent of endovenous methods, subfascial endoscopic perforating vein surgery (SEPS) was the established technique for perforator closure and remains the gold standard against which outcomes comparison is made. In a large meta-analysis of SEPS including 1140 limbs with 526 ulcers, Tenbrook et al. demonstrated overall ulcer healing and recurrence rates of 88% and 13%, respectively, with a low rate of complications (1% DVT, 6% wound infection, 7% paresthesia) [73].

While RCT on perforator treatment are lacking, there are many prospective observational studies that support the benefit of perforator closure in chronic venous disease. Lawrence et al. treated 86 IPVs in 75 ulcers refractory to best practice conservative wound care management and achieved an ulcer closure rate of 93% (80/86). No ulcer healed without at least one perforator closure strongly suggesting an active contribution of the perforator reflux to the disease process [74]. Masuda et al. achieved healing in 67.6% of refractory ulcers with isolated perforator reflux after IPV closure with ultrasound-guided sclerotherapy [61]. Van Gent et al. attempted to evaluate perforator closure effect upon venous ulcer healing in an RCT of SEPS with compression versus compression alone for treatment of venous ulcers. The study was confounded by permission of concurrent or prior superficial vein surgery in the majority of subjects undergoing SEPS and failed to demonstrate improved ulcer healing or decreased recurrence. However, when the data was reexamined from the perspective of completed SEPS versus incomplete SEPS due to missed incompetent perforators detected on duplex US, the authors found a statistically significant higher ulcer recurrence rate in the subjects with incomplete SEPS [75, 76].

Restoration of Iliocaval Patency While catheter-directed iliofemoral thrombolysis in acute DVT setting has been shown to relieve venous obstruction, preserve valve function, and reduce risk of post-thrombotic syndrome [77], the venous ulcer patient typically presents years after the initial thrombotic event with chronic organized thrombus not amenable to thrombolysis. In these patients, stenting of pelvic venous outflow occlusions is associated with good patency rates, low risk of complications, and increased healing of refractory ulcers. Neglen et al. reported a series of 982 iliac stents placed for both NIVL and thrombotic occlusions, noting primary, assisted primary, and secondary cumulative patencies of 79%/100%/100% for NIVL and 57%/80%/86% for CTO at 72 months. There was no associated mortality; early thrombotic complications occurred in 1.5%, late thrombotic complications in 3%, and overall ulcer healing in 58% at 5 years [78]. Raju analyzed 1500 iliac stent cases from retrospective case series and reported 90–100% patency for nonthrombotic and 74–89% patency for post-thrombotic disease at 3–5 years, with 58–89% ulcers healed [79]. In a recent review of 16 studies on endovenous stenting

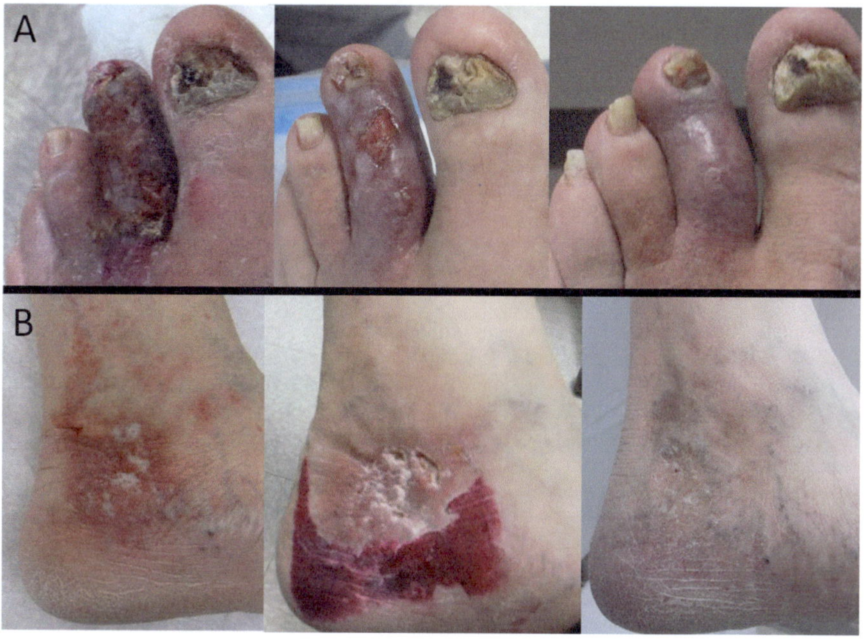

Fig. 16.11 Examples of ulcer response to endovenous treatment: (**A**) *left* second toe ulcer of 15-month duration, compression therapy complicated by location of the lesion. This patient was treated with EVLA of the left GSV only and subsequently healed the ulcer within 3 months. (**B**) Patient with recurrent *left* medial ankle ulcers for over many years. He was treated with EVLA of the left GSV with sclerotherapy of varicose veins around the ankle. The ulcer healed, and the patient continues without recurrence for over 5 years

in chronic venous disease, Saeger et al. reported ulcer healing rate of 56–100% in lesions that had previously failed conservative management [80]. Figure 16.11 presents examples of refractory venous ulcers that healed after endovenous treatment.

Conclusion

Correcting underlying venous obstruction and reflux is an important component of successful venous ulcer management, particularly in the stabilization of healing ulcers. Endovenous techniques for saphenous ablation, perforator closure, and pelvic venous outflow obstruction clearance have become first-line therapies for addressing correctable components of chronic venous insufficiency. These minimally invasive therapies are easy and safe to perform, outpatient based, and able to address the underlying pathophysiology of venous hypertension. They serve as important adjunctive treatments to wound management in the care of the venous ulcer patient.

References

1. Meissner M. Lower extremity venous anatomy. Semin Interv Radiol. 2005;22(3):147–56.
2. Caggiati A, Bergan J, Gloviczki P, et al. Nomenclature of the veins of the lower limbs: an international interdisciplinary consensus statement. J Vasc Surg. 2002;36:416–22.
3. Caggiati A, Bergan J, Gloviczki P, et al. Nomenclature of the veins of the lower limb: extensions, refinements and clinical application. J Vasc Surg. 2005;41(4):719–24.
4. Ludbrook J. The musculovenous pumps of the human lower limb. Am Heart J. 1966;71(5):635–41.
5. Recek C. Calf pump activity influencing venous hemodynamics in the lower extremity. Int J Angiol. 2013;22:23–30.
6. White J, Katz M, Cisek P, et al. Venous outflow of the leg: anatomy and physiologic mechanism of the plantar venous plexus. J Vasc Surg. 1996;24:819–24.
7. Yamaki T, Nozaki M. Patterns of venous insufficiency after an acute deep vein thrombosis. J Am Coll Surg. 2005;201:231–8.
8. Caps M, Manzo R, Bergelin R, et al. Venous valvular reflux in veins not involved at the time of acute deep vein thrombosis. J Vasc Surg. 1995;22:524–31.
9. Kahn S, Ginsberg JS. Relationship between deep venous thrombosis and the postthrombotic syndrome. Arch Intern Med. 2004;164:17–26.
10. Kahn S, Comerota A, Cushman M, et al. The postthrombotic syndrome: evidence-based prevention, diagnosis, and treatment strategies: a scientific statement from the American Heart Association. Circulation. 2014;130:1636–61.
11. Ziegler S, Schillinger M, Maca TH, et al. Post-thrombotic syndrome: after primary event of deep venous thrombosis 10 to 20 years ago. Thromb Res. 2001;101:23–33.
12. Gabriel F, Labios M, Gil J, et al. Incidence of post-thrombotic syndrome and its association with various risk factors in a cohort of Spanish patients after one year follow-up following acute deep venous thrombosis. Thromb Haemost. 2004;92:328–36.
13. Laurikka J, Sisto T, Tarkka M, et al. Risk indicators for varicose veins in forty to sixty-two year olds in the Tampere Varicose Vein Study. World J Surg. 2002;26:648–51.
14. Fowkes F, Lee AJ, Evans CJ, et al. Lifestyle risk factors for lower limb venous reflux in the general population: Edinburgh Vein Study. Int J Epidemiol. 2001;30:846–52.
15. Callum M. Epidemiology of varicose veins. Br J Surg. 1994;81:167–73.
16. Cornu-Thenard A, Boivin P, Baud J, et al. Importance of the familial factor in varicose vein disease. J Dermatol Surg Oncol. 1994;20:318–26.
17. Markovic J, Shortell C. Genomics of varicose veins and chronic venous insufficiency. Semin Vasc Surg. 2013;26:2–13.
18. Tassiopoulos A, Golts E, Oh D, et al. Current concepts in chronic venous ulceration. Eur J Vasc Endovasc Surg. 2000;20:227–32.
19. Labropoulos N, Mansour M, Kang S, et al. New insights into perforator vein incompetence. Eur J Vasc Endovasc Surg. 1999;18:228–34.
20. Delis K, Husmann M, Kalodiki E, et al. In situ hemodynamics of perforating veins in chronic venous insufficiency. J Vasc Surg. 2001;33:773–82.
21. Gloviczki P, Comerota A, Dalsing M, et al. The care of patients with varicose veins and associated chronic venous diseases: clinical practice guidelines of the Society for Vascular Surgery and the American Venous Forum. J Vasc Surg. 2011;53:2S–48S.
22. Valencia I, Falabella A, Kirsner R, et al. Chronic venous insufficiency and venous leg ulceration. J Am Acad Dermatol. 2001;44:401–21.
23. Porter J, Moneta G, et al. Reporting standards in venous disease: an update. J Vasc Surg. 1995;21:635–45.
24. Gillet J, Perrin M, Allaert F. Clinical presentation and venous severity scoring of patients with extended deep axial venous reflux. J Vasc Surg. 2006;44:588–94.
25. Lunois R, Mansilha A, Jantet G. International psychometric validation of the chronic venous disease quality of life questionnaire (CIVIQ-20). Eur J Endovasc Surg. 2010;40:783–9.

26. Rabinovich A, Kahn S. The postthrombotic syndrome: current evidence and future challenges. J Thromb Haemost. 2017;15:230–41.
27. Coleridge-Smith P, Labropoulos N, Partsch H, et al. Duplex ultrasound investigation of the veins in chronic venous disease of the lower limb – UIP consensus document. Part 1. Basic principles. Eur J Endovasc Surg. 2006;31:83–92.
28. Meissner M, Moneta G, Burnand K, et al. The hemodynamics and diagnosis of venous disease. J Vasc Surg. 2007;46:4S–24S.
29. Nicolaides A, Hussein M, Szendro G, et al. The relationship of venous ulceration with ambulatory venous pressure measurements. J Vasc Surg. 1993;17:414–9.
30. Eberhardt R, Raffetto J. Chronic venous insufficiency. Circulation. 2005;111:2398–409.
31. Word R. Medical and surgical therapy for advanced chronic venous insufficiency. Surg Clin N Am. 2010;90:1195–214.
32. Goodyear S, Nyamekye I. Radiofrequency ablation of varicose veins: best practice techniques and evidence. Phlebology. 2015;30(25):9–17.
33. Carradice D, Leung C, Chetter I. Laser: Best practice techniques and evidence. Phlebology. 2015;30(25):36–41.
34. Neumann H, van Germert M. Ins and outs of endovenous laser ablation: afterthoughts. Lasers Med Sci. 2014;29:513–8.
35. Lawrence P, Chandra A, Wu M, et al. Classification of proximal endovenous closure levels and treatment algorithm. J Vasc Surg. 2010;52:388–93.
36. Rasmussen L, Lawaetz M, Bjoern L, et al. Randomized clinical trial comparing endovenous laser ablation, radiofrequency ablation, foam sclerotherapy, and surgical stripping for great saphenous varicose veins. Brit J Surg. 2011;98:1079–87.
37. Dermody M, O'Donnell T, Balk E. Complications of endovenous ablation in randomized controlled trials. J Vasc Surg Venous Lym Dis. 2013;1:427–36.
38. Weiss M, Hsu J, Neuhaus I, et al. Consensus for sclerotherapy. Dermatol Surg. 2014;40:1309–18.
39. Frullini A, Cavezzi A. Sclerosing foam in the treatment of varicose veins and telangiectases: history and analysis of safety and complications. Dermatol Surg. 2002;28:11–5.
40. Guex JJ. Complications and side-effects of foam sclerotherapy. Phlebology. 2009;24:270–4.
41. Willenberg T, Smith P, Shepherd A, et al. Visual disturbances following sclerotherapy for varicose veins, reticular veins and telangiectasias: a systematic literature review. Phlebology. 2013;28:123–31.
42. Morrison N, Neuhardt D. Foam sclerotherapy: cardiac and cerebral monitoring. Phlebology. 2009;24:252–9.
43. Alder G, Lees T. Foam sclerotherapy. Phlebology. 2015;30:18–23.
44. Guex JJ. Foam sclerotherapy: an overview of use for primary venous insufficiency. Semin Vasc Surg. 2005;18:25–9.
45. Myers K, Roberts S. Evaluation of published reports of foam sclerotherapy: what do we know conclusively? Phlebology. 2009;24:275–80.
46. Biemans A, Kockaert M, Akkersdijk G, et al. Comparing endovenous laser ablation, foam sclerotherapy, and conventional surgery for great saphenous varicose veins. J Vasc Surg. 2013;58:727–34.
47. Gibson K, Kabnick L. A multicenter, randomized, placebo-controlled study to evaluate the efficacy and safety of Varithena (polidocanol endovenous microfoam 1%)for symptomatic, visible varicose veins with saphenofemoral junction incompetence. Phlebology. 2017; 32(3):185–93.
48. Todd K, Wright D, et al. The VANISH-2 study: a randomized blinded, multicenter study to evaluated the efficacy and safety of polidocanol endovenous microfoam 0.5% and 1.0% compared with placebo for the treatment of saphenofemoral junction incompetence. Phlebology. 2014;29(9):608–18.
49. van den Bos R, Arends L, Kockaert M, et al. Endovenous therapies of the lower extremity varicosities: a meta-analysis. J Vasc Surg. 2009;49:230–9.
50. Tang T, Kam J, Gaunt M. ClariVein – early results from a large sing-centre series of mechanochemical endovenous ablation for varicose veins. Phlebology. 2017;32(1):6–12.

51. Bishwai M, Bernstein R, Boter M. Mechanochemical ablation in patients with chronic venous disease: a prospective multicenter report. Phlebology. 2014;29(6):397–400.
52. Lane T, Bootun R, Dharmarajah B, et al. A multi-centre randomised controlled trial comparing radiofrequency and mechanochemical occlusion chemically assisted ablation of varicose veins – final results of the Venefit versus Clarivein for varicose veins trial. Phlebology. 2017; 32(2):89–98.
53. Morrison N, Gibson K, McEnroe S, et al. Randomized trial comparing cyanoacrylate embolization and radiofrequency ablation for incompetent great saphenous veins (VeClose). J Vasc Surg. 2015;61:985–94.
54. Proebstle T, Alm J, Dimitri S, et al. The European multicenter cohort study on cyanoacrylate embolization of refluxing great saphenous veins. J Vasc Surg Venous Lym Dis. 2015;3:2–7.
55. Koromatz I, Kilic H, Gokalp F, et al. Ablation of the great saphenous vein with nontumescent n-butyl cyanoacrylate versus endovenous laser therapy. J Vasc Surg Venous Lym Dis. 2017;5:210–5.
56. Gibson K, Ferris B. Cyanoacrylate closure of incompetent great, small and accessory saphenous veins without the use of post-procedure compression: initial outcomes of a post-market evaluation of the VenaSeal system (the WAVES study). Vascular. 2017;25(2):149–56.
57. O'Donnell T, Passman M, Marston W, et al. Management of venous leg ulcers: clinical practice guidelines of the Society for Vascular Surgery and the American Venous Forum. J Vasc Surg. 2014;60:3S–59S.
58. Marsh P, Price B, Holdstock J, et al. One-year outcomes of radiofrequency ablation of incompetent perforator veins using the radiofrequency stylet device. Phlebology. 2010;25:79–84.
59. Shi H, Liu X, Lu M, et al. The effect of endovenous laser ablation of incompetent perforating veins and the great saphenous vein in patients with primary venous disease. Eur J Vasc Endovasc Surg. 2015;49:574–80.
60. Proebstle T, Herdmann S. Early results and feasibility of incompetent perforator vein ablation by endovenous laser treatment. Dermatol Surg. 2007;33:162–8.
61. Masuda E, Kessler D, Lurie F, et al. The effect of ultrasound-guided sclerotherapy of incompetent perforator veins in venous clinical severity and disability scores. J Vasc Surg. 2006;43:551–7.
62. Lawrence P, Alktaifi A, Rigberg D, et al. Endovenous ablation of incompetent perforating veins is effective treatment for recalcitrant venous ulcers. J Vasc Surg. 2011;54:737–42.
63. Hagar E, Washington C, Steinmetz A, et al. Factors that influence perforator vein closure rates using radiofrequency ablation, laser ablation or foam sclerotherapy. J Vasc Surg Venous Lym Dis. 2016;4:51–6.
64. Kabnick L, Ombrellino M. Ambulatory phlebectomy. Semin Interv Radiol. 2005;22(3):218–24.
65. Labropoulos N, Waggoner T, Sammis W, et al. The effect of venous thrombus location on the development of post-thrombotic signs and symptoms. J Vasc Surg. 2008;48:407–12.
66. Marsten W, Fish D, Unger J, et al. Incidence of and risk factors for iliocaval venous obstruction in patients with active or healed venous leg ulcers. J Vasc Surg. 2011;53:1303–8.
67. Neglen P, Thrasher T, Raju S, et al. Venous outflow obstruction: an underestimated contributor to chronic venous disease. J Vasc Surg. 2003;38:879–85.
68. Iida O, Nanto S, Uematsu M, et al. Influence of stent fracture on the long-term patency in the femoral-popliteal artery: experience of four years. J Am Coll Cardiol Intv. 2009;2:665–71.
69. Raju S. Treatment of iliac-caval outflow obstruction. Sem Ther. 2015;28:47–53.
70. Gohel M, Barwell J, Taylor M, et al. Long term results of compression therapy alone versus compression plus surgery in chronic venous ulceration (ESCHAR): randomised controlled trial. BMJ. 2007 Jul 14;335(7610):83. Epub 2007 Jun 1.
71. Mauck K, Asi N, Undavalli C, et al. Systematic review and meta-analysis of surgical interventions versus conservative therapy for venous ulcers. J Vasc Surg. 2014;60:60S–70S.
72. Kheireseid E, Bashar K, Aherne T, et al. Evidence for varicose vein surgery in venous leg ulceration. Surgeon. 2016;14(4):219–33.

73. Tenbrook J, Iafrati M, O'Donnell T, et al. Systematic review of outcomes after surgical management of venous disease incorporating subfascial endoscopic perforator surgery. J Vasc Surg. 2004;39:583–9.
74. Lawrence P, Akjtaifi A, Rigberg D, et al. Endovenous ablation of incompetent perforating veins is effective treatment for recalcitrant venous ulcers. J Vasc Surg. 2011;54:737–42.
75. van Gent W, Hop W, van Praag M, et al. Conservative versus surgical treatment of venous leg ulcers: a prospective, randomized, multicenter trial. J Vasc Surg. 2006;44:563–71.
76. van Gent W, Wittens C. Influence of perforating vein surgery in patients with venous ulceration. Phlebology. 2015;30(2):127–32.
77. Haig Y, Enden T, Klew N, et al. Post-thrombotic syndrome after catheter-directed thrombolysis for deep vein thrombosis (CaVenT): 5-year follow-up results of an open-label, randomised controlled trial. Lancet. 2016;3:e64–71.
78. Neglen P, Hollis B, Olivier J, et al. Stenting of venous outflow in chronic venous disease: long-term stent-related outcome, clinical, and hemodynamic result. J Vasc Surg. 2007;46:979–90.
79. Raju S. Best management options for chronic iliac vein stenosis and occlusion. J Vasc Surg. 2013;57:1163–9.
80. Seager M, Busuttil A, Dharmarajah B, et al. Editor's choice – a systematic review of endovenous stenting in chronic venous disease secondary to iliac vein obstruction. Eur J Endovasc Surg. 2016;51:100–20.

Index

D.P. Orgill (ed.), *Interventional Treatment of Wounds*,
https://doi.org/10.1007/978-3-319-66990-8

Q

R

MIX
Papier aus verantwortungsvollen Quellen
Paper from responsible sources
FSC® C105338

If you have any concerns about our products,
you can contact us on
ProductSafety@springernature.com

In case Publisher is established outside the EU,
the EU authorized representative is:
Springer Nature Customer Service Center GmbH
Europaplatz 3, 69115 Heidelberg, Germany

Printed by Libri Plureos GmbH
in Hamburg, Germany